Nanomaterials: Biomedical, Environmental, and Engineering Applications

Scrivener Publishing
100 Cummings Center, Suite 541J
Beverly, MA 01915-6106

Publishers at Scrivener
Martin Scrivener (martin@scrivenerpublishing.com)
Phillip Carmical (pcarmical@scrivenerpublishing.com)

Nanomaterials: Biomedical, Environmental, and Engineering Applications

Edited by

Suvardhan Kanchi, Shakeel Ahmed, Myalowenkosi I. Sabela and Chaudhery Mustansar Hussain

Scrivener Publishing

WILEY

This edition first published 2018 by John Wiley & Sons, Inc., 111 River Street, Hoboken, NJ 07030, USA and Scrivener Publishing LLC, 100 Cummings Center, Suite 541J, Beverly, MA 01915, USA

For more information about Scrivener publications please visit www.scrivenerpublishing.com.

Wiley Global Headquarters
111 River Street, Hoboken, NJ 07030, USA

For details of our global editorial offices, customer services, and more information about Wiley products visit us at www.wiley.com.

Library of Congress Cataloging-in-Publication Data

ISBN 978-1-119-37026-0

Cover image: Pixabay.Com
Cover design by Russell Richardson

Set in size of 11pt and Minion Pro by Exeter Premedia Services Private Ltd., Chennai, India

10 9 8 7 6 5 4 3 2 1

Contents

Preface

Nanostructure science and technology is a broad and interdisciplinary area of research and development that has been growing explosively in the past decades. Nanomaterials can be obtained either naturally or incidentally or can be manufactured. They are crystalline or amorphous of organic or inorganic materials having sizes in the range of 1-100 nm, which exist in unbound state or as an aggregate or agglomerate. Nanomaterials are classified as nanostructured and nanophase/nanoparticle materials. Their properties are significantly different and they can be significantly improved relative to those of their coarser-grained counterparts. Most benefits of nanomaterials depend on the fact that it is possible to tailor the essential structures of materials at the nanoscale to achieve specific properties. Hence, the evolution of nanotechnology represents an ever improving process in the design, discovery, creation, and novel utilization of artificial nanoscale materials. Research on variety of chemical, mechanical, and physical properties is beginning to yield a glimmer of understanding on how this interplay manifests itself in the properties of these new materials.

To meet the major challenges in environmental sustainability, these nanomaterials in various hierarchical fashions are stimulating various important practical applications in the environmental sector. Their applications involve addressing the existing environmental problems, preventive measures for future problems resulting from the interactions of energy and materials with the environment.

In comparison to their larger counterparts, nanomaterials also have unique physico-chemical and biological properties. Therefore, nanomaterials properties, such as size, shape, chemical composition, surface structure and charge, aggregation and agglomeration, and solubility, have been investigated for advancement of diagnostic biosensors, drug delivery, and biomedical imaging.

The contents of the book includes mainly the fundamentals of nanoparticles, state-of-the-art in synthesis and characterization of nanomaterials and their influence of nanomaterials on the analytical systems (macro to micro & lab-on-a-chip) for biomedical and environmental applications. The evolution in the nanotechnology world clearly signifies a need for broader understanding and, therefore, we hope this book with contribute to this effort.

Part I

SYNTHESIS AND CHARACTERIZATION

1

Synthesis, Characterization and General Properties of Carbon Nanotubes

Falah H. Hussein[1*], Firas H. Abdulrazzak[2] and Ayad F. Alkaim[3]

[1]College of Pharmacy, Babylon University, Hilla, Iraq
[2]Chemistry Department, College of Education for Pure Sciences, Diyala University, Diyala, Iraq
[3]College of Science for Women, Babylon University, Hilla, Iraq

Abstract
Carbon is among the most abundant elements found on Earth, forming different carbonaceous materials by bonding with various atoms, starting with hydrogen and ending with most of the elements on the periodic table. Besides, carbon atoms can react with each other to form different structures by using various types of hybridization: sp, sp^2, and sp^3. The most important hybridization for carbon atoms is sp^2, which can form amazing and rare structures such as graphite, graphene, and fullerene. These carbonaceous nonomaterials have drawn great attention throughout the world as a result of their particular nano- and micro-structures, their unique physiochemical properties, and their potential unprecedented application in many fields. The most important nanostructures made of carbon material are carbon nanotubes (CNTs); the molecular structure of carbon nanotubes consists of pristine carbon atoms linked together to look like a polymer in a hexagonal arrangement in a monolayer of carbon atoms. This new carbon material consists of CNTs, which appear to become a reality for science, thanks to Iijima who synthesized one type of carbon nanotube and called it a single wall in 1991 with Ichihashi. This was a challenge and temptation at the same time due to its physiochemical properties being unknown to some extent, and the variety of types of single-walled carbon nanotubes (SWNTs), double-walled carbon nanotubes (DWNTs), few-walled carbon nanotubes (FWNTs), and multi-walled carbon nanotubes (MWNTs). Extensive studies and research were done on these materials due to their many specific physiochemical properties and representing

**Corresponding author*: abohasan_hilla@yahoo.com

Suvardhan Kanchi, Shakeel Ahmed, Myalowenkosi I. Sabela and Chaudhery Mustansar Hussain (eds.) Nanomaterials: Biomedical, Environmental, and Engineering Applications, (3–60)

The most abundant element in nature. There are three primary methods that are used for the synthesis of CNTs: chemical vapor deposition (CVD), arc-discharge, and laser ablation. In recent years, carbon nanotubes have been prepared under different labels for the various techniques used, and in fact represent the development of methods and techniques for the three methods mentioned above, with new titles. In any industrial application, the most important issues in the production process are represented by substrate cost, quality, and yield of product. The economic feasibility of the production of carbon nanotubes is seen in the CVD method, whereby hydrocarbon is pyrolyzed or dissociated in the presence of suitable metal catalysts. This has attracted attention due to the possibility of producing nanotubes on a large commercial scale. For various kinds of deposition processes, many materials are used as carbon sources, such as ROH or many unsaturated hydrocarbons, which are used as sources of energy in addition to many industrial purposes; thus, a lot of these sources are at risk of depletion in the near future in addition to the high cost of these materials compared with many other materials that can be used for the same purpose. Therefore, many attempts have used natural hydrocarbon precursors, which are interesting because of the possibility of the synthesis of CNTs from the bank of hydrocarbon compounds that are being renewed by nature that is available and low cost, such as essential oils, sucrose, or plant and animal waste. In this work, the waste from date palms is used as a source of carbon to synthesize CNTs. It is rare to find literature or books, which deal with carbon nanotubes without mentioning lijima, but the story of carbon nanotubes started before that; therefore, a section specifically about their history before lijima has been included here. A variety of techniques are used to characterize the surface chemistry or structure of CNTs after covalent functionalization. These characterizations may be classified to qualitative, semi-quantitative, and quantitative analyses.

Keywords: carbon nanotubes, synthesis, chemical vapor deposition

1.1 Introduction

The molecular structure of carbon nanotubes (CNTs) consists of pristine carbon atoms linked together to look like polymer in a hexagonal arrangement of a monolayer of carbon atoms [1–3]. The carbon atoms react with each other to form different structures using various types of hybridizations: sp, sp^2, and sp^3.

The most important hybridization for carbon atoms is sp^2, which can form amazing and rare structures such as graphite, graphene, and fullerene [1]. The most important nanostructures made of carbon material are CNTs. The CNTs appear to become a reality for science, thanks to Iijima [4], who synthesized the single-wall carbon nanotubes in 1991 with

Ichihashi [5]. This was a challenge and temptation at the same time due to its physiochemical properties [6], being unknown to some extent, and the variety of types. The common types are single-walled carbon nanotubes (SWNT), double-walled (DWNT), few-walled (FWNT), and multi-walled (MWNT). Extensive studies and research were done with these materials due to their many specific physiochemical properties and representing the most abundant element in nature.

Generally, there are three primary methods that are used for the synthesis of CNTs: chemical vapor deposition (CVD) [7], arc-discharge [8], and laser ablation [9]. In recent years, CNTs have been prepared under different labels for various techniques [10, 11]. The economic feasibility of the production of carbon nanotubes is seen in the CVD method, whereby hydrocarbon is dissociated in the presence of suitable metal catalysts. This has attracted attention due to the possibility of producing nanotubes on a large commercial scale [12]. For various kinds of deposition processes, many materials are used as carbon sources, such as ROH or many unsaturated hydrocarbons, which are used as sources of energy in addition to many industrial purposes. It is rare to find a literature or a book that deals with CNTs without mentioning lijima, but the story of CNTs started before that; therefore, a specific section deals with the history before lijima.

1.2 The History of Carbon Nanotubes

The first event where CNTs appeared was the Paris Universal Exposition [13] in 1889 in a patent by Edison that proposed the use of filaments in light bulbs. The filaments consisting of carbon atoms that were formed during thermal decomposition experiments that involved passing of cyanogens over red-hot porcelain. This may represent the first mention of the possibility for the preparation of CNTs. At that time, it was impossible to identify nanostructures because the resolutions of optical microscopes were only able to see filaments of a few micrometers, which prevented finding out more about these structures. Thus, the decision to synthesize CNTs remained hidden and without confirmation. But the evidence for the process and conditions of pyrolysis refer to MWNTs. The decision still remained hidden until specific, advanced technology appeared able to scan on the nanoscale. In 1939, the Siemens company succeeded in producing the first version of transmission electron microscopy, which opened new horizons to discover many details about CNTs. The first recorded attempt to study CNTs was done by two Russian researchers, Radushkevich and Lukyanovich [14] in 1952. The two researchers published the carbon filaments in the Journal of Physical Chemistry of Russia, which were produced from the decomposition of carbon monoxide on the surface of iron at 600 °C. The images that were obtained from transmission electron microscopy (TEM) showed tubular structures with diameters around 50 nm. They inferred from these images that the dissolution of carbon in iron resulted in the formation of iron carbide at first, and then the deposition of carbon over the iron carbide, which led to the formation of a graphene sheet. In 1953, two Russian scientists Tesner and Echeistova [13] published that lampblack particles of carbon were exposed during the burning of methane, benzene, or cyclohexane at temperatures above 977 °C. These results were not available globally due to the cold war and the article being published in the Russian language, which prevented Russian publications from reaching America and Europe. It is believed that Russian scientists succeeded in preparing CNTs before this time, but their publication depended on the discovery of TEM as we reported earlier. The first version of TEM had a resolution only in the nanometer range, which prevented scientists from finding out the nature of graphene sheets in CNTs, whether to be their concentric, herringbone, bamboo, or platelet. In 1953, Davis *et al.* [14] reported that carbon nanofibers had been grown from the reaction of CO and Fe_2O_4 at 450 °C in a brickwork blast furnace. The product was identified using electron micrographs and XRD spectroscopy, which postulated that iron and iron carbide behave as a support to precipitate carbon atoms in layers of carbon that varied in thickness from 10 to 200 nm. Hofer *et al.* (1955) found that the diameter of the carbon layers was (0.01–0.2) μm at 390 °C [15]. In 1958, Hillert and Lange [16] reported two textures of graphene filaments: the first was a concentric composition that was determined by electron diffraction, and the second was a bamboo composition. In 1973, Baker *et al.* [17] showed that during the chemical vapor deposition for C_2H_2 onto surfaces that contained iron, cobalt, and chromium, filaments of graphene were deposited onto the surfaces of the catalyst.

In 1976, Oberlin *et al.* [18] prepared carbon fibers that had various external shapes and contained a hollow tube with a diameter ranging from 20 to more than 500 Å along the fiber axis. This work referred to MWNTs without referring to the tubular form, as in CNTs. All of these attempts did not attract any real attention. However, the real revolution in the carbon field occurred when researchers became interested in this new allotropic form of carbon in 1985. During this year, Kroto *et al.* [19] published in *Nature* Journal the formation of clusters consisting of carbon atoms in ball shapes, which were called Fullerene C_{60}. In 1991, the schematic for CNTs was completed when Iijima [4] repeated the reaction that was done by Kroto and his colleagues. Mostly, the aim was to study the reaction by a characterization process. The surprise was the identification of carbon structures in the form of C_{60} and other fullerenes, when Arc-Discharge was done in graphite with Ar gas atmosphere. Iijima reported the preparation of a new type of finite carbon structure filaments of graphene consisting of needle-like tubes. After that, on April 23, 1993, Iijima and Ichihashi succeeded in synthesizing single-wall CNTs [5], which represented the first paper about the synthesis of SWNTs. At the same time, on May 24, Bethune *et al.* from IBM in California published [20] a second paper about SWNTs. The discovery of SWNTs was incidental without any preparation in advance in both cases. The SWNTs were formed during failed attempts to produce MWNTs, with different transition metals. Perhaps the most important reason [21] for the late appearance of this material was that filaments of graphene represented a byproduct from the production processes of the coal and steel industries that hindered them. These filaments also represented an important problem for cooling systems in nuclear reactors; thus, the study of these materials was limited to prevent or at least reducing their formation.

1.3 Graphene

The first publication on graphene was in 1947 by P. R. Wallace [22], who studied the band structure and explained the semimetallic behavior of this material. A typical example of a sp^2 hybridized crystal structure graphite represents one of the softest materials, consisting of bonding and anti-bonding π- and π^*-orbitals. It consists of carbon atoms bonded with three neighboring atoms in a honeycomb lattice with a lattice constant or the distance between carbon atoms a = 0.142 nm [23]. From Figures 1.1 and 1.2, this value is compared with single (C–C = 0.147 nm) and double (C=C = 0.135 nm) bands between carbon atoms representing their average. The distances between carbon atoms refer to the unit cell of a lattice structure that consists of two atoms of carbon. The lattice vectors can be defined as

$$a_1 = \frac{a}{2}\left(3, \sqrt{3}\right) \tag{1.1}$$

$$a_2 = \frac{a}{2}\left(3, -\sqrt{3}\right) \tag{1.2}$$

The length of the lattice spacing (a) can be found by the equation:

$$a = \left|\vec{a_1}\right| = \left|\vec{a_2}\right| = \sqrt{3}\, a_{c-c} = 0.246 \text{ nm} \tag{1.3}$$

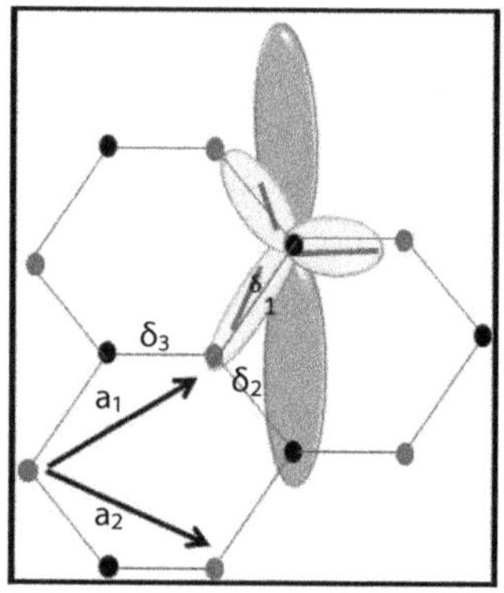

Figure 1.1 Honeycomb lattice structure of graphene, consisting of two triangular lattices a_1 and a_2, which are the lattice unit vectors, and δ_1, δ_2, δ_3, which are the nearest-neighbor vectors.

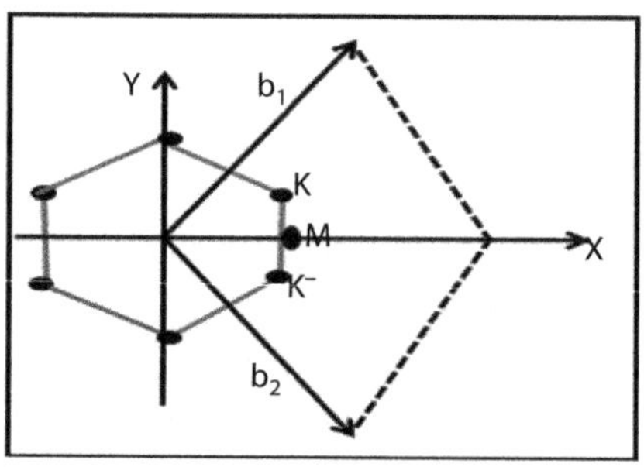

Figure 1.2 Honeycomb lattice structure of graphene, the Brillouin zone. The Dirac cones are located at the K and K⁻ points.

The reciprocal honeycomb lattice vectors are given as

$$b_1 = \frac{2\pi}{3a}\left(1, \sqrt{3}\right) \tag{1.4}$$

$$b_2 = \frac{2\pi}{3a}\left(1, -\sqrt{3}\right) \tag{1.5}$$

The Brillouin zone of the reciprocal lattice in graphene refers to the planes mediating for vectors to the nearest reciprocal lattice points as bounded. The distribution was the same form as the original hexagons of the honeycomb lattice, but rotated as compared to them by a vector $\pi/2$. Figure 1.2 shows that the Brillouin zone for graphene consists of six points in the corner, divided into two equivalent groups with about three points known by the symbols K and K⁻. The values of K and K⁻ can be explained [24] by two equations:

$$K = \frac{2\pi}{3a}\left(1, \frac{1}{\sqrt{3}}\right) \tag{1.6}$$

$$K^{-} = \frac{2\pi}{3a}\left(1, -\frac{1}{\sqrt{3}}\right) \tag{1.7}$$

The vectors of the three nearest neighbors in real space can be represented by the following equations.

$$\delta_1 = \frac{a}{2}\left(1, \sqrt{3}\right) \tag{1.8}$$

$$\delta_2 = \frac{a}{2}\left(1, -\sqrt{3}\right) \tag{1.9}$$

$$\delta_3 = -a(1, 0) \tag{1.10}$$

The positions of the second six nearest are located in the following equations:

$$\delta_1^{-} = \mp a_1 \tag{1.11}$$

$$\delta_2^{-} = \mp a_2 \tag{1.12}$$

$$\delta_3^{-} = \mp(a_2 - a_1) \tag{1.13}$$

Graphene can take on many forms, and every one of these forms is characterized by specific and unique physiochemical properties, as shown in Figure 1.3.

Graphene represents a two-dimensional (2-D) material, sp^2 in nanocarbon systems, which can be understood when recalling the graphene edge energy γ. The edge energy for the graphene scheme includes the position of armchair (A) to zig-zag (Z) and all the intermediate orientation chiral angles. Saito *et al.* [23] found that the inter-sheet distance in a multi-sheet nanotube is 0.344 nm, which is close to the value of the distance between two layers of graphene in graphite, which equals 0.335 nm [24].

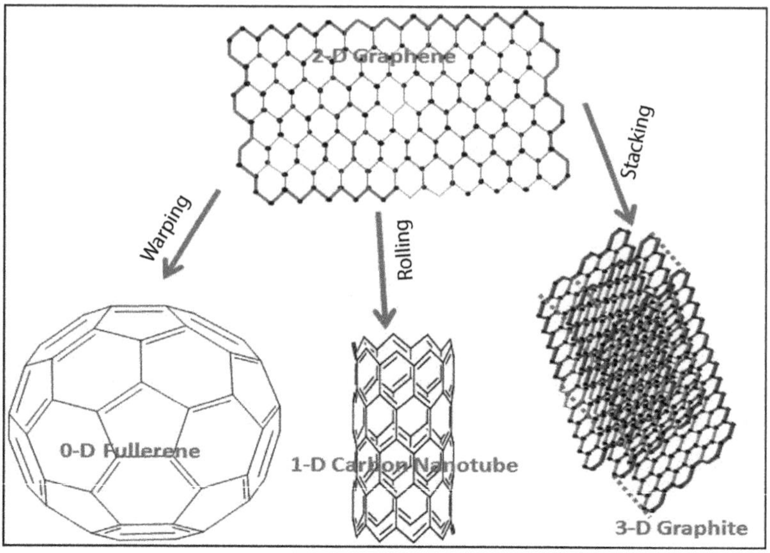

Figure 1.3 The structure of graphene in nature.

1.4 Graphite

This three-dimensional material consists of many sheets of graphene bonded with each other by weak van der Waals forces, which occur as a result of the π-orbitals that are distributed over all the surfaces of the sheets. Kiselev *et al.* reported that graphite was discovered by Borrowdale in Cambria, England, in the 16th century [24]. The literature refers to graphite as a stack of many 2-D graphene layers combined through layer-by-layer orientation to form a 3-D structure. The distance between the layers is approximately $d = 0.34$ nm [25], with the arrangements of carbon atoms in two layers bonded from the centers of the hexagons for one of these two layers. This organization makes the translation between the layers possible with two probabilities. The first happens if the translation between the layers produces a rhombohedra configuration; thus, 6 atoms per unit cell will extend in three dimensions along the z-axis, which produces β-graphite. The second probability occurs if the stacking between the layers behaves like a hexagon; in this case, 4 atoms per unit cell will extend in two dimensions along the z-axis, which produces α-graphite [26]. Generally, the crystalline α-graphite occurs more often in nature compared to β-graphite. Although different in terms of the crystal structure, these two forms have identical physical properties. The alpha forms can be converted into the beta by mechanical treatment, while the opposite process is more difficult which requires heating above 1000 °C.

1.5 Fullerene

The 0-D graphitic allotope (fullerene) was discovered in 1985 by Kroto *et al.* [19]; its most prominent representative is the C_{60} molecule, which has the form of a football and is also called a "buckyball." It consists of a graphene sheet, where some hexagons are replaced by pentagons, which causes a crumbling [27–28] of the sheet and the final formation of a graphene spherical. Its existence had been predicted before, by Ozawa and Ōsawa [28], in 1970, when described fullerenes as a class of closed-cage molecule, containing 12 pentagonal structures with the complete ball structure of hexagons [29]. The number of hexagons in the structure can be determined by using a simple relation [30], which is

$$\text{Hexagons} = [(\text{carbon atoms}) - 20]\,/2 \tag{1.13}$$

The most common consists of a polygon with 60 vertices and 32 faces, 12 of which are pentagonal and 20 hexagonal. Fullerenes are characterized by high reactivity and strain energies, which decrease during saturation of the pi-bonds. The steric hindrance with reduced Pi-bonds causes a reduction in the electrophilic. The activity of fullerenes behaves like electrophiles in nucleophilic reactions and can be a legend in organometallic reactions. Fullerenes without functional groups behave positive effects and act as antioxidants, while functional groups can be converted into a highly toxic material. Fullerenes in the environment can be dangerous because they are soluble in organic solvents such as benzene, toluene, or chloroform.

1.6 Rehybridization

Common factors between graphene, carbon nanotubes, and fullerenes of all types include hybridization, which is represented by sp^2 and the carbon atoms; thus, the length and angle between the carbon atoms may be the same. But the truth is the opposite of this because the linear bond in space will behave differently in a tubular structure or in a circular ball. Theoretically [31–32], if the sheet of graphene is rolled or contorted into CNTs or fullerenes, the length of the sigma band should be reduced in spite of using the same hybridization and the same carbon atoms. The π bond is distributed over a 2-D sheet of graphene up and down the sheet in equal value, while with regard to the distribution for 0-D and 1-D, the structures will change outside and inside when the outer sites are much higher than the inner cities.

From Figure 1.4, two regains can be seen: the first inside the rings and the second outside the rings. The part inside the rings looks like a continuous dark color, which refers to the δ bond only without the clouds of π bonding. The change in the arrangements of the δ and π bonds makes the surface able to capacitance all of π with δ bond, so that it shows two different bonds on the surfaces that are referred by two different colors. This is caused by the appearance of two hybridizations sp^2 and sp^3 that are mixed together and can be seen by using Raman spectroscopy as a Δ and G band [3,33]. However, the degree of hybridization could be obtained by the equation

$$\text{Degree of hybridization} = sp^{2+\eta}, \tag{1.14}$$

where η refers to a number between 0 and 1; in this description, one can specify the ratio between the sp^2 and sp^3 hybridization. The important factor that play a major role in enhancing the distribution was the tilting angle

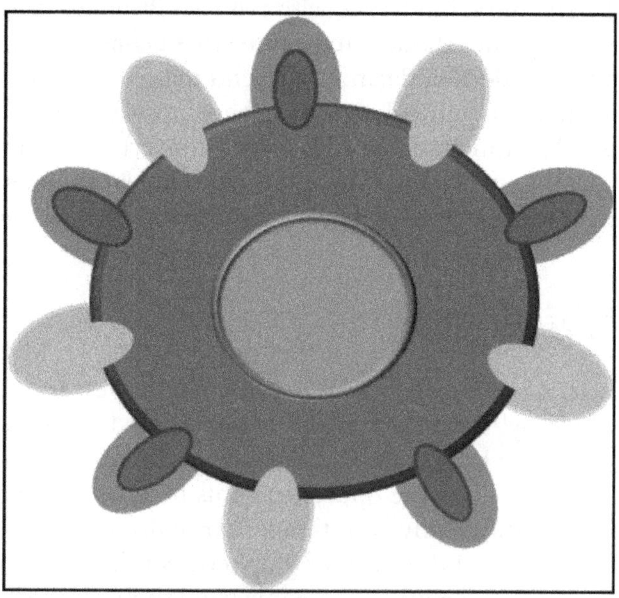

Figure 1.4 Distribution sigma δ (blue color) and pi π (bright color) bonds.

(δ) contributing to the bending of the π-orbitals outside the CNTs [20], which depend on the diameter (d) and chirality of the curved wall:

$$\delta = a/2\sqrt{3d} \tag{1.15}$$

while a refers to a lattice constant.

1.7 Structure of Carbon Nanotubes (CNTs)

The most promising materials from nanotechnology are CNTs, which refer to one-dimensional material consisting of carbon atoms only bonded with each other. The sp^2 hybridization in a graphene sheet or graphite is closely related to the honeycomb arrangement or the carbon atoms making a network of hexagons. As mentioned before in the rehybridization section, the p orbital on the carbon atoms form an extended π system that allows for a lattice of graphite to conduct. The simplest images of a CNT can be imagined as a sheet of graphene that has been rolled up to form a seamless cylinder with a hollow core [32,33], which may be opened or closed from two ends such as fullerenes. CNTs have two types or structures. The first is single-walled carbon nanotubes (SWNTs), which are made up of a monolayer of carbon atoms in a graphene sheet rolled into a cylinder structure. The SWNTs behave as either metal or semiconductor depending on the tube's diameter, the direction of the wrap, and the helicity [33]. The second type is multi-walled carbon nanotubes (MWNTs), graphene sheets rolled into a cylinder. Recently, few-walled carbon nanotubes (FWNTs) [34], which are a special kind of MWNT that consist of two to six layers of graphene sheets, can be considered as an intermediate structure between SWNTs and MWNTs. They have a diameter in the range of nanometers from 0.3 up to 100 nm [35], but their length might reach to more than 18 cm [34]. The diameter of a typical single-walled CNT (SWNT) is around 1 nm and for multi-walled CNTs (MWNTs) it could reach 10 nm [35], while for FWNTs their diameter is around 4–7 nm [36–37].

1.8 Classification of CNTs

A classification of the material represents the common ways to understand and make the studies more clear and easy. A carbon nanotube was classified according to many physical and chemical properties such as chirality, conductivity, or number of graphene layers [34–37].

1.8.1 Classification by Chirality

The chirality of a carbon atom refers to molecules that are non-super impossible on their mirror image, or chiral molecules are those that include different groups attached to the central atom. For carbon nanotubes, this type of classification depends on how the carbon sheet is wrapped into a tube; however, the chiral [33] can be described by the chiral vector which indicates the direction in which the tube rolls up:

$$C_h = n\mathrm{a}_1 + m\mathrm{a}_2 \tag{1.16}$$

where a_1 and a_2 are the unit vectors of graphene and n and m are integers. The values of n and m have important indicators for the electronic properties of CNTs. Figure 1.5 shows that two different categories of nanotubes depend on the simple expression $C_\mathrm{h} = (n, m)$: the first being achiral. This includes two types: one refers to $(n = m)$ the nanotube that has the characteristics of an armchair nanotube within $(\theta = 30°)$, and the other appears when $(m = 0)$; the nanotube in this case is called a zigzag nanotube within $(\theta = 0°)$. The second category of nanotubes is chiral nanotubes that occur when $(\mathrm{m} \neq \mathrm{n} \neq 0)$.

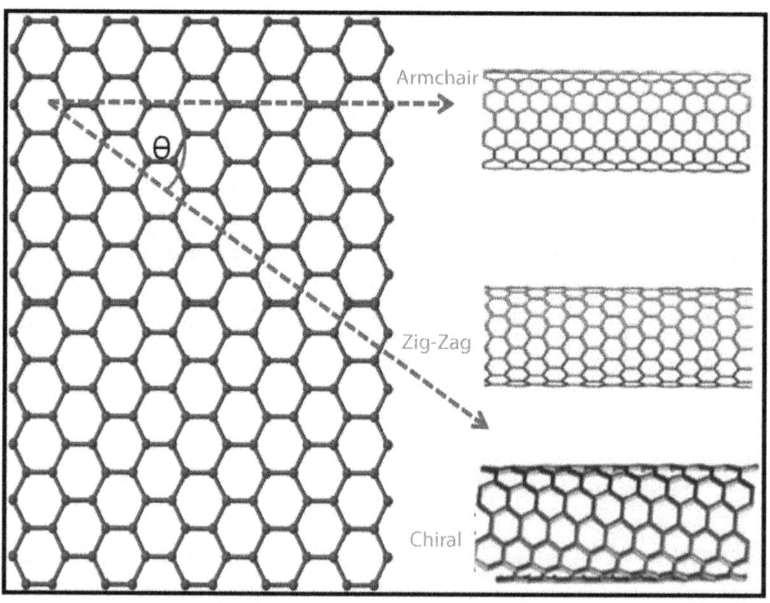

Figure 1.5 Graphene map chirality of (n, m) chiral vectors that give three structures armchair, zig-zag and chiral nanotubes

1.8.2 Classification by Conductivity

According to these phenomena, carbon nanotubes include two types: metallic and semiconducting, which are mainly affected by the chirality [33] of the CNT, when the chiralities are determined by the n and m values. It is mathematically possible to predict the type of carbon nanotube according to two probabilities; the first is when n-m is a multiple of 3 or an armchair, then the nanotube is metallic; the second refers to n-m not being a multiple of 3 or a zig-zag or chiral, then the nanotube is a semiconductor.

1.8.3 Classification by Layers

These types of classifications depend on the number of graphene layers that form a tubular structure and which commonly include two types:

i. Single-walled carbon nanotubes: This type consists of one layer of graphene (SWNTs).
ii. Multi-walled carbon nanotubes. Many layers of graphene sheet are wrapped around to form it (MWNTs).

In recent years, two other types have been added, which are double-walled carbon nanotubes (DWNTs) [35], which consist of two layers of graphene, and few-walled carbon nanotubes (FWNTs) [34], which consist of (2–6) layers of graphene sheets.

1.9 Crystal Structures of Carbon Nanotubes

Carbon nanotubes can be defined as a sheet of graphene that is wrapped from side to side, producing a tubular structure; this expression refers to the transformation of the material from 2-D to 1-D. The two characteristic morphologies depend on establishing a complete understanding of the crystal structures of carbon nanotubes, which are SWNTs and MWNTs. The graphene layer consists of a hexagonal carbon network; the nature of how the sheet is wrapped will decide the physical and chemical properties of the carbon nanotubes [35–39]. Figure 1.6 shows [40] that (XRD) patterns on a *(Rigaku Rotalflex) (RU-200B)* X-ray diffractometer for SWNT and MWNT were measured by using Cu Kα radiation (wavelength 0.15405 nm) with a Ni filter. The tube current was 100 mA with a tube voltage of 40 kV. The 2θ angular regions between 10° and 80° were explored at a scan rate of 5°/min. For all XRD tests, the resolution in the 2θ scans was kept at 0.02°.

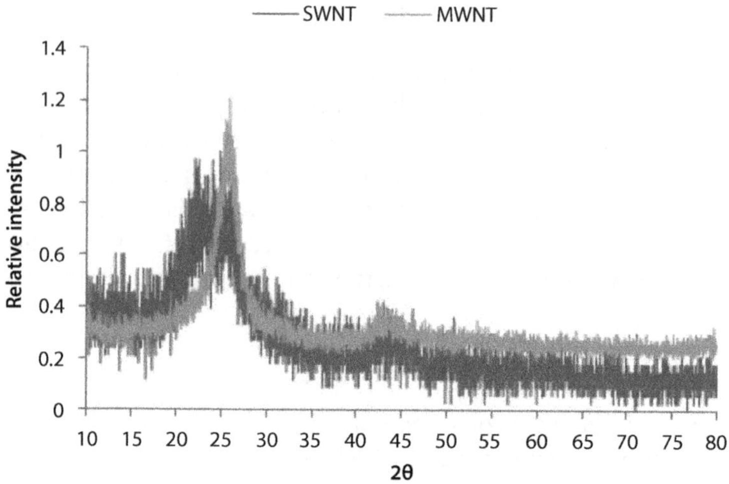

Figure 1.6 The X-ray diffraction patterns of SWNT (red color) and MWNT (green color).

The red spectrum refers to SWNT that consists of one sheet of graphene; therefore, one isolated tube cannot be seen easily by using X-ray diffraction. The absence of the repeating planes prevents or at least reduces the ability to detect one tube of SWNTs; thus, many noises can be seen. The green spectrum of MWNTs, which are many monolayers of graphene repeated in the same center with different radii, makes the Bragg equation very sensitive for these structures. Thus, creating the typical peaks shown clearly with MWNTs at $2\theta = 25.3°$, with the Miller index (002) and a spacing value equal to 0.35 nm. It is possible that the preparation conditions or the process of purification does not allow for the filaments of the tubes to be isolated. In the best conditions, carbon nanotubes consist of micron-size aggregates, referring to many groups of CNTs together due to Van der Waals interaction [41–42]. Further research has found that the methods of preparing carbon nanotubes have an influence on the degree of crystallization of the as-grown carbon nanotubes. The common literature is interested in the fact that XRD forms a scattering angle of between 15° and 30°, which refers to the Miller index (002). The wider root of the (002) peak centered at 23° is induced by the disordered carbon, and the higher sharp peaks centered at 26° mostly on the characterization and identification of carbon nanotubes [43]. By comparing the relative magnitude of the (002) profiles of the graphite and disordered carbon, XRD can provide some information on the average degree of crystallization of the entire sample. Khani and Morad [41] reported that after treating the MWNTs with different oxidants, a clear decrease in the nanotube diameters along the tube walls was observed. The decrease in the degree of crystallization starts with the full width at half maximum (FWHM) widening of the XRD diffraction peaks. The particle size (d_{002}) calculated by Bragg's law increases depending on the kind of oxidants; the procedure can be performed using a mixture of HNO_3/H_2SO_4 on the surface of the MWNTs with an outer diameter 10 to 20 nm. However, the diffraction patterns of pristine and oxidized MWNTs are similar. Therefore, the MWNTs that undergo the oxidation process are able to preserve the first features of their structures, even though some narrowing of their outer diameters and decreasing in the crystallization occurs. Generally, the observed narrow and sharp reflections have suggested good crystallinity and structural integrity. Also, the crystal structures of the CNTs, which represent one of their physical properties, are influenced by the diameters of the tubes with ratios of defects and deformations on their surfaces [43–45].

1.10 Synthesis Methods

The main methods reported commonly depend on the synthesis of carbon nanotubes including three types. All of these methods are economically feasible for large-scale production; however, they all produce many byproducts that all need the purification process. The purification techniques still have to be developed. Improvements include varying the temperature, the catalyst composition, and other process parameters. Consequently, the average diameter and length of the carbon nanotubes can be varied.

1.10.1 Arc-Discharge

Iijima [4] used the arc-discharge method to produce fullerenes, when an electric arc between two graphite rods is placed in an inert atmosphere. Carbon evaporation is initiated by a high-intensity electric current passing through the two rods, which are placed near to each other approximately 1 mm in order to initiate the arc production. Figure 1.7 shows a simple scheme for this method, which includes a direct current of 50 to 100 amp. Driven by approximately 20 V, thus creating a high temperature and low pressure (between 50 and 700 mbar) [5], the high yield production of the carbon nanotubes depends on the homogeneity of the plasma arc and the temperature of the deposit on the two electrodes. Normally, multiwalled nanotubes will be produced if the two electrodes include graphite only without a catalyst. If holes are bored into the graphite rods and then filled with appropriately proportional composites of graphite powder and

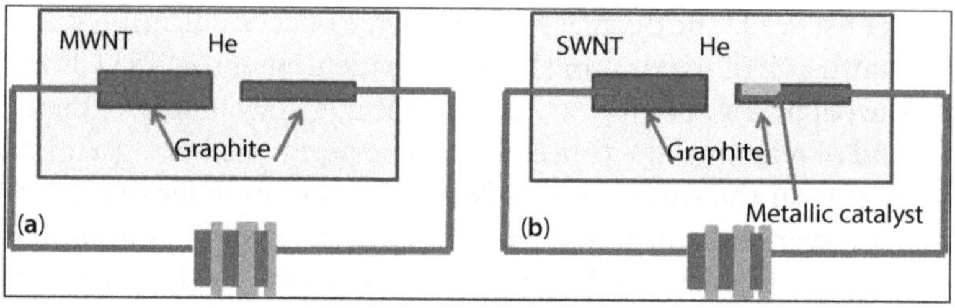

Figure 1.7 The arc discharge system for the synthesis of A-MWNTs and B-SWNTs.

catalytic materials, the SWNTs can be produced [8]. Recent investigations have shown that it is also possible to create nanotubes with the arc method in liquid nitrogen.

The two carbon rods are different in size; the depositing process takes place on the big rod. The products created using this method are usually short tubes with diameters ranging from 0.6 to 1.4 nm for single-walled and 10 nm for multi-walled carbon nanotubes. This method is relatively easy to implement, and will produce a yield of 30%. The most important parameter that influences the various activities involved in this method is the efficient cooling system [4] of the cathode, which has been shown to be essential in controlling the quality. Generally, the types and the qualities of the product depend on many parameters such as the metal concentration, the inert gas pressure, kind of gas, current, and the system geometry. The disadvantage of using this technique is that it requires mixture of components than can separate the nanotubes from the soot and the catalytic metals from the crude product.

1.10.2 Laser Ablation

The second way of producing high-quality CNTs from carbon plasma is by using a laser beam, typically a YAG or CO_2 laser, where intense laser pulses ablate graphite as a source of carbon [9,44]. Figure 1.8 shows graphite placed into a furnace heated to 1200 °C in the presence of an inert gas such as helium, and then it is directed toward a cold collector that causes the vapor to quickly condense into large clusters. The result of the product depends on the catalyst. In absence of catalyst, the product will be SWNTs, whereas MWNTs will be formed in presence of catalyst. This method was first discovered by Guo *et al.* at Rive University in 1995 [44]. The tubes produced by this method are in the form of a mat of ropes 10–20 nm

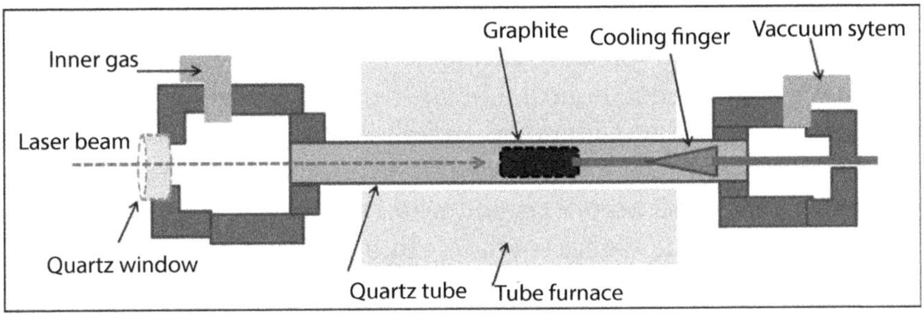

Figure 1.8 The laser ablation system for the synthesis of CNTs.

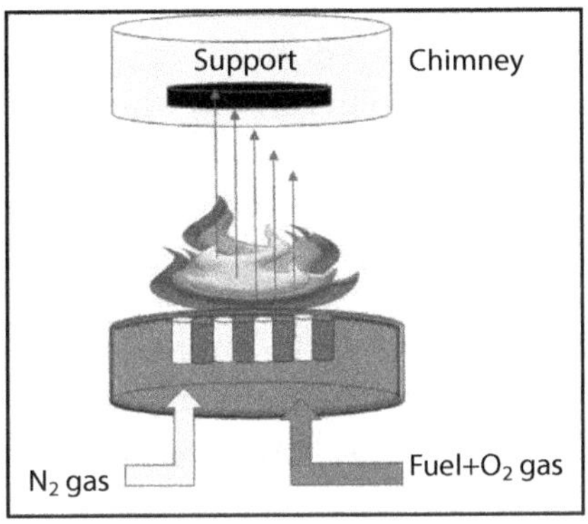

Figure 1.9 Schematic diagram for the flame reactor to the formation of carbon nanotubes.

in diameter and up to 100 microns or more in length. The advantage of this method is high-quality SWNT, diameter control, the investigation of growth dynamics, and the production of new materials.

1.10.3 Flame Methods

The flame by hydrocarbon in gaseous or liquid phase provides two of the most important conditions for the growth of CNTs, which are energy and a source of free radical carbon. The most important difference between CVD and the flame method, is that high concentrations of intermediate radicals formed in the flame medium.

Figure 1.9 shows the combustion of hydrocarbon with oxygen in atmospheric pressure is an exothermic reaction that produces high heat with a rich carbon radical atmosphere suitable for CNT growth. The process includes a mixture of hydrocarbon and oxygen in equivalence rations, which was required to produce carbon atoms in a free radical phase with the heat which needed to build a tubular structure of carbon. The common name for this reactor was premixed flame.

Vander Wal *et al.* [45] synthesized CNTs using various premixed flames with ethane, ethylene, acetylene, and propane, as fuel and sources of carbon-free radicals. The flames method can be done by changing the ways of mixing the fuel and oxidizer; thus, it can be classified into three types: premixed, non-premixed (diffusion), and partially premixed.

The parameters that influence in the nature and yield of carbon nanotubes [46–47] are gas flow rates, nature of catalyst, the fuel molecular constitution, the flame temperature, and growth times. The flame medium is characterized by complex homogeneous gas phase kinetics that lead to the formation of nano-structured solid carbon, which influence the configuration of flame.

Gulder reported that [47] fuel molecular constitution and flame temperature are the two factors dominating the soot and carbon nanotube formation in laminar diffusion flames. Li Ming *et al.* [48] used stainless grid flame supplied by propane-air to synthesized CNTs on the surfaces, which are covered with iron, chromium, and nickel oxide in a nitrogen atmosphere. Diener *et al.* [49] synthesized (SWNTs) by flames when subliming the bis(cyclopentadienyl) into an inert gas feed line that mixes with the hydrocarbon fuel and oxygen at the burner surface with used iron and nickel as catalysts. The growth of the SWNTs in the flame was related to catalyze by the presence of metals. This homogeneous gas phase kinetics is closely coupled with the heterogeneous kinetics of gas–surface interactions leading to the formation of nano-structured solid carbon.

1.10.4 Chemical Vapor Deposition

The catalytic chemical vapor deposition (CVD) of carbon was already reported in 1959 [51]; however, only in 1993, carbon nanotubes were formed using this method [44]. Today, the most popular CNT technique, the CVD, may probably be the oldest technique of growing CNTs as filaments and fibers [51–52]. The CVDs refer to the process of forming a thin film by deposition chemical reactions to build high-quality layers of a designated material by using a special chamber containing one or more heated objects to be coated.

CVD seems the most promising method for possible industrial applications due to the relatively low growth temperature, high yields, and high purities with many specific properties that can be achieved during its production. The vapor in the CVD means that the process implies the sources used in the deposition method are in the gaseous state. The precursor that uses gases supplied from gaseous containers or other sources stored as liquids. Occasionally, solid sources could be used that undergo sublimation at low temperatures as compared with the process of precipitation [53].

In CVD, the synthesis of carbon nanotubes depends on the pyrolysis of hydrocarbons over the catalyst particle or without a catalyst [7]. The catalyst material may be solid, liquid, or gas and can be placed inside the furnace or fed in continuously from outside. Figure 1.10 shows the general structure of the CVD system. The carbon source is typically a hydrocarbon material, possibly a gas such as acetylene or ethylene, or a liquid such as different types of alcohol, which are usually supplied to the reactor by evaporation using a suitable method. The carrier gases are used to input the carbon clouds into the reactor. Sometimes a mixture of carrier gas (inert gas) and hydrogen is used as a reducing agent. The concentration of reactants in the mixture is determined by accurate flow meters. The operating temperature inside the quartz tube ranges from 500 °C to 1200 °C. Inside the tube, there are support materials that are covered with a suitable catalyst that behaves as an active site for the growth of carbon nanotubes.

The four main parameters that decided the type of CNTs, i.e., whether SWNTs or MWNTs, are the atmosphere of the reactor, the hydrocarbon source, the catalyst, and the growth temperature. Generally a low temperature in the range of 600–900 °C yields MWNTs, whereas a higher temperature of more than 900 °C during the reaction mostly yields SWNT growth.

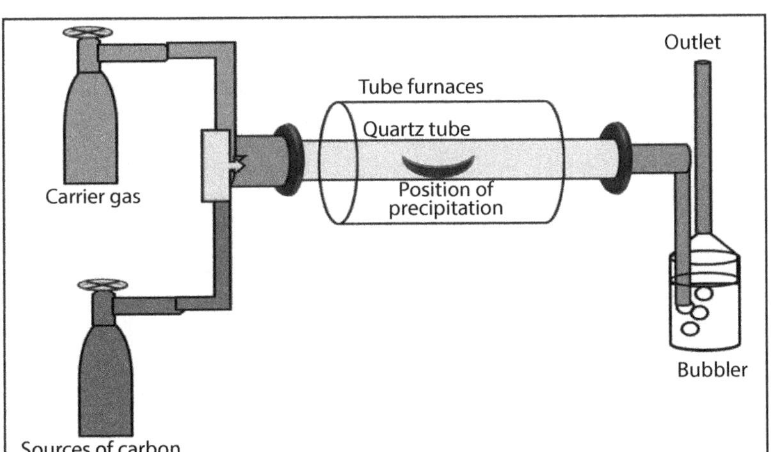

Figure 1.10 Typical CVD apparatus for the production of carbon nanotubes.

1.11 The Purification Process of CNTs

The process of producing carbon nanotubes by any of the available methods, mostly the synthesized material, contains a large amount of impurities. These can be in the form of metal particles as catalyst or support for precipitation, unconverted carbon such as amorphous carbon, and fullerenes [54–55]. The ability and the activity [56] of the CNTs to be used in nanoscience for either biological or chemical applications requires optimum removal of impurities. Each method used for purification has one or more disadvantages, such as non-selectivity damaging of nanotubes, formation of toxic wastes, and the lengthy procedures. For this reason, CNTs have numerous methods based on filtration, chromatography, and oxidations with gas or liquid. The common methods involve the treatment of the CNTs with oxidizing one acid or a mixture of acids and bases [57–58]. The treatments, mostly non-destructive and scalable, lead to the removal of various non-CNT materials without damaging the tubes to any significant extent. The typical method [59] is extremely fast, very simple to use, and offers a convenient way to remove these kinds of impurities from CNTs. One of the reagents used for this purpose is Piranha mixture [60], with a composition of either acidic (H_2SO_4/H_2O_2) or basic (NH_4OH/H_2O_2). Martinez *et al.* [61] reported that synthesized SWNTs were purified by a combination of air treatment/acid microwave, leading to high efficiency with high metal removal percentages in short time as compared with the acid reflux treatments. Gomez *et al.* used a new method for purification, which involve treatment with microwave followed by gas-phase chlorination. This method is able to removed and clean the carbon shells that encase the residual metal catalyst. Rasel *et al.* [63] use mixture of hydrogen peroxide with KOH and HCl to purify MWNTs. The method (HCl/H_2O_2) showed 100% purification yield as compared to HCl and KOH/H_2O_2 with purification yields 93.46% and 3.92%, respectively. Stancu *et al.* [64] reported different methods that were used for the purification of MWNT synthesized by the arc discharge method. The metal catalyst was removed by treatment with acids, while the amorphous carbon was removed by using two approaches. The first approach was the weak oxidation performed by refluxing the MWCNTs in strong acid for 6 h and the second method was the oxidation with air for 10 minutes. Ebbesen *et al.* and Vivekchand *et al.* reported mostly high-temperature oxidation in the air purification strategy of MWNTs [65–66], which did not satisfy for use with SWNTs due to the catalyst metal particles present in the material. Mahalingam *et al.* [67] reported the review of the past and recent developments until 2012 in the chemical oxidation, physical separation, for purification of CNTs with combinations of chemical and physical techniques to develop and enhance the process. We must distinguish between two terms, which is the separation and purification process of CNTs; the first refer to isolated specific types of CNTs from pure sample. The second term refers to the steps to remove all the interference materials from synthesized CNTs. Naoki Komatsu and Feng Wang [68] published a review including the separation methods that are commonly used such as electrophoresis, centrifugation, chromatography, selective solubilization, and selective reaction. Hou *et al.* [69] reported that purification methods can be classified into three categories: chemical, physical, and a combination of both. The chemical methods depend on the chemical reaction represented by the oxidation process that is accrued by the gas phase, liquid phase, and electrochemical oxidation. The physical methods that depends on the physical properties of CNTs to separate them from impurities such as filtration, centrifugation, solubilization, and high temperature annealing. Other physical techniques [70–71] that are effective in removing metal particles entrapped by carbon layers include the magnetophoretic technique, supercritical fluid carbon dioxide extraction, and a mechanically ejecting technique.

The products after purifying were mostly characterized by many techniques such as thermal gravimetric analysis, scanning electron microscope, transmission electron microscope, energy dispersive X-ray spectroscope, X-ray photoelectron spectroscopy (XPS), and Raman spectroscopy.

1.12 Mechanism of Growth CNTs

The optimum environment that is needed for growing and controlling the particle size for catalytic particles must allow the control and prediction of the diameter and chirality of the carbon nanotubes. Despite numerous studies on the synthesis of carbon nanotubes, the mechanism for growth is still in its early stages. This section includes the most common and accepted mechanism that is dependent on understanding the mechanism of forming the tubular structure of carbon nanotubes.

1.12.1 The Model for Carbon Filament Growth

This model was derived from the concepts of vapor–liquid–solid theory, which in turn is used for explaining the mechanism of the growth of CNTs. The credibility of this hypothesis arises from a TEM image of the synthesized product which shows two probabilities. The first of them is

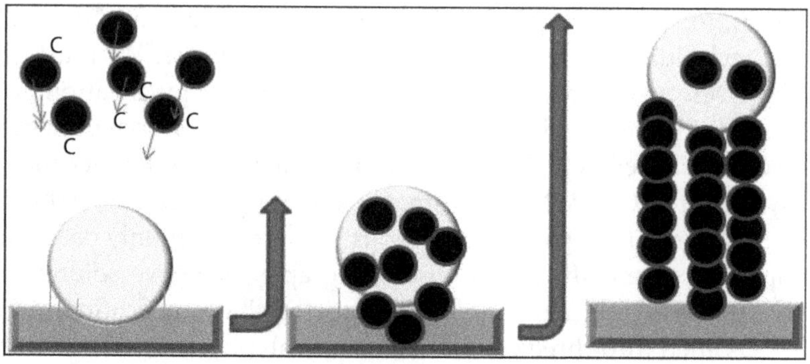

Figure 1.11 A tip growth model of driving force carbon diffusion.

related to the appearance of a nanoparticle catalyst at the end of the carbon filament, while the other shows the nanoparticle catalyst at the base of the filament [72].

1.12.1.1 Tip Growth Model

The clouds of hydrocarbon diffuse through the catalytic particle, whether or not the decomposition of the carbon source on the exposed surface of the metal catalyst results in the formation of hydrogen and carbon species. Figure 1.11 shows that the carbon dissolves in catalytic particles until reaching a supersaturated state, and then continues building in the top direction. In this case, the bonding between catalytic particles and the support surfaces is more for the surfaces and the particles of carbon atoms; thus, the catalytic particle always sits on the top of the growing nanotube.

1.12.1.2 Base Growth Model

Bottom or root carbon diffuses through a catalytic particle, as shown in Figure 1.12. In this case, the bonding between the catalyst and support is more than with particles of carbon; thus, the catalytic particle stays on the growth substrate. The carbon species dissolve in the particle and diffuses through it until a supersaturated state happens; they precipitate on top of the metal particle in the form of graphene tubes.

The process of diffusion and precipitation of carbon atoms depends on the dimensions of the catalyst, the temperature, and the hydrocarbons and gases involved in the process. At the same time, these details directly affect

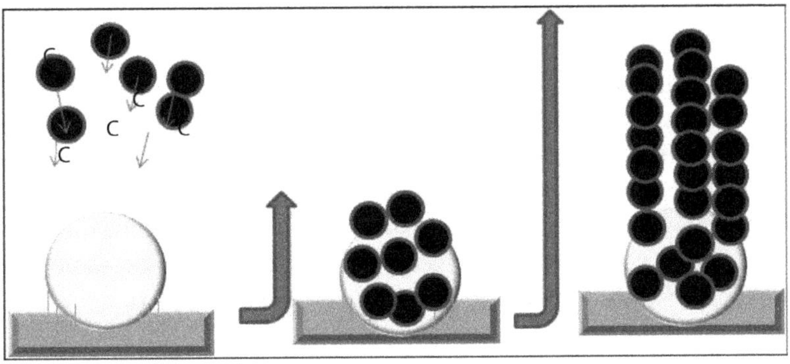

Figure 1.12 The base growth model of carbon diffusion.

the type of carbon nanotube synthesis. The two proposed models postulate that increasing the diameters of the catalyst particles increases the number of walls that form one tube. Thus, the product mostly refers to multi-walled carbon nanotubes, while decreasing the diameters changes the types to few- and single-walled carbon nanotubes. The two probabilities, the density or concentration of the catalyst per area of support, play an important role in determining the nature of the growth, which will be explained in more detail in the catalyst effect section.

Generally, the most desirable mechanism in CVD synthesis is root growth, since CNTs produced in this way are longer, more symmetrical, and better aligned than those produced by the tip growth mechanism [73]. The mechanism of SWNT production is usually root growth, but MWNTs can be produced by both growth mechanisms [74].

Experimentally, the oxidation state of the catalyst determined the types of growth; thus, the catalyst in oxidized form stays on the substrate (root growth), while the catalyst in reduced form separates from the substrate (growth tip).

1.12.2 Free Radical Condensate

This section refers to an important point, that is, ability for hydrocarbon dissociation is not essential in a catalyst for the growth of CNTs. Vander Wal *et al.* [75] suggested that catalytic behavior can be explained by electron donation to the support when creating d-vacancies, which acts as an active site to exit the hydrocarbon dissociation. Reilly and Whitten [76] completed this view when assuming that the donor or acceptor electrons enhance the formation and condensation of free radicals. Free radicals form during the process of hydrocarbon pyrolysis by breaking the bonds between the carbon and other atoms, which produce different fragments of free radicals allowing for the rapid rearrangement of carbon bonds. In this case, the catalyst particle's role simply is to provide an interface where carbon rearrangement can occur and act as a template for growth. In some cases, metal catalysts are without d-vacancies, which do not produce active sites to dissolve carbon, so neither saturation nor precipitation is possible. These catalysts are characterized by high melting points, such as Al_2O_3, having demonstrated the ability to catalyze CNT formation.

1.12.3 Yarmulke Mechanism

This mechanism was proposed by Dai *et al.* [77], which is supported by molecular dynamics simulations [78]. The proposal depends on representing the graphene as a cap collected on the surface of the particles with the chemical nature of its edges strongly bonded to the stimulator. The graphene cap tends to reduce the total capacity of the particle surface, due to the fact that the base plane of graphite has an extremely low surface energy. It also adds extra carbon atoms, and a fullerene cap is formed. Particles rise to the surface and create a hollow tube with a continued diameter growing out of the particle.

All the literature proposing a mechanism for this reaction may be a variation in terms of technique, precursor, carrier gas, catalyst, and temperature of precipitation, but all of it agrees on a set of basic principles that explain the overall process:

i. Nucleation, which is the crucial process that defines the CNT diameter and the number of walls.
ii. Growth, the second step which includes the change in diameter and the wall number of the carbon nanotubes.
iii. Termination, the third step, which is caused by catalyst deactivation, a lack of reactants due to high transport resistances, and other usually unwanted phenomena.

The growth rate of CNTs is defined by growth kinetics, activation energy, and transport resistance, which is the topic of many research groups. It is important to point out that the second step deals with the growth of tube structure, is supposed to be a fixed action unless the synthesis parameters change dramatically, or unexpected defects take place in the CNT structure.

1.13 Properties of Carbon Nanotubes

In this section, the electronic and mechanical properties are explained to understand this structure in addition to the deformation and defects that are included to complete this part.

1.13.1 Electronic Properties of Carbon Nanotubes

After 1991, when Iijima discovered CNTs, this discovery spread quickly. Carbon nanotubes as a new component in the 20th century excited every scientist, especially when there was a technological device that could achieve this purpose. One of these attempts tended to classify CNTs according to the number of walls forming them, which included SWNTs, FWNTs, and MWNTs, as mentioned previously. The histological [79] way that gave more precise details was through the chiral vector C_h, which refers to how the axis of the rolled tube is rotated in comparison with the initial unit vector of the graphene sheet.

The diameter of the tubes d_t can be obtained from the chiral vector:

$$d_t = \frac{a}{\pi}\sqrt{n^2 + m^2 + nm} = 0.0783(n^2 + m^2 + nm)^{1/2}, \qquad (1.17)$$

where $a = a_1 = a_2 = 0.246$ nm which refers to the basis vector of the graphene network. The structure of the hexagonal symmetry will always be limited between the ranges of angle $0 \leq |\theta| \leq 30$; thus, the tubes' chiral angle θ is defined as the angle between C_h and a_1. The chiral angle θ, which is the angle of the hexagons' tilt compared to the tubes, can be mathematically expressed as the equation

$$\theta = \cos^{-1}\left(2n + m/2\sqrt{n^2 + m^2 + nm}\right). \qquad (1.18)$$

The first person to predicate this phenomenon was Saito *et al.* [31]. After that, many attempts were made to study CNTs closely to create a new and modern view of these structures, later measured directly using scanning tunneling microscopy (STM) by Wildoer *et al.* [80]. The number of hexagons in one cell of carbon nanotubes can be expressed by the equation below:

$$N = 2(n^2 + m^2 + nm)/d_R, \qquad (1.19)$$

where d_R refers to the diameter of carbon nanotubes.

1.13.2 Mechanical Properties of CNTs

The materials on the nanoscale show new and varied physiochemical properties, for example, CNTs have attracted considerable attention due to their fundamental characteristics measurements and possible applications. These properties represent the main causes of much behavior such as conductivity. The mechanical properties can be understood as the nature of the bonds that form these materials, when the σ-bond is a strong chemical bond and plays an important role in the impressive mechanical properties of CNTs. The out-of-plane bond that is represented by a relatively weak π-bond enhances the interaction between the layers in MWNTs, and between SWNTs in SWNT bundles. The bonding is not purely sp^2 in nanotubes, as bending the graphene sheet inside the tube re-hybridizes the σ and π orbitals, yielding a mixture of hybridization [30].

There are several methods that could be available to predict the mechanical properties, depending on the covalent bond in the CNTs. One of the models that include these properties was the semi-empirical model. This model was proposed by Oleinik and Pettifor [79] and depends on the tight-binding approach, which applies to hydrocarbon systems. The nature and distribution of the defect directly influence the mechanical properties of CNTs, which relate to the methods used for preparing CNTs. The mechanical properties of CNTs are represented by their inelastic behavior such as fracture and plastic yielding, and their elastic properties, deformability through buckling, twisting, and flattening.

Electronic wire represents the most important applications [81] for the mechanical properties of CNT, their conductance between electrodes due to their electronic properties, as well as their mechanical deformations. The mechanical deformations can change the electronic property of nanotubes from a semiconductor to a metal, and vice versa [74]. The mechanical properties of the nonmaterial represent one of the most significant challenges in nanoscience due to the difficulty of measuring the mechanical properties of individual constituents that comprise the nanosystem.

1.14 Applications of Carbon Nanotubes

The applications of carbon nanotubes may represent the most important reason for the huge research with this material. The application includes adsorption of different poisoning materials and chemical compound, synthesis composite for a variety of applications and in the field of energy to produce and store it.

1.14.1 Fuel Cells

The unique electrical and structural properties of CNTs have proven useful in fuel cell applications [82–86]. The high surface/volume ratios make carbon nanotubes potentially useful as an additive [83] or as an anode material [84]. The useful properties of CNTs as a catalyst support [85], low resistance, high mechanical strength, and chemical stability are essential for catalytic electrodes in fuel cells such as lithium-ion battery systems. Carbon nanotubes have a large surface area and high conductivity, which can be used for many applications. For example, Pt can disperse to a higher degree on the surfaces of CNT, which acts as a support as well as a size reduction of the Pt particles with the production of huge amounts of active sites. Carbon nanotube films produced on a Si (100) substrate without any metal catalyst are used as electrodes in galvanic cells where the kinetics of hydrogen evolution influence the quantity of hydrogen stored in the nanotube [86].

The reaction starts on the anode side when hydrogen enters the fuel cell chamber from the gas channel, which transfers to the catalyst through the specific type of layers synthesized for this purpose. On the surfaces of the catalyst, the hydrogen is converted into positive protons and negative electrons, which act as an electrical power supply while the protons transfer to the cathode through the membrane layers. The two parts electrons and protons will react with oxygen to form water and heat.

The methods for preparing the electrodes for fuel cells with existing CNTs were done by using many strategies. The first method synthesizing CNT/metallic particle hybrids on pressed porous stainless steel pellets [83–84], by CVD on a nickel catalyst. An impregnation of the pellets is with a highly dispersive colloidal solution of nickel acetate in ethanol with heat treatment. This technology can simplify the fuel cell design as in this hybrid structure, the catalytic electrode, gas diffusion layer, and current collector are combined in one step without any complication of the synthesis process. The use of MWNTs as a platinum support for proton exchange membrane fuel cells has been investigated as a way of reducing the cost of fuel cells [86] through an increased utilization of platinum. Carbon nanotubes were selectively grown directly on the carbon paper by chemical vapor deposition with electrodeposited cobalt catalyzing the growth of the carbon nanotube. The as-prepared carbon nanotubes were employed as the support for the subsequent platinum catalyst, which is electrodeposited on the carbon nanotube. Nanotubes come with a variety of band gaps, high surface area, good conductivity, controllable porosity, and appropriate electrochemical stability under fuel cell operating conditions. The conductivities raise many intriguing possibilities for additional nanodevices

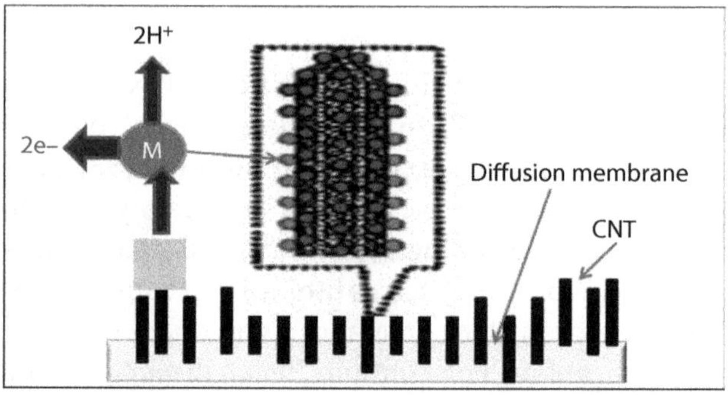

Figure 1.13 Schematic diagram of M/CNTs showing the higher distribution of M on the surfaces of CNTs with the reaction in the fuel cell.

with the increased stability of catalyst nanoparticles deposited on CNT-based support materials. Typically, when metal nanoparticles decorate carbon [86–87] nanotube, soot is prepared. This latter process allows catalyst decoration only for the active area exposed to the fuels, thus improving efficiency and reducing the cost of electrode manufacture. This architecture also functions as the gas diffusion layer, reducing the number of components required for the fuel cell device. Figure 1.13 shows the actions that can be carried out by CNTs to enhance the activities of fuel cells when representing the best material to distribute the metal in fuel cells and preventing the agglomerate.

1.14.2 Solar Cells

The photovoltaic or solar cells that produce electricity from the sun's rays use a photovoltaic process that represents renewable power. In 1839, a French physicist Alexandre-Edmond Becquerel [88] observed that there was a light-dependent voltage between two electrodes immersed in an electrolyte. In 1876, the same effect was demonstrated in selenium. In 1941, the first silicon-based solar cell was demonstrated, followed by the real beginning of modern solar cell research in 1954. This was similar to a battery when it supplies DC power, yet unlike it's due to the fact that the voltage supplied by the cell altered by changes in the resistance of the load.

Semiconductor material can be *p*-type (hole carriers), which has impurities with an extra electron, or *n*-type (electron carriers), which has impurities with one fewer electron. The system that includes them together is a solar cell with a very large *p*–*n* junction (or diode). The activities of semiconductor silicon can be explained briefly. The holes from the *p*-type side diffuse to the n-type side, the excited electrons diffuse toward the p-type, missing the electrons and leaving behind charged ions. This process causes the production of an electric field, which makes it easy for the current to flow in one direction, but hard to flow in the opposite direction. The band gap of silicon is 1.11 eV [89]; visible light can break silicon bonds and create free electrons and holes missing electrons. When sunlight collides with the surfaces of a solar cell, incident photons absorb their energy by electrons in the lower p-type layer. The absorbent photons cause the electrons to be transferred across the barrier into the upper n-type layer and escape out into the circuit that produces a DC current. Due to the need for producing green sources of energy, there has been a huge interest in looking for routes for improving efficiency in solar cells. The most common [90] cells being used commercially today are silicon-based solar cells. The most important factors that affect solar cell performance are light intensity, wavelength, the angle of incident light, the surface condition of the solar cells (cleanness), and the temperature of the solar cells [91].

The CNTs allow a current capacity four times larger than Cu, which is the best material. The MWNTs can absorb in the aggregated pores, inside the tube and/or on the external walls. These properties make CNTs very useful in numerous applications [125], particularly the semiconducting type that represents ideal solar cells. The SWNTs are very attractive for solar cell applications for many reasons: (1) the ability to absorb light with very low energy near the IR spectral range (800–1800 nm), which is not possible for most organic compounds that are used as a sensitizer in solar cells [126]. (2) The high carrier mobility and lower band-gap value of individual SWNTs [127–128] makes them the best sensitizer compared with many materials used for this purpose.

Michael *et al.* [129] fabricated flexible, transparent conducting electrodes by printing films of SWNTs networks on plastic, proving the use of these tools as transparent electrodes for efficient, flexible, polymer-fullerene, bulk-heterojunction solar cells. This printing method provides relatively smooth, homogeneous films with a transmittance of 85% at 550 nm. Huda *et al.* [130] showed that CNTs have the ability to separate carriers whereby they can form heterojunctions with conducting polymers. In addition, CNTs can transfer electrons or holes efficiently and exhibit good photovoltaic properties, in spite of the efficiency of polymer solar cells being limited to a few percent, much lower than Si-based solar cells.

The proposed rules of CNTs can lead to an increase in the efficiency of solar cells. Prashant *et al.* [97] found a good alignment between CNTs that can further enhance their photoconductivity on illumination. This may be attributed to the active surface area of the CNTs increasing their ability to absorb huge concentrations of energy from solar photons [98], while π electrons are delocalized in nature giving a high electronic polarizability. Scarselli *et al.* [99] assumed that conduction due to sp^2-hybridized carbon atoms also exhibits faster phonon transport than any other material. Khatri *et al.* [100] proposed that a heterojunction component was formed between CNTs, and incorporated into silicon. This skim behaves as an ideal separation charge due to the behavior of a highly conductive percolated network for charge transport, and as a transparent electrode for light illumination and charge collection. Jia *et al.* [101] found that the stability of synthesized connections in CNT/Si heterojunctions for a modest cell is the primary requirement for efficiency and an improvement in activity.

1.14.3 Dye-sensitized Solar Cells

Lee *et al.* [102] fabricated dye-sensitized solar cells (DSCs) using TiO_2-coated multi-walled carbon nanotubes (TiO_2-CNTs). They introduced CNTs into DSCs to improve solar cell performance, although a reduction in series resistance has attracted much attention in this field. TiO_2-CNTs were obtained by using the Sol–Gel method, with TiO_2 content only 0.1 wt.% of CNTs producing a cell with a more than 50% increase in conversion efficiency. The activity can relate to an increase in the short circuit current density, an increase in the absorbance of light, and interconnectivity between the TiO_2 particles and the CNTs in the porous TiO_2 film. Arman *et al.* [103] synthesized three types of counter electrodes consisting of TiO_2 and Pt. The modification was made by using MWNTs fabricated as follows: counter electrodes Pt, MWNT-counter electrodes, and mixed Pt-MWNT-counter electrodes. The results show that an enhanced efficiency was obtained by using the Pt MWNT-counter electrodes, when the energy conversion efficiency increased to about 18% in comparison with standard DSSCs.

1.15 Characterization of CNTs

Many techniques were used to characterize and understand the structure and nature of carbon nanotubes. In this section the common methods were explained briefly.

1.15.1 Raman Spectroscopy

Raman spectroscopy is a technique that investigates a sub-category of a material vibration condition using monochromatic light. The activities of this technique are represented in its ability to convey the information about the characteristic vibrations of the material, both optical and electronic. During irradiation, the spectrum of the scattered radiation is measured at 90° with an appropriate spectrometer. The intensities of the Raman lines are 0.001% of the intensity of the source, which could be Stokes scattering. This can be shown by using common materials for this purpose; CCl_4 when irradiating a sample of carbon tetrachloride with an intense beam from an argon ion laser have a wavelength of 488.0 nm (20492 cm^{-1}). The emitted radiation as shown in Figures 1.14 and 15 produces three types of scattering signals: the first two types are Stokes and anti-Stokes scattering that represent less than 1% of the scattering radiation. The third type is Rayleigh scattering, which accounts for more than 99%. The first type refers to the indicator for Raman spectroscopy, but not all of it because the anti-Stokes lines are appreciably less intense that the corresponding Stokes lines. Thus, only the Stokes part of the spectrum is generally used which is independent of the excitation wavelength.

The Raman spectrum is represented by the wavenumber shift $\Delta\upsilon$, which is defined as the difference in wavenumbers (cm^{-1}) between the observed radiation and that of the source.

The Stokes and anti-Stokes types are different from the Rayleigh radiation in terms of their frequencies corresponding to $\pm\Delta E$, the energy of the first vibrational level of the ground state. If the bond was infrared active [103], the energy of its absorption would also be ΔE. Thus, the Raman frequency shift and the infrared absorption peak frequency are identical. Rayleigh scattering has a considerably higher probability of occurrence than Raman because the most probable event is the energy transfer of molecules in the ground state and re-emission by the return of these molecules to the ground state (>99%). The relative population of the two Stokes emissions is much favored over anti-Stokes. The ratio of anti-Stokes to Stokes intensity increases with temperature because a larger fraction of the molecules is in

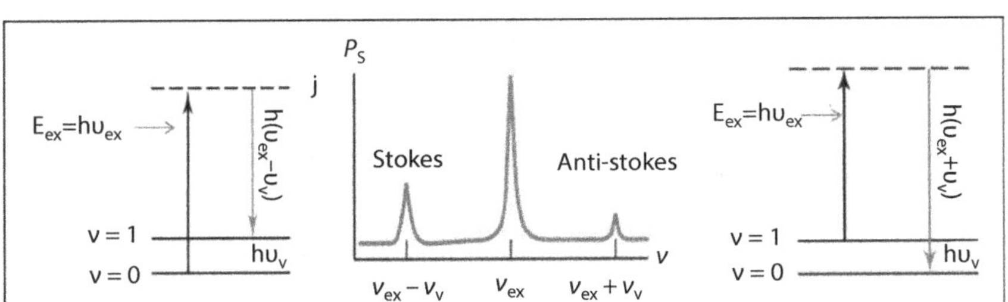

Figure 1.14 Schematic of the Stokes and anti-Stokes transition with a Raman shift.

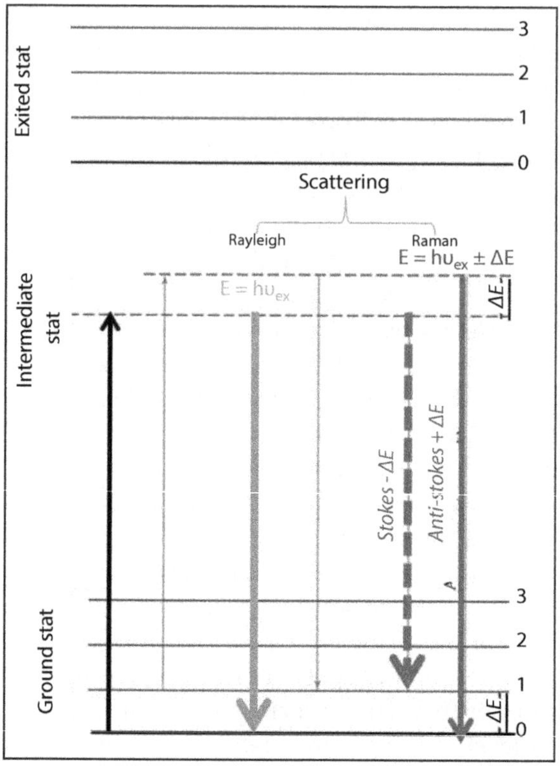

Figure 1.15 Schematic diagram showing the types of transition of the electrons and the Rayleigh and Raman scattering.

the first vibrationally excited state under these circumstances. The Raman spectroscopy recognized by the energy shifts observed should be identical [104] to the energies of its infrared absorption bands. That provided the vibrational activities involved are active with both infrared absorption and Raman scattering. The differences between a Raman spectrum and an infrared spectrum depend on the real conditions between them, that is, the dipole moment. Infrared absorption requires a vibrational mode of the molecule has a change in dipole moment or the charge distribution associated with it. Scattering involves a momentary distortion of the electrons distributed around a bond in a molecule, followed by re-emission of the radiation as the bond returns to its normal state. The distorted form of the molecule is temporarily polarized, which momentarily develops an induced dipole that disappears upon relaxation and re-emission. The Raman activity of a given vibrational mode may differ markedly from its infrared activity. The intensity of the Raman peak depends in a complex way on the polarizability of the molecule, the intensity of the source, and the concentration of the active group. The power of the Raman emission increases with the fourth power of the frequency of the source. The advantage can rarely be taken of this relationship because of the likelihood that ultraviolet irradiation will cause decomposition by the light. Raman intensities are usually directly proportional to the concentration of the active species. Polarization is a property of a beam of radiation and describes the plane in which the radiation vibrates, which is required for excited Raman spectra. The scattered radiation is found to be polarized to various degrees depending on the type of vibration responsible for the scattering. The depolarization ratio P is defined as

$$p = \frac{I_{\perp}}{I_{\shortparallel}} \tag{1.24}$$

Experimentally, the depolarization ratio may be obtained by inserting a polarizer between the sample and the monochromator. The depolarization ratio is dependent on the symmetry of the vibrations responsible for scattering. Thus, polarized band: $p = <0.76$ for totally symmetric modes (A_{1g}), depolarized band: $p = 0.76$ for B_{1g} and B_{2g} nonsymmetrical vibrational modes, and anomalously polarized band: $p = >0.76$ for A_{2g} vibrational modes.

The Raman spectra of many carbon materials containing a variable amount of sp^2 structures as a type of symmetric model have been extensively studied [107]. Raman spectroscopy is one of the most extensively employed methods for the characterization of carbon nanotubes, and which is a tool for the characterization of carbon nanotubes and functionalized carbon nanotubes [158], attracting a lot of attention in recent years. Theoretically, it is possible to predict morphological characteristics such as the diameter of the tubes and experimentally a powerful method for determining the degree of structural ordering or the presence of contaminants [104–108]. The variety of carbon materials arise from the strong dependence of their physical properties on the ratio of sp^2 such as graphite to sp^3 such as diamond [109]. There are many forms of sp^2-bonded carbons with various degrees of graphitic ordering, ranging from single crystals of graphite, to nanocrystals, to glassy carbon [110].

As shown in Figure 1.16, the most distinguished Raman features in CNTs are the radial breathing modes (RBMs), caused by the higher frequency of disordered D, the G graphite network, and the G' (second-order Raman scattering from D-band variation) modes. The D, G and G^- modes are found in graphite; and the RBM is specific to CNTs and is representative of

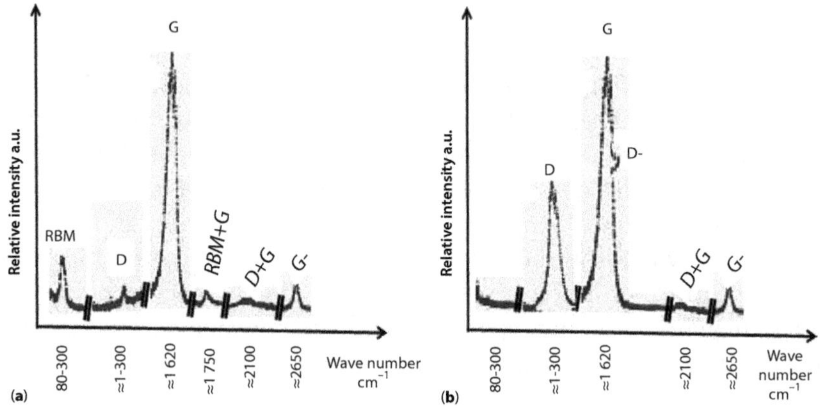

Figure 1.16 Skim of typical Raman spectroscopy for (a) SWNT and (b) MWNT.

the isotropic radial expansion of the tube. The RBM frequency is inversely proportional to the diameter of the tube, making it an important feature for determining the diameter distribution in a sample. The RBM bands are a useful diagnostic tool for confirming the presence of CNTs in a sample. The composite of CNTs with different materials has been evaluated by using Raman spectroscopy, which shows the state of dispersion and the polymer–filler interactions, reflected by shifts or width changes of the peaks. The sensitivity of some bands of CNTs to an application of mechanical distortion of the composite has also been used to quantify the load transferred from the matrix to the nanotubes and the interfacial adhesion [109].

1.15.1.1 G band

The G band as shown in Figure 1.16 is a tangential shear mode of carbon atoms assigned to the in-plane vibration of the C–C bond that corresponds to the stretching mode in the graphite plane [111]. In simple graphite, a single mode is observed at 1580 cm^{-1} while in CNTs this mode transforms into two modes as a result of the confinement of wave vectors along the circumference. The position of the G-band can be used to monitor the energy state change due to the environment. The frequency of the high-energy branch G^+ does not differ with diameter, while the lower energy peak G^- becomes more regular for smaller diameter CNTs. One of the important aspects of CNTs [112] is either metallic or semiconducting with a variable and direct band gap. The metallic tubes are easily recognized by the broad and the asymmetric line shape of the G^- band. The frequency down shift of the G^- band is particularly strong for metallic tubes, with down shifts of greater than 100 cm^{-1} for smaller diameter tubes, whereas the G^+ frequency remains essentially constant with diameter for metallic and semiconductor tubes.

1.15.1.2 D Band

The second peak is the D band, which is a longitudinal optical (LO) phonon and known as the disordered or defect style because a defect is required to scatter flexibly in order to maintain momentum. This property may relate to scattering from that defect and amorphous carbon impurities present in preparing CNTs. This style is usually located between 1250 and 1450 cm^{-1} and has a linear according to the laser excitation energy [113]. The D band is present in all carbon allotropes, including sp^2 and sp^3 amorphous carbon. This band is activated from the first-order scattering process of sp^2 carbons by the presence of in-plane substitution hetero-atoms, vacancies, grain boundaries, or other defects, and by finite size effects. All of these characteristics reduce the crystal symmetry [114] of the lattice network. When observed in MWNTs, the D band is generally represented by a defect in the tubes. This band can be used to observe the complete building of a perfect structure of nanotubes. It can also be used to qualitatively characterize the chemical functionalization of the tube. Sidewall functionalization damages the tube, thus increasing the D band intensity, thus use to evaluate the quality using the D/G band intensities. For high-quality samples without defects and amorphous carbon, the D/G ratio is often less than 2%. The D-band width for CNTs is generally 10 to 20 cm^{-1}.

The D to G band intensity ratio (I_D/I_G) is the intensity of the disorder mode divided by the intensity of the graphite mode. This ratio is commonly used to evaluate the distortion on the surfaces of CNTs, an increase in the ID/IG ratio indicates an increase in the number of defects on the sidewall of the G' Band [114]. The G-band frequency is close to twice that of the D band and is found from 2500 to 2900 cm^{-1}. This is a second-order process from two-zone boundary LO phonons, or it may be attributed to the overtone of the D band. This band is commonly used to evaluate the load transfer between SWNTs and other types. The G-band is an intrinsic property of the nanotube and graphite, and is present even in defect-free nanotubes for which the D band is completely absent.

1.15.1.3 Radial Breathing Mode

The radical breathing mode (RBM) constitutes evidence for the existence of CNTs in a sample, and represents the borderline between a planar structure and a cylindrical structure. The RBM is used to characterize between graphene and carbon nanotubes due to a very important point that is not present in graphite. This mode is found between 75 and 300 cm^{-1} from the excitation line, and is associated with the symmetric transmission carbon atoms in the radial direction. The RBM [111–112] frequency (ω_r) is inversely proportional to the nanotube diameter with the relationship

$$\omega_r = 224(cm^{-1})/d_t(nm). \tag{1.24}$$

Tube diameters between 0.8 and 1.3 nm give nearly identical results. Most single-grating Raman spectrometers have cutoff frequencies between 100 and 120 cm^{-1}, which limits the range of tube diameters to smaller than 2 to 2.5 nm. Larger tubes can be measured with high Rayleigh rejection multi-grating systems that allow frequencies of less than 100 cm^{-1}. Due to the resonance behavior of the Raman intensity, several laser lines should be used to determine the extent of the diameter distribution.

1.15.2 X-Ray Diffraction

X-ray diffraction (XRD) is one of the most important non-destructive tools for analyzing all kinds of matter ranging from fluids, to powders and crystals, from research, to production and engineering. This technique uses X-ray diffraction on powder or microcrystalline samples, where ideally every possible crystalline orientation is represented equally. The resulting orientation averaging causes the three-dimensional reciprocal space that is studied in single crystal diffraction to be projected onto a single dimension. X-rays can be obtained from different sources, including basically either X-ray generators or synchrotron facilities [116–117]. In the first case, the wavelength depends on the metal used as an anode. For copper, the characteristic spectral line used is that of a wavelength 0.154 nm. For X-ray synchrotron radiation, besides a much higher radiation flux, a tuning of the λ-values is possible. The simplest and probably the most frequently used implication of the scattering theory is Bragg's law. By considering crystals as reflection layers for X-rays, Bragg derived the following equation [117]:

$$n\lambda = 2d_{hkl}\sin\theta, \tag{1.25}$$

where λ is the wavelength of the X-rays, 2θ is the diffraction angle, n is an integral number which refer to order of diffraction, and d represents the distance between the successive identical in the crystal. Many materials do not appear as single crystals but in a polycrystalline state and therefore the diffraction spots transform into circles due to the different orientation of the crystallites. A common alternative process includes fixing the sample in the horizontal position and moving both the source and the detector by $-\theta$ and θ, respectively. The different crystallographic planes in a crystal are characterized by the Miller indexes (hkl). The three integral numbers were related to the reciprocal values of the intersection of a given plane with the crystallographic unit cell axes being an indispensible method for the characterization and quality control of structural materials. The equation that used was the Debye–Scherrer equation [117]:

$$d = K\lambda/\beta \cos\theta, \tag{1.26}$$

where d is the average crystallite size, λ is the X-ray wavelength in nanometers (nm) equal to (0.15405 nm), and β is the peak width of the diffraction peak profile at half the maximum height resulting from a small crystal (FWHM) size in radians. The K is a constant related to the crystallite shape mostly equal to 0.94. Carbon nanotubes basically adopt two characteristic morphologies, either possessing a single wall or having multiple walls. SWNTs are made from a single graphene layer, which is a hexagonal carbon network, where the way in which the layer is rolled up determines the chirality of the nanotube and controls the electronic properties. MWNTs consist of concentric single-walled tubes, where each individual tube may have a different chirality.

The XRD pattern for CNTs generally shows two characteristic peaks at $2\theta \approx 26\theta$. When compared to normal graphite at $2\theta = 26.5°$, this peak shows a downward shift due to an increase in the sp^2; C = C layers spacing [118] and ≈43° appear, which can be attributed to the diffraction from the C(001) and C(002) planes of the carbon nanotubes. The second peak is more intense in MWNTs than in SWNTs [118]. One of the most important uses of XRD is ascertaining the quality and crystalline nature of nanotubes as opposed to amorphous carbon materials, as well as the purities of synthesized CNTs.

1.15.3 X-ray Photoelectron Spectroscopy

The X-ray photoelectron spectroscopy (XPS) techniques is among a group of techniques that depends on the photoelectron effect. These techniques includes Electron Spectroscopy for Chemical Analysis (ESCA), and Ultraviolet Photoelectron Spectroscopy (UPS) or Photoemission Spectroscopy (PES). The technique provide information about chemical composition and structure of a surface. The method was developed in 1960 by Kai Siegbahn and his research group at the University of Uppsala, Sweden [119]. The idea behind this technique can be related to the levels of energy for every shells of electrons such 1s, 2s, 2p, etc. which represent the identified spectra of the shell. Every ejected photoelectron has kinetic energy KE, which is identified by equation:

$$KE = hu - BE. \tag{1.27}$$

The value of hu refers to photon energy and BE = energy necessary to remove a specific electron from an atom, which is mostly equal to orbital energy. The BE for conducting and isolating samples can be measured by XPS or ESCA spectra, which is the identification for the metals and compounds. The in XPS, the energy spectrum depends on the anode used to produce the X-rays, meaning the photoelectric lines move in position when the same sample is analyzed but using a different anode to produce the X-rays, these lines provide the bulk of the chemical information found in the spectra, and it is this chemical information that makes XPS such a powerful technique. The photoelectric line positions with respect to a binding energy scale are independent of the X-rays used to excite the sample, while Auger line positions are invariant with respect to the X-ray anode only when plotted against a kinetic energy scale. The surface consist of an atoms layer which influenced by 2–10 atomic layers that are below it (0.5–3 nm). After the radiation by X-ray which penetrates with a depth ~1 μm, many electrons will be emitted. The typical process for the XPS spectrum that include two axes which are intensities of photoelectrons versus EB or KE. The technique can be for elemental identification, chemical state of element, relative composition of the constituents in the surface region, valence band. The advantages of XPS analysis includes higher sensitive at monolayer surface, ability to analyze a wide range of solids, and relatively non-destructive capabilities. It disadvantages are related to high cost, long analysis time and poor spatial resolution. The limitation of XPS [120] It major limitation, from the operational point of view is that it requires not less than ~5 mg sample. This is due to the comparatively large analysis area of ~10 μm diameter that is required. In an analysis of sample such as graphene, the characterization peak of carbon corresponding to C=C is expected at 284 e V. Table 1.1: shows common values of band that predicted existence in carbon nanotubes.

For example, the synthesized carbon nanotubes from natural petroleum gas were tested with X-ray photoelectron spectroscopy. The nature of different groups that were covalently linked to the nanotube surface refer to the existence of C=C which refer to nanotubes or graphene sheets. Figure 1.17a shows the photoemission C1s peaks were studied between 282 and 292 ev, a dominant peak at 284.5 eV regarding the sp2 hybridized C=C bonds in extensive conjugated systems[121–122] which mostly refer

Table 1.1 Binding energy for different functional groups.

Functional group		Binding energy (eV)
hydrocarbon	C–H, C–C	285.0
amine	C–N	286.0
alcohol, ether	C–O–H, C–O–C	286.5
Cl bound to C	C–Cl	286.5
F bound to C	C–F	287.8
carbonyl	C=O	288.0

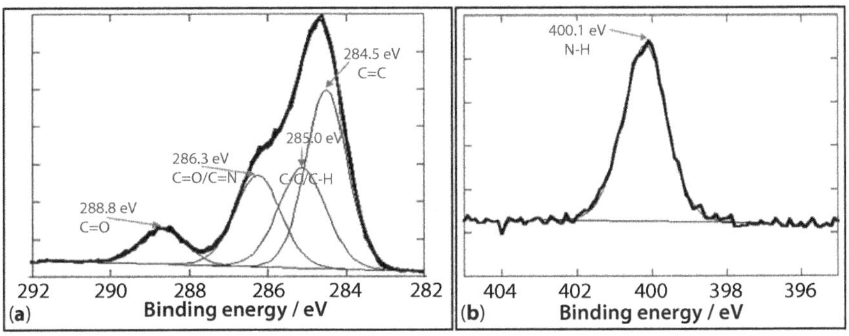

Figure 1.17 XPS of synthesized MWNTs. (a) C 1s spectra between 282 and 292 eV, (b) N–H spectra between 396 and 404 eV. Arrows show possible positions of carbon peaks as described in the text.

to graphene sheet in carbon nanotubes. The same figure includes a peak at 285.0 eV, which is characteristic of sp^3-hybridized C–C bonds present at defective locations [123] and tubular structure asymmetry, which related to C–H and C–C [124]. Two additional photoemission peaks are observed at 286.3 and 288.8 ev. The first at 286.3 ev is attributed to carbon atoms bonded to oxygen atoms C–O which bonded with C–N. The second at 288.8 ev is characteristic of carbon atoms pertaining to carbonyl groups C=O [125]. Figure 1.17b shows N 1s 400.1 ev spectra which corresponds to N-H where N is bonded to C=C groups [126].

1.15.4 Thermo Gravimetric Analysis

Thermo gravimetric analysis (TGA) is a technique that studies the weight of materials as they change with temperature or time. The methods depend on the idea which is that after decomposition by heating, the decomposition temperature and change in weight is a characteristic property of each material. The data obtained from a TG experiment are displayed as a thermal curve with a diagram displaying the units of weight on the *y* axis, and the *x* axis may be in units of either temperature or time. The process that causes a change in the weight of the materials in this technique was desorption, drying, dehydration, desolvation, vaporization, decomposition, solid–solid reactions, and solid–gas reactions, the whole of this process causing a reduction in the weight of the sample. There are other processes that cause increases in the weight of the samples such as adsorption, absorption, and oxidation, in addition to solid–gas reactions, which may cause increasing the weight of the sample. The change in the weight of the sample was made by using thermo balance, which is characterized by a high degree of precision in three actions: the change in the weight of the sample, the temperature of the reaction, and the change in temperature.

The other part of this apparatus consists of computerized furnaces which are characterized by their ability to make changes in the temperature to a high degree of sensitivity so as to make the change in heat constant. The maximum temperature is selected so that the specimen weight is stable at the end of the experiment, implying that all the chemical reactions are completed. For this work, which is dealing with carbon nanotubes, when all of the carbon is burnt off, metal oxides are left behind. The evaluation of a single TG curve is shown in Figure 1.18. The reactions corresponding to the mass losses can be determined, or confirmed, by a simultaneous evolved gas analysis (EGA),

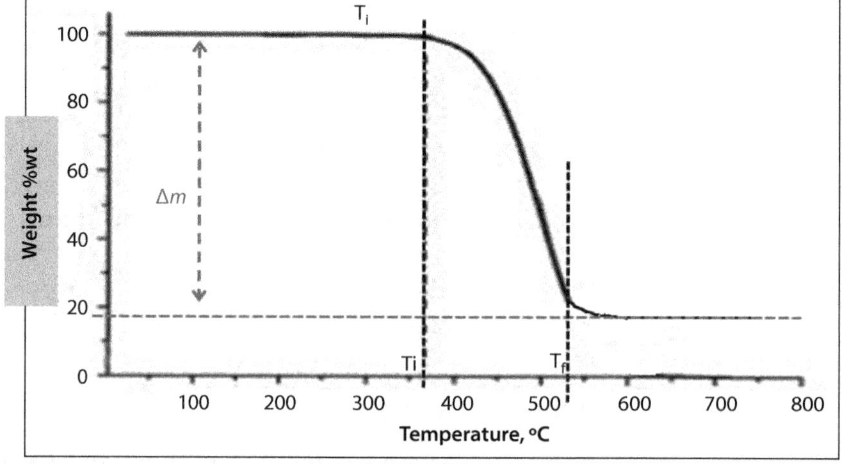

Figure 1.18 The evaluation of a single TGA curve.

where T_i and T_f are the initial and final temperatures of decomposition. In most cases, the TGA analysis is performed in an oxidative atmosphere (air or oxygen and inert gas mixtures) with a linear temperature slope.

The oxidation rates of carbon nanotubes measured in air at atmospheric pressure within the TGA are unique for each CNT sample of different walls. The oxidation temperature [127] can be defined by the temperature of the maximum in the weight loss rate ($\delta_m/\delta T_{max}$) and the weight loss onset temperature (T_{onset}). The former refers to the temperature of the maximum rate of oxidation, while the latter refers to the temperature when the oxidation has just begun. The first term $T_o = \delta m/\delta T_{max}$ is preferred for two reasons:

1. The gradual initiation of transition (sometimes up to 100 °C) may make it difficult to determine T_{onset} precisely. Gradual onset is believed to be due to the nanotubes being contaminated with amorphous carbon and other types of carbonaceous impurities that oxidize at temperatures lower than that of the nanotubes. In these cases, T_{onset} describes the properties of the impurities rather than the nanotubes.
2. Weight loss due to carbon oxidation is often imposed on the weight increase due to catalyst oxidation at low temperatures.

A typical analysis [128] using a TGA measurement of an as-produced nanotube material in air generally shows one peak in the dm/dT curve. An analysis of purified nanotube material in air may produce more than one peak that may relate to many causes: one reason for which is related to the deformation found on the surfaces of carbon nanotubes. The ether group is probably arises from the synthesis or purification process. In addition to various components in the nanotube material such as amorphous carbon, nanotubes, and graphitic particles, the TGA can depend on an evaluation of the purities of synthesized carbon nanotubes, the nature of the surfaces of the tubular structures, and the types of CNTs.

1.15.5 Transmission Electron Microscopy

Transmission electron microscopy (TEM) represents the most important requirement in the science of nanotechnology. This tool now obtains very high-quality images for the investigation of many physical and chemical properties with a resolution reaching 100–1000 keV. This includes the size, density, and nature of surfaces, as well as their electronic and magnetic properties. Chemically, they are represented by the strength of the bond between the components of the samples in addition to the change that occurred for the materials [129] after the reaction. The process depends on electrons, whereby one type of ionizing radiation is capable of removing one of the tightly bound inner-shell electrons from the attractive field of the nucleus. The resolution ρ of the TEM can be found by using a simple equation, which is Abbe's theory of images formation for a incoherent electron beam:

$$\rho = \frac{0.61\lambda}{\sin\alpha}, \tag{1.28}$$

when ρ directly influences the wavelength of the incident light λ, and the maximum value of the angle a between the incident and deflected beam in the limit of the lens diffusion. The incident light should be concentric in the fixed ring of the wavelength, which requires a higher efficiency lens not yet found; however, this problem can be reduced by using many lenses to raise the activity for the TEM resolutions. Hans Bush showed in 1927 that a magnetic coil can focus an electron beam to the same extent that glass lens can produce. In 1932, Ernst Ruska and Max Knoll succeeded in taking the first images from a TEM. In this case, they accelerated the electrons by 100–1000 kV, which could reach the speed of light and the magnitude to magnitude to increase the resolution of the TEM. In 1950, Raymond used an X-ray detector with an electron probe known as EDS spectrometry, which is commonly used by TEM to analyze many materials.

The process of analyzing the sample includes specific arrangements to prepare the sample due to many reasons such scattering caused by a strong interaction between the electrons of the beam and the atoms of the samples. One should take care with the thickness of the sample, which influences the efficiency of the system, and which depends on the material's properties, the acceleration voltage, and the requirements of the individual investigation method. The intensity needed for the test should be enough to allow for the transmittance of electrons up to 100 nm. Thus, there are some notes that deal with the disadvantages, as follows:

1. A long time is required for the preparation of the sample to be examined.
2. Only a small part of the sample can be examined.
3. The electron beams used in these techniques cause damage to samples such as living objects, biomolecules, and inorganic substances.

Kroto *et al.* [19] reported that (TEM) represents the ideal methods for carbon nanomaterial research due to the ability of carbon atoms to form different structures such as diamond, graphite, fullarene, carbon nanofibers, and MWNTs [130–131]. Carbon nanofibers and any type of carbon nanotubes look similar when observed with scanning electron microscopy. It is almost impossible to distinguish between carbon nanofibers and MWNTs unless observed using TEM, as the former are solid filled 1-D nanostructures and the latter are hollow concentric 1-D nanotubules. TEM gives direct insight into the nanostructure of carbon materials. The absence of TEM observations can lead to wrong conclusions in the case of carbon nanomaterials. It is the most important and most reliable technique for correctly identifying the nature and form of carbon nanomaterials in academic research and industry. From TEM observations, it can be seen whether the nature of the CNT walls are well crystallized or not [132–133], in addition to giving direct insight into the microstructure of these materials and informing about the nature or form of the material. The high resolution transmission electron microscopy (HR-TEM) observation of the formation of carbon nanfibers and SWNT is very important to understanding the orientations of carbon atoms in CNTs; whether they are forming metallic ones or semiconductors [133–135].

1.15.6 Scanning Electronic Microscopy

This is a microscope that produces an image by using electrons instead of light to form an image that scans the surface of a specimen inside a vacuum chamber. A beam of electrons is focused on a spot volume of the specimen, resulting in the transfer of energy to the spot, excluding electrons from the specimen itself. The removed electrons, also known as secondary electrons, are attracted and collected by a positively biased grid or detector, and then translated into a signal.

These bombarding electrons are used in many applications such as topography and morphology, chemistry, crystallography, and orientation of grains. In a scanning electron microscope (SEM), they probe very carefully with electrons, with an energy up to 40 kV focusing on the surface of the sample. The working mechanism of this system depends on the number of phenomena that occur on the surface which comes under the influence of electrons. Those most important to the microscope and the emission of secondary electrons with energies of a few tens of volts and the re-emission or reflection of electrons with a high energy counterattack from the primary beam. The emission intensity of each of the secondary electrons is very sensitive, as is the counterattack of the angle at which the electron beam hits the surface, i.e., to the topographic features on the sample. The electron current that is emitted and amplified is collected. Using variations in the signal output power, the electron investigation is also scanned across the sample to change the brightness of the impact of the cathode ray tube, which is scanned in synchronization with the investigation. Consequently, there is direct correspondence *in situ* between the scanning electron beam across the sample and the fluorescent image on the cathode ray tube. The working mechanism for this system depends on the use of electrons instead of light to form an image. A beam of electrons is produced at the top of the microscope by heating a metallic filament. The electron beam follows a vertical path through the column of the microscope. This column fixes the direction of the path directly through electromagnetic lenses that focus and draw the line toward the beam down toward the sample. As soon as it hits the sample, other electron backscatter or the secondary ones are ejected from the sample. Detectors collect the secondary or backscattered electrons, and convert them into a signal that is sent to a viewing screen in order to produce an image of the sample in the measured region.

The magnification produced by SEM is the ratio between the dimensions of the final image display and the field scanned on the specimen. Usually, the magnification range of SEM is between 10 and 200,000 X, and the resolution (resolving power) is between (4 to 10) nm (40–100) Angstroms. Field Emission Scanning Electron Microscopy (FESEM) is a modified technique that has a wider scope of activity compared with SEM without any enhancement by field emission, a high-resolution imaging technique providing topographical and structural information in plain view or in cross-section. In the last few years, many instruments joined SEM to create a system more active for analysis, often in conjunction with SEM; Energy Dispersive X-Ray Spectroscopy (EDX) is used to qualitatively and quantitatively analyze the elements present in the selected area of the SEM image. Together, the FE-SEM and EDX capabilities allow irradiation by a focused electron beam, imaging secondary or backscattered electrons and an energy analysis of X-rays. Typical SEM applications include plan view and cross-sectional imaging for process development and failure analysis. EDX applications include specific defect analysis or compositional analysis.

1.15.7 Scanning Helium Ion Microscopy

This SHIM technique also refers as rHeIM or HIM is capable of making observation at sub-nanometer resolution. The advantage of using helium ion as the emitting source instead photons or electrons is the ability to obtain scans that are not feasible by conventional microscopes. This is due to the short De Broglie wavelength of the helium ions, which is inversely proportional to their momentum, providing a very high source brightness.

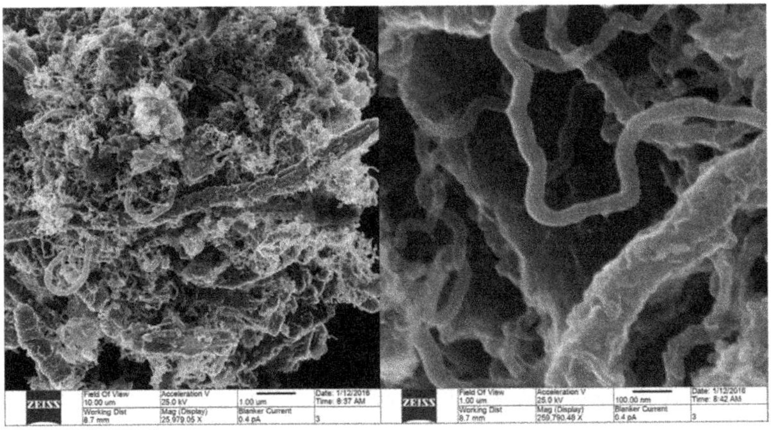

Figure 1.19 Typical HIM image for synthesized CNTs.

The device depends on interacting the helium ion beam with the sample, which is concerned with small volume, thus providing sharp images, a large depth of materials. The ion source consists of a needle supplied with high voltage under vacuum and low temperature. The concentric electric field causes many helium atoms to convert into ions which accelerated away from the needle. The accelerated ions will emit at 1 A° in size forming brightness beam of 4×10^9 A/cm^{2}sr. From Figure 1.19, the images of HIM for the samples show the presence of the catalyst with MWNTs in addition to clear images to determine the diameter of the tubes.

1.16 Composite of CNTs/Semiconductors

Continuous changes in the production techniques of composites have attracted the attention of researchers in the various branches of science. These techniques aim to preserve their beneficial properties and try to increase their efficiency with the introduction of new standards to this component, which may not be already owned or efficiently in few capacities and are intended to be introduced to the composites [135–140]. One of their most important properties is the production of nanomaterials along with the improvement of their physiochemical properties, due to the unique importance in the technology of its applications. It may have been their low cost and small dimensions that represented the primary concern of huge practical applications of various metal oxides such as TiO_2, SnO_2, ZnO, Fe_2O_3, MnO_2, and RuO_2 with CNTs, which were reported in a lot of the literature [141–148]. The methods for preparing composites with carbon nanotubes include many ways of combining semi-conductors with carbon nanotubes such as mechanical mixing [149], sol–gel [150–153], chemical vapor deposition [154], and electro-spinning methods [155]. The common denominators that combine these ways are that all of these methods produce *in situ* dipping for semi-conductors with CNTs, except for mechanical mixing, which is not *in situ* dipping. The simplest methods have included first CNTs treated chemically to enhance the activity [150–159] of the surfaces before dispersing in the solutions of the semi-conductors, followed by removing the solvents. The aims behind the activation process were the creation of many reactive points at the locations where the reaction is desired to achieve the purpose of the synthesis of hybrid composites, which was to offer new advantages. The CNT surface serves as a template where many types of semiconductors are absorbed or linked by bonds [160–161]. The hybrid composites between CNTs and semiconductors show more activity, which enhances the activities produced from CNTs. The most cases related the activity to increasing the spectrum of the absorbance of the light from the semiconductors or reducing its band gap. The two cases lead to the same results, which is a new semiconductor activity as compared with it alone. There are different mechanisms between semiconductors and CNTs regardless of the aims behind the synthesis composite such as fuel cells, hydrogen production, photocatalytic degradations, or sensitizers. All share a particular object of this stimulus, which is CNTs of higher surface areas and good conductivity can withdraw the exiton electron from the semiconductor to CNTs. This behavior prevents the recombination of e^-/h^+ and [162] increases the rate of the reactions due to the dispersion of the electrons into more regions to increase the probability of a photoreaction. Our previous works include two sections: Firstly, the adsorption with CNTs by available adsorption sites of CNT bundles, which involved the external surface, interstitial and groove areas, and the inner pores of the CNTs tubes. Secondly the increase in adsorption and photocatalytic activities of binary and ternary composites [163]. The binary composites as depicted in Figure 1.20, relate activity to the formation of OH in high concentration and conductivity, while the agglomerations of TiO_2 is lowered.

The ternary composites as we reported in our previous work [40] when Pt–TiO_2 NPs/CNTs were synthesized utilizing sonochemical/hydration–dehydration techniques. The Pt was loaded on TiO_2 by a photodeposition method to achieve electron–hole pair separation and promote the surface reaction. The activity of ternary composites as shown in Figure 1.21 was related to three causes. Firstly, the Pt nanoparticles that are photodeposited on TiO_2 forming a Schottky barrier at the Pt–TiO_2 interface based on the difference between the Pt and the electron affinity of the TiO_2 conduction

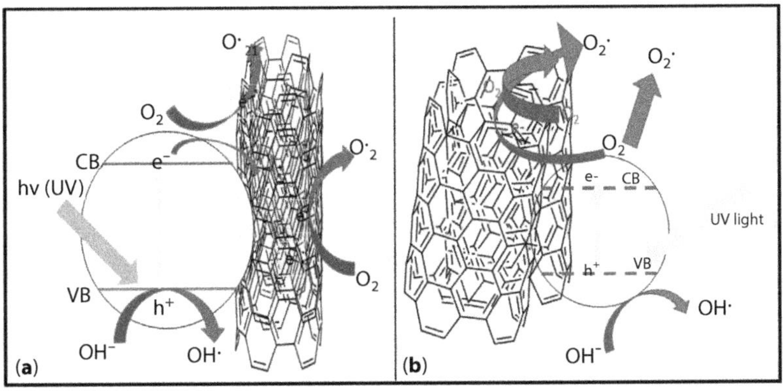

Figure 1.20 Schematic of a proposed model for (a) TiO_2/MWNT and (b) TiO_2/SWNT mechanisms.

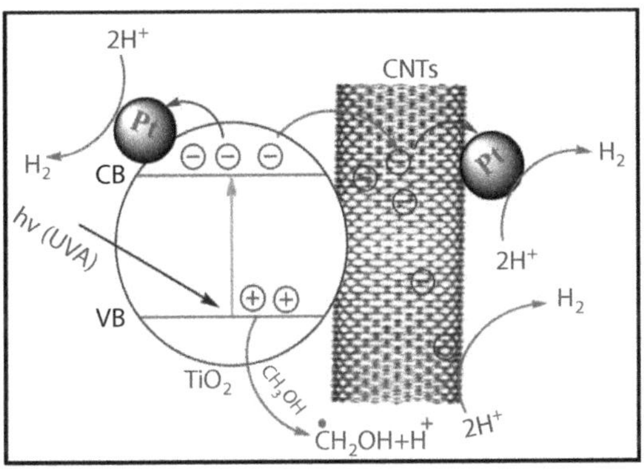

Figure 1.21 Schematic diagram for the mechanism of the reactions for the ternary composite (Pt-TiO_2/fCNTs).

band. Secondly, the excited electrons transferred from the low electron conductivity of the TiO_2 phase to the high electron conductivity of the carbon phase in the TiO_2/CNT composites. Lastly, the TiO_2 particles well-mixed with the fCNTs network create local potential differences in the TiO_2 phase that spread through the sample, resulting in more effective e−/h+ separation within the entire sample.

1.17 Recent Updates on Synthesis of CNTs

Carbon nanotubes (CNTs) were synthesized by flame fragments deposition (FFD) of natural gas. In this method, natural gas was used as a carbon source for synthesizing CNTs and as a source for the required energy. The deposition of CNTs was done at low temperatures (160 °C). The natural gas was fed into a homemade instrument. The instrument consists of an internal burner to burn the natural gas in the existence of oxygen gas to maintain the continuity of the flame of the burner while nitrogen gas is used to keep the flame at a suitable form. In addition, nitrogen gas is used to cool the synthesized sample. Gases flow rates are controlled by specific gauges. The synthesization was carried on without using a catalyst [164–166].

References

1. Popov, V. Carbon nanotubes: properties and application. *Mater. Sci. Eng. R.*, 43, 3, 61, 2004.
2. Dresselhaus, M., Jorio, A., Saito, R. Characterizing graphene, graphite, and carbon nanotubes by Raman spectroscopy. *Annu. Rev. Condens. Matter Phys.*, 1, 89, 2010.
3. Dai, H. Carbon nanotubes: Synthesis, integration, and properties. *Acc. Chem. Res.*, 35, 12, 1035, 2002.
4. Iijima, S. Helical microtubules of graphitic carbon. *Nature.*, 354, 56, 1991.
5. Iijima, S., Ichihashi, T. Single-shell carbon nanotubes of 1-nm diameter. *Nature.* 363, 603, 1993.
6. Kenan, S., Yiying, Z., Jiangsha, M., Emily, C., Navid, T. Structural polymer-based carbon nanotube composite fibers: understanding the processing structure performance relationship. *Materials.*, 6, 2543, 2013.
7. Kumar, M., Ando, Y. Chemical vapor deposition of carbon nanotubes: A review on growth mechanism and mass production. *J. Nanosci. Nanotechnol.*, 10, 6, 3739, 2010.
8. Ando, Y., Zhao, X. Synthesis of carbon naotubes by arc-discharge methods. *New Diam. Front. C Tec.*, 16, 3, 125, 2006.
9. Scott, C., Arepalli, S., Nikolaev, P., Smalley, R. Growth mechanisms for single-wall carbon nanotubes in a laser-ablation process. *Appl. Phys. A.*, 72, 5, 573, 2001.
10. Teo, K., Chhowalla, M., Amaratunga, G., Milne, W., Pirio, G., Legagneux, P., Wyczisk, F., Olivier, J., Pribat, D. Characterization of plasma-enhanced chemical vapor deposition carbon nanotubes by Auger electron spectroscopy. *Am. Vac. Sci. Technol B.*, 20, 1, 116, 2002.
11. Szabó, A., Perri, C., Csató, A., Giordano, G., Vuono, D., Nagy, J. Synthesis methods of carbon nanotubes and related materials. *Materials.*, 3, 5, 3092, 2010.
12. Awasthi, K., Kumar, R., Raghubanshi, H., Awasthi, S., Pandey, R., Singh, D., Srivastava, O. Synthesis of nano-carbon (nanotubes, nanofibres, graphene) materials. *Bull. Mater. Sci.*, 34, 4, 607, 2011.

13. Radushkevich, L., Lukyanovich, V. About the structure of carbon formed by thermal decomposition of carbon monoxide on iron substrate. *Zurn. Fisic. Chim.*, 26, 88, 1952.
14. Davis, W., Slawson, R., Rigby, G. An unusual form of carbon. *Nature.*, 171, 756756, 1953.
15. Hofer, L., Sterling, E., McCartney, J. Structure of carbon deposited from carbon monoxide on iron, cobalt and nickel. *J. Phys. Chem.*, 59, 11, 1153, 1955.
16. Hillert, M., Lange, N. The structure of graphite filaments. *Z Kristallogr.*, 111, 1, 24, 1958.
17. Baker, R., Harris, P., Thomas, R., Waite, R. Formation of filamentous carbon from iron, cobalt and chromium catalyzed decomposition of acetylene. *J. Catal.*, 30, 86, 1973.
18. Oberlin, A., Endo, M., and Koyama, T. Filamentous growth of carbon through benzene decomposition. *J. Cryst. Growth*, 32, 3, 335, 1976.
19. Kroto, H., Heath, J., Brin, S., Curl, R., Smally, R. C_{60}: Buckminsterfullerene. *Nature.*, 318, 162, 1985.
20. Bethune, D., Kiang, C., Vries, O., Gorman, G., Savoy, R. Cobalt catalysed growth of carbon nanotubes with single-atomic-layer walls. *Nature.*, 7, 363, 1958.
21. Pierson, H. *Handbook of Carbon, Graphite, Diamond and Fullerenes.*Norwich: William Andrew Publishing, 1993.
22. Wallace, P.R. The band theory of graphite. Phys. Rev., 71, 9, 622, 1947.
23. Saito, R., Dresselhaus, M., Dresselhaus, G. *Physical Properties of Carbon Nanotubes.* 1st ed. World Scientific Publishing Company, 259, 1998.
24. Kiselev, N., Hutchison, J., Ryabenko, A., Rakova, E., Chizhov, P., Zhigalina, O., Artemov, V., Grigoriev, V. Two structural types of carbon bi-filaments. *Carbon.*, 43, 1897, 2005.
25. Bandow, S., Kokai, F., Takahashi, K., Yudasaka, M., Qin, L.C., Iijima, S., Interlayer spacing anomaly of single-wall carbon nanohorn aggregate. *Chem. Phys. Lett.*, 321, 514, 2000.
26. Kekulé, A. Bulletin de la Societe Chimique de Paris vol. 3 no. 2, pp. 98 (1865); *Annalen der Chemie und Pharmazie,* vol. 137, no. 2, pp. 129, 1866.
27. Pop, E., Varshney, V., Roy, A. Thermal properties of graphene: Fundamentals and applications. *MRS Bull.*, 37, 1273, 2012.
28. Ōsawa, E., Ozawa, M. Carbon blacks as the source materials for carbon nanotechnology. *Carbon Nanotechnology*, Dai, L. (ed.), Elsevier: Dordrecht, Chapter 6, 127, 2006.
29. Palser, A.H.R. Interlayer interactions in graphite and carbon nanotubes. *Phys. Chem.*, 1, 4459, 1999.
30. Yadav, B., Kumar, R. Structure, properties, and applications of fullerenes. *Int. J. Nanotechnol. Appl.*, 2, 1, 15, 2008.
31. Yuy, O., Jing-Cui, P., Hui, W., Zhi-Hua, P. The rehybridization of electronic orbitals in carbon nanotubes. *Chin. Phys. B.*, 17, 3123, 2008.
32. Saito, R., Fujita, M., Dresselhaus, G., Dresselhaus, M. Electronic structure of chiral graphene tubules. *Appl. Phys. Lett.*, 60, 18, 2201, 1992.

33. Dittmer, S. Development of a method for highly localized growth of carbon nanotubes. *PhD Thesis, Chalmers University of Technology*, 5, 12, 116, 2008.
34. Wang, X., Li, Q., Xie, J., Jin, Z., Wang, J., Li, Y., Jiang, K., Fan, S. Fabrication of ultra long and electrically uniform single-walled carbon nanotubes on clean substrates. *Nano Lett.*, 9, 9, 3137, 2009.
35. Cheng, Q., Hang, Q., Bo, G., Yuan, C., Qi, Q., Lu, C., Otto, Z., Jie, L. Fabrication of small diameter few-walled carbon nanotubes with enhanced field emission property. *J. Nanosci. Nanotechnol.*, 6, 5, 1346, 2006.
36. Gruneis, A., Rummeli, M.H., Kramberger, C., Barreiro, A., Pichler, T., Pfeiffer, R., Kuzmany, H., Gemming, T., Buchner, B. High quality double wall carbon nanotubes with a defined diameter distribution by chemical vapor deposition from alcohol. *Carbon.*, 44, 15, 3177, 2006.
37. Murakami, Y., Miyauchi, Y., Chiashi, S., Maruyama, S. Direct synthesis of high-quality single-walled carbon nanotubes on silicon and quartz substrates. *Chem. Phys. Lett.*, 377, 49, 2003.
38. Wang, T., Huang, J., Kim, P., Lieber, C. Atomic structure and electronic properties of single-walled carbon nanotubes. *Nature.*, 391, 62, 1997.
39. García-Gutiérrez, M., Nogales, A., Hernández, J., Rueda, D., and Ezquerra, T. X-ray scattering applied to the analysis of carbon nanotubes polymers and nanocomposites. *Optical Pure Appl.*, 40, 2, 195, 2007.
40. Lijie, C., Bingqing, W., Cailu, X., Ji, L., Dehai, W., Sishen, X., Weiy, Z., Yubo, L., Zuqin, L., Dongsheng, T. Crystallization behavior of the amorphous carbon nanotubes prepared by the CVD method. *J. Cryst. Growth*, 233, 823, 2001.
41. Abdulrazzak, F.H., Hussein, F.H., Alkaim, A.F., Ivanova, I., Emeline, A.i.V., Bahnemann, D.W. Sonochemical/hydration–dehydration synthesis of Pt–TiO2 NPs/decorated carbon nanotubes with enhanced photocatalytic hydrogen production activity. *Photochem. Photobiol. Sci.*, 15, 1347, 2016.
42. Khani, H., Morad, O. Influence of surface oxidation on the morphological and crystallographic structure of multi-walled carbon nanotubes via different oxidants. *J. Nanostructure Chem.*, 3, 73, 2, 2013.
43. Rols, S., Almairac, R., Henrard, L., Anglaret, E., Sauvajol, J-L. Diameter distribution of single wall carbon nanotubes in nanobundles. *Eur. Phys. J. B.*, 18, 201, 2000.
44. Domingo, C. Espectroscopía Raman de nanotubos de carbon. *Opt. Pura Apl.*, 40, 175, 2007.
45. Guo, T., Nikolaev, P., Thess, A., Colbert, D., Smalley, R.E. Catalytic growth of single-walled nanotubes by laser vaporization. *Chem. Phys. Lett.*, 243, 1, 49, 1995.
46. Vander, R.L., Hall, L.J., Berger, G.M. Optimization of flame synthesis for carbon nanotubes using supported catalyst. *J. Phys. Chem. B.*, 106, 13122, 2002.
47. Shaijumon, M.M, Ramaprabhu, S. Studies of yield and nature of carbon nanostructures synthesized by pyrolysis of ferrocene and hydrogen adsorption studies of carbon nanotubes. *Int. J. Hydrog. Energy.*, 30, 311, 2005.

48. Gulder, Q.L. Influence of hydrocarbon fuel structural constitution and flame temperature on soot formation in laminar diffusion flames. *Combust. Flame.*, 78, 179, 1989.
49. Yuan, L., Saito, K., Hu, W., Chen, Z. Ethylene flame synthesis of well-aligned multi-walled carbon nanotubes. *Chem. Phys. Lett.*, 346, 23, 2001.
50. Diener, M.D., Nichelson, N., Alford, J.M. Synthesis of single-walled carbon nanotubes in flames. *J. Phys. Chem. B*, 104 (41), 9615, 2000.
51. Walker, P., Rakszawski, J., Imperial, G. Carbon formation from carbon monoxide-hydrogen mixtures over iron catalysts: I. Properties of carbon formed. *J. Phys. Chem.*, 63, 2, 133, 1959.
52. Yacamn, M., Yoshida, M., Rend, L., Santiesteban, J. Catalytic growth of carbon microtubules with fullerene structure. *Appl. Phys. Lett.*, 62 , 6, 657, 1993.
53. Endo, M., Takeuchi, K., Kobori, K., Takahashi, K., Kroto, H., Sarkar, A. Pyrolytic carbon nanotubes from vapor-grown carbon fibers. *Carbon.*, 33, 873, 1995.
54. Michael, J., Peter, A., Colbert, D., Smith, K., Smalley, R.E. Gas-phase production of carbon single-walled nanotubes from carbon monoxide via the HiPco process: A parametric study. *American Vacuum Society., J. Vac. Sci. Technol. A.*, 19, 4, 1800, 2001.
55. Leela, M.R.A, Ramaprabhu, S. Hydrogen storage properties of nanocrystalline Pt dispersed multi-walled carbon nanotubes. *Int. J. Hydrogen Energy.*, 32, 3998, 2007.
56. Park, T., Banerjee, S., Hemraj-Benny T., Stanislaus, S.W. Purification strategies and purity visualization techniques for single-walled carbon nanotubes. *J. Mater. Chem.*, 2006, 16, 141, 2006.
57. Abdulrazzak, F.H., Esmail, S.K., Dawod, H.A., Abbas, A.M., Almaliki, M.K.K. X-ray analysis for purification process of synthesized multi-walled carbon nanotubes by chemical vapor deposition. *IJTAS.*, 8, 37, 2016.
58. Abdulrazzak, F.H. Enhance photocatalytic degradation of cobalamin by TiO_2 with single walled carbon nanotubes. *Int. J. Multidiscip. Curr. Res.*, 4, 119, 2016.
59. Mgheer, T.A., Abdulrazzak, F.H. Oxidation of multi-walled carbon nanotubes in acidic and basic Piranha mixture. *Frontiers Nanosci. Nanotechnol.*, 2, 155, 2016.
60. Dillon, A.C., Gennett, T., Jones, K.M., Alleman, J.L., Parilla, P.A., Heben, M.J. A simple and complete purification of single-walled carbon nanotube materials. *Adv. Mater.*, 11, 16, 1999.
61. Chia J.S.Y, Tan M.T.T., Chin J.K., Khiew P.S., Lee H.,A parametric study on the synthesis of graphene using Piranha-like thermal exfoliation. *IPCBEE.*, 48, 143, 2012.
62. Martinez, M.T., Callejas, M.A., Benito, A.M., Maser, W.K., Cochet, M., Andres, J.M., Schreiber, J., Chauvet, O., Fierro, J.L.G. Microwave single walled carbon nanotubes purification. *Chem. Commun.*, 1000, 100, 2002.
63. Gomez, V., Irusta, S., Olawale, B., Adams, W., Hauge, R.H., Dunnill, C.H., Barron, A.R. Enhanced purification of carbon nanotubes by microwave and chlorine cleaning procedures. *RSC Adv.*, 6, 11895, 2016.

64. Das, R., Eaqub Ali, Md., Abd Hamid, S.B., Annuar, M.S.M., Ramakrishna, S. Common wet chemical agents for purifying multiwalled carbon nanotubes. *J. Nanomater.*
65. Stancu, M., Ruxana, G., Ciuparu, D., Dinescu, A. Purification of multiwall carbon nanotubes obtained by AC arc discharge method. *Optoelectron. Adv. M [FZJ].*, 5, 8, 846, 2011.
66. Ebbesen, T.W., Ajayan, P.M., Hiura, H., Tanigaki, K. Purification of nanotubes, *Nature.*, 367, 519, 1994.
67. Vivekchand, S.R.C., Jayakanth, R., Govindaraj, A., and Rao, C.N.R., *Small.*, 1, 10, 920, 2005.
68. Mahalingam, P., Parasuram, B., Maiyalagan, T., Sundaram, S. Chemical methods for purification of carbon nanotubes: A review. *J. Environ. Nanotechnol.*, 1, 1, 53, 2012.
69. Komatsu, N., Wang, F. A comprehensive review on separation methods and techniques for single-walled carbon nanotubes. *Materials.*, 3, 3818, 2010.
70. Hou, P.X., Liu, C., Cheng, H.M. Purification of carbon nanotubes. *Carbon.*, 46, 2003, 2008.
71. Thien, L., Hernadi, K., Ljubovic, E., Garaj, S., Forro, L. Mechanical purification of single-walled carbon nanotube bundles from catalytic particles. *Nano Lett.*, 2, 1349, 2002.
72. Yang, Y.L., Xie, L.M., Chen, Z., Liu, M.H., Zhu, T., Liu, Z.F. Purification and length separation of single-walled carbon nanotubes using chromatographic method. *Synth. Met.*, 155, 455, 2005.
73. Pettifor, D., Oleinik, H., Analytic bond-order potentials beyond Tersoff–Brenner. II. Application to the hydrocarbons. *Phys. Rev. B.*, 59, 13, 8500, 1999.
74. Yang, L., Han, J. Electronic structure of deformed carbon. *Phys. Rev. Lett.*, 85, 154, 2000.
75. Peng, S., O'Keeffe, J., Wei, C., Cho, K., Kong, J., Chen, R., Franklin, N., and Dai, H. Carbon nanotube chemical and mechanical sensors. *Conference Paper for the 3rd International Workshop on Structural Health Monitoring.*
76. Van der, R., Tichich, M., Curtis, V. Substrate-support interactions in metal-catalyzed carbon nanofiber growth. *Carbon.*, 39, 2277, 2001.
77. Reilly, P., Whitten, W. The role of free radical condensates in the production of carbon nanotubes during the hydrocarbon CVD process. *Carbon.*, 44, 1653, 2006.
78. Dai, H., Rinzler, A., Nikolawv, P., Thess, A., Colbert, T., Smalley, R. Single-wall nanotubes produced by metal-catalyzed disproportionation of carbon monoxide. *Chem. Phys. Lett.*, 260, 471, 1996.
79. Shibuta, Y., Maruyama, S. Molecular dynamics simulation of formation process of single-walled carbon nanotubes by CCVD method. *Chem. Phys. Lett.*, 382, 381, 2003.
80. Pettifor, D., Oleinik, H., Tersoff–Brenner. Analytic bond-order potentials beyond. II. Application to the hydrocarbons. *Phys. Rev. B.*, 59, 13, 8500, 1999.

81. Wildöer, G., Venema, L., Rinzler, A., Smalley, R., Dekker, C. Electronic structure of atomically resolved carbon nanotubes. *Nature.*, 391, 59, 1998.
82. Yang, L., and Han, J. Electronic structure of deformed carbon. *Phys. Rev. Lett.*, 85, 154, 2000.
83. Larminie, J., Dicks, A. *Fuel Cell Systems Explained.* New York: Wiley, 291, 2002.
84. Kim, D., Lee, J., Lee, G., Overzet, L., Kozlov, M., Aliev, A., Park, Y., Yang, D. Carbon nanotubes based methanol sensorfor fuel cells application. *J. Nanosci. Nanotechnol.*, 6, 1, 2006.
85. Zhang, W., Ravi, S. Application of carbon nanotubes in polymer electrolyte based fuel cells. *Rev. Adv. Mater. Sci.*, 29, 1, 2011.
86. Prosini, P., Pozio, A., Botti, S., Ciardi, R. Electrochemical studies of hydrogen evolution, storage and oxidation on carbon nanotube electrodes *J. Power Sources.*, 118, 1, 265, 2003.
87. Endo, M., Kim, Y., Hayashi, T., Nishimura, K., Matushita, T., Miyashita, K., Dresselhaus, M. Vapor-grown carbon fibers (VGCFs): Basic properties and their battery applications. *Carbon.*, 39, 9, 1287, 2001.
88. Khantimerov, S., Kukovitsky, E., Sainov, N., Suleimanov, N. Fuel cell electrodes based on carbon nanotube/metallic nanoparticles hybrids formed on porous stainless steel pellets. *Int. J. Chem. Eng.*, 4, 157098, 2013.
89. Yang, J. A novel electrode catalyst for proton exchange membrane fuel cell using aligned carbon nanotube. *Fuel Cell Seminar, Palm Springs, CA*, 2005.
90. Bradley, K., Cumings, J., Star, A., Gabriel, J., Gruner, G. Infrared and X-ray photoelectron spectroscopic studies of the reactions of hydrogen-terminated crystalline Si(111) and Si(100) surfaces with Br, I, and ferrocenium in alcohol solvents. *Nano Lett.*, 106, 14, 3639, 2003.
91. Shao, Z., Joghee, P., Hsing, I. Preparation and characterization of hybrid Nafion-silica membrane doped with phosphotungustic acid for high temperature operation of PEMFC. *J. Membr. Sci.*, 229, 43, 2004.
92. Zhang, W., Sherrell, P., Minett, I., Razal, M., Chen, J. Carbon nanotube architectures as catalyst supports for proton exchange membrane fuel cells. *Energy Environ Sci.*, 3, 9, 1286, 2010.
93. Bergeron, B., Marton, A., Oskam, G., Meyer, G. Dye-sensitized SnO_2 electrodes with iodide and pseudohalide redox mediators. *J. Phys. Chem. B.*, 109, 935, 2005.
94. Zhou, Y., Liu, Y., Cheng, J., Lo, Y. Bias dependence of sub-band gap light detection for core–shell silicon nanowires. *ACS Nano Lett.*, 12, 11, 5929, 2012.
95. Levitsky, I., Euler, W. Photoconductivity of single wall carbon nanotubes under CW NIR illumination. *Appl. Phys. Lett.*, 83, 1857, 2003.
96. Michael, W., Topink, A., McGehee, D., Prall, H., Dennler, G., Sariciftci, S., Hu, L., Gruner, G. Organic solar cells with carbon nanotube network electrodes. *Appl. Phys. Lett.*, 88, 23, 233506, 2006.
97. Huda, A., Zeid, A., Joseph, G., Saikh, M. Use of carbon nanotubes (CNTs) with polymers in solar cells. *Molecules.*, 19, 11, 17329, 2014.

98. Kamat, P. Meeting the clean energy demand: Nanostructure architectures for solar energy conversion. *J. Phys. Chem. C.*, 111, 7, 2834, 2007.
99. Liu, Y., Lu, S., Panchapakesan, B. Alignment enhanced photoconductivity in single wall carbon nanotube films. *Nanotechnology.*, 20, 3, 2009.
100. Scarselli, M., Scilletta, C., Tombolini, F., Castrucci, P., Crescenzi, M., Diociaiuti, M., Casciardi, S., Gatto, E., and Venanzi, M. Photon harvesting with multi wall carbon nanotubes. *Superlattices Microstruct.*, 46, 1, 340, 2009.
101. Khatri, I., Adhikari, S., Aryal, H., Soga, T., Jimbo, T., Umeno, M. Improving photovoltaic properties by incorporating both single walled carbon nanotubes and functionalized multiwalled carbon nanotubes. *Appl. Phys. Lett.*, 94, 9, 930509, 2009.
102. Jia, Y., Wei, J., Wang, K., Cao, A., Shu, Q., Gui, X., Zhu, Y., Zhuang, D., Zhang, G., Ma, B., Wang, L., Liu, W., Wang, W., Luo, J., Wu, D. Nanotube-silicon heterojunction solar cells. *Adv. Mater.*, 20, 23, 4594, 2008.
103. Lee, T., Alegaonkar, P., Yoo, J. Fabrication of dye sensitized solar cell using TiO_2 coated carbon nanotubes. *Thin Solid Films.*, 515, 12, .5131, 2007.
104. Tuinstra, F., Koenig, L. Raman spectrum of graphite. *J. Chem. Phys.*, 53, 1126, 1970.
105. Nemanich, R., Solin, S. First- and second-order Raman scattering from finite-size crystals of graphite. *Phys. Rev. B.*, 20, 392, 1979.
106. Saito, R., Kawarada, H. Optical properties and Raman spectroscopy of carbon nanotubes. In *Carbon Nanotubes: Synthesis, Structure, Properties, and Applications Top. Appl. Phys.*, 80, 213, 2001.
107. Wang, Y., Alsmeyer, D.C., McCreer, R.L. Raman spectroscopy of carbon materials: Structural basis of observed spectra. *Chem. Mater.*, .2, 557, 1990.
108. Graupner, R. Raman spectroscopy of covalently functionalized single-wall carbon nanotubes. *J. Raman Spectrosc.*, 38, 673, 2007.
109. Brar, V., Samsonidze, G., Dresselhaus, G., Dresselhaus, M., Saito, R., Swan, K. Second-order harmonic and combination modes in graphite, single-wall carbon nanotube bundles, and isolated singlewall carbon nanotubes. *Phys Rev. B.*, 66, 155418, 2002.
110. Park, Y., Choi, Y., Kim, K., Chung, D., Bae, D., An, K. High yield purification of multiwalled carbon nanotubes by selective oxidation during thermal annealing. *Carbon.*, 39, 655, 2001.
111. Graupner, R. Raman spectroscopy of covalently functionalized single-wall carbon nanotubes. *J. Raman Spectrosc.*, 38, 673, 2007.
112. Brar, V., Samsonidze, G., Dresselhaus, G., Dresselhaus, M., Saiton R., Swan, K. Second-order harmonic and combination modes in graphite, single-wall carbon nanotube bundles, and isolated singlewall carbon nanotubes. *Phys. Rev. B.*, 66, 155418, 2002.
113. Park, Y., Choi, Y., Kim, K., Chung, D., Bae, D., An, K. High yield purification of multiwalled carbon nanotubes by selective oxidation during thermal annealing. *Carbon.*, 39, 655, 2001.

114. Ferrari, A., Robertson, J. Resonant Raman spectroscopy of disordered, amorphous, and diamond-like carbon. *Phys. Rev. B.*, 64, 75414, 2001.
115. Ferrari, A., Robertson, J. Interpretation of Raman spectra of disordered and amorphous carbon. *Phys. Rev. B.*, 61, 14095, 2000.
116. Calleja, F., Vonk, C. X-Ray Scattering of Synthetic Polymers. 18th edn, Harvard., 1989.
117. Kittel, C. Introduction to Solid State Physics. 7th ed., Wiley, 1996.
118. Dresselhaus, M., Eklund, P. Phonons in carbon nanotubes. *Adv. Phys.*, 49, 705, 2000.
119. Siegbahn, K. Nordling, C. Fahlman, A.. Nordberg, R Hamrin K., Hedman, J. Johansson G., Bergmarch, T. Karlsson, S.E. Lindgren I. Lindberg B., *ESCA: Nova Acta Regiae Sot. Sci. Ups. Ser. IV*, 20, 1967.
120. Kevin A. Wepasnick & Billy A. Smith & Julie L. Bitter & Howard Fairbrother, D., Chemical and structural characterization of carbon nanotube surfaces. *Anal. Bioanal. Chem.*, 396, 1003, 2010.
121. Yang, D.Q., Rochett, J.F., Sacher, E. controlled chemical functionalization of multiwalled carbon nanotubes by kiloelectronvolt argon ion treatment and air exposure. *Langmuir.*, 21, 8539, 2005.
122. Li, M., Boggs, M., Beebe, T.P., Huang, C.P. Oxidation of single walled carbon nanotubes in dilute aqueous solutions by ozone as affected by ultrasound. *Carbon.*, 46, 466, 2008.
123. Ramana, G., Kumar, V., Naresh, R., Prabhakar, K.V.P., Jain, P.K, Balaji, P. Mechanical properties of multi-walled carbon nanotubes reinforced polymer. *Indian J. Eng. Mater. Sci.*, 17, 331, 2010.
124. Dilip, C., Nath, V., Sahajwalla, D. Analysis of carbon nanotubes produced by pyrolysis of composite film of poly (vinyl alcohol) and modified fly ash. *Mater. Sci. Appl.*, 3, 103, 2012.
125. Xia, W., Wang, Y., Bergstraszer, R., Kundu, S., Muhler, M. High-density and well-aligned carbon nanotubes formed by surface decomposition of SiC. *Appl. Surf. Sci.*, 254, 257, 2007.
126. Yang, K., Gu, M., Guo, Y., Pan, X., Mu, G. Effects of carbon nanotube functionalization on the mechanical and thermal properties of epoxy composites. *Carbon.*, 47, 1723, 2009.
127. Mansfield, E., Kar, A., Hooker, S. Applications of TGA in quality control of SWCNTs. *Anal. Bioanal. Chem..* 369, 3, 1071, 2009.
128. Pang, L., Saxby, J., Chatfield, S. Thermogravimetric analysis of carbon nanotubes and nanoparticles. *J. Phys. Chem.*, 97, 27, 6941, 1993.
129. Hirsch, P., Horne, R., Whelan, M. Direct observation of the arrangement and motion of dislocations in aluminum. *Phil. Mag.*, 86, 4553, 2006.
130. Dresselhaus, M., Dresselhaus, G., Eklund, P. *Science of Fullerene and Carbon Nanotubes*. Academic Press, 1996.
131. Bandow, S., Asaka, S., Saito, Y., Rao, A., Grigorian, L., Richter, E., Eklund, P.C. Effect of the growth temperature on the diameter distribution and chirality of single-wall carbon nanotubes. *Phys. Rev. Lett.*, 80, 3779, 1998.

132. Milne, W.I., Teo, K.B.K., Mann, M. Carbon nanotubes as electron sources. *Physica Status Solidi (A).*, 203, 1058, 2006.
133. Somani, P., Somani, S., Umeno, M. Planer nano-graphenes from camphor by CVD. *Chem. Phys. Lett.*, 430, 56, 2006.
134. Zhu, H., Suenaga, K., Hashimoto, A., Urita, K., Hata, K., Iijima, S. Atomic-resolution imaging of the nucleation points of single-walled carbon nanotubes, *Small*, 12, 1180, 2005.
135. Bonetta, S., Bonetta, S., Motta, F., Strini, A., Carraro, E. Photocatalytic bacterial inactivation by TiO_2-coated surfaces. *AMB Express.*, 3, 1, 59, 2013.
136. Yin, W., Chen, S., Yang, X. Gong, Y. Yan, Y., Wei, S. Effective band gap narrowing of anatase TiO_2 by strain along a soft crystal direction. *Appl. Phys. Lett.*, 96, 22, 221901, 2010.
137. Sai, G., Gui, B. Electronic structures and optical properties of TiO_2: Improved density-functional-theory investigation. *Chin. Phys. B.*, 1, 5, 057104, 2012.
138. Paola, A., Bellardita, M., Palmisano, L. Brookite, the least known TiO_2 photocatalyst. *Catalysts.*, 3, 36, 2013.
139. Drew, K., Vinodgopal, K., Vinodgopal, P. Boosting fuel cell performance with a semiconductor photocatalyst: TiO_2/Pt-Ru. *J. Phys. Chem. B.*, 109, 24, 11851, 2005.
140. Hunger a, M., Hüsken, G., Brouwers, H.J.H. Photocatalytic degradation of air pollutants: From modeling to large scale application. *Cem. Concr. Res.*, 40, 313, 2010.
141. Satoh, N., Nakashima, T., Yamamoto, K. Metastability of anatase: size dependent and irreversible anatase-rutile phase transition in atomic-level precise titania. *Sci. Rep.*, 3, 1959, 1, 2013.
142. Xiao, P., Sheppard, D., Rogal, J., Henkelman, G. Solid-state dimer method for calculating solid-solid phase transitions. *J. Chem. Phys.*, 140, 174104, 2014.
143. Weller, H. Colloidal semiconductor Q-particles: Chemistry in the transition region between solid state and molecules. *Chem. Int. Ed. Engl.*, 32, 1, 41, 1993.
144. Anantram, M., Leonard, F. Physics of carbon nanotube electronic devices. *Rep. Prog. Phys.*, 69, 507, 2006.
145. Avramov, P., Yakobson, B., Scuseria, G. Effect of carbon network defects on the electronic structure of semiconductor single-wall carbon nanotubes. *Phys. Solid State.*, 46, 6, 1168, 2004.
146. Girifalco, L., Hodak, M., Lee, R. Carbon nanotubes, buckyballs, ropes, and a universal graphitic potential. *Phys. Rev. B.*, 62, 13104, 2000.
147. Wang, X., Xia, B., Zhu, X., Chen, J., Qiu, S., and Li, J. Controlled modification of multiwalled carbon nanotubes with ZnO nanostructures. *Solid State Chem.*, 181, 4, 822, 2008.
148. Liu, J., Li, X., Dai, L. Water-assisted growth of aligned carbon nanotube-ZnO heterojunction arrays. *Adv. Mater.*, 18, 3, 1740, 2006.
149. Fan, X., Tan, F. MWCNTs hybrids with selectively ferromagnetic or super-paramagnetic properties. Mater. Sci. Eng. *A.*, 454, 37, 2007.
150. Wang, Z., Chen, G., Xia, D. Coating of multiwalled carbon li-ion battery. *Power Sources.*, 184, 2, 432, 2008.

151. Tasviri, M., Pourb, H., Ghourchianb, H., Gholami, M. Amine functionalized TiO_2 coated on carbon nanotube as a nanomaterial for direct electrochemistry of glucose oxidase and glucose biosensing. *Mol. Catal. B: Enzym.*, 68, 2, 206, 2011.
152. Kuo, C. Prevenient dye-degradation mechanisms using UV/TiO_2/carbon nanotubes process. *Hazard. Matter.*, 163, 1, 239, 2009.
153. Feng, W., Feng, Y., Wu, Z., Fujii, A., Ozaki, M., Yoshino, K. Optical and electrical characterizations of nanocomposite film of titania adsorbed onto oxidized multiwalled carbon nanotubes. *J. Phys: Condens Matter.*, 17, 4361, 2005.
154. Fan, W., Gao, L., Sun, J. Anatase TiO_2-coated multi-wall carbon nanotubes with the vapor phase method. *J. Am .Ceram. Soc.*, 89, 731, 2009.
155. Frontera, P., Trocino, S., Donato, A., Antonucci, P.L., Lo Faro, M., Squadrito, G., Ner, G. Oxygen-sensing properties of electrospun CNTs/PVAc/TiO_2 composites. *Electron. Mater. Lett.*, 10, 1, 305, 2014.
156. Balasubramanian, K., Burghard, M. Chemically functionalized carbon nanotubes. *Small.*, 1, 2, 180, 2005.
157. Niyogi, S., Hamon, M.A., Hu, H., Zhao, B., Bhowmik, P., Sen, R., Itkis, M.E., Haddon, R.C. Chemistry of single-walled carbon nanotubes. *Acc. Chem. Res.*, 35, 1105, 2002.
158. Kan, Z., Zeda, M., Wonchun, O. Degradation of rhodamine B by Fe-carbon nanotubes/TiO_2 composites under UV light in aerated solution. *Chin. J. Catal.*, 31, 7, 751, 2010.
159. Zhang, W., Zhang, Z., Zhang, Y. The application of carbon nanotubes in target drug delivery systems for cancer therapies. *Nanoscale Res. Lett.*, 6, 555, 2011.
160. Denisyuk, I.Y., Fokina M.I. A review of high nanoparticles concentration composites: semiconductor and high refractive index materials. *Nanocatalyst*, Intech, 109, 2014.
161. Kim, Y., Park, H. Light-harvesting multi-walled carbon nanotubes and CdS hybrids: Application to photocatalytic hydrogen production from water. *Energy Environ. Sci.*, 4, 685, 2011.
162. Ahmed, M. K., Halah, T.M., Ayad, F.A., Falah, H.H. Adsorption of Congo red on multiwall carbon nanotubes: Effect of operational parameters. *J. Chem. Pharm. Sci.*, 9, 3, 2016.
163. Firas, H.A. Enhance photocatalytic activity of TiO_2 by carbon nanotubes. *Int. J. ChemTech. Res.*, 9(3), 431, 2016.
164. Falah, H.,H., Ban, S.H., Massar, B.M., Zeyad, H.N., Ghassan, J.M. Pharmaceutical application of carbon nanotubes synthesized by flame fragments deposition method. *J. Environ. Anal. Chem.*, 4(4), 1, 2017.
165. Jassam, A.M., Hussein, F.H., Abdulrazzak, F.H., Alkaim, A.F., Joda, B.A. Synthesis and characterization of carbon nanotubes by modified flame fragments deposition method. *Asian J. Chem.*, 29(12), 2804, 2017.
166. Abdulrazzak, F.H., Abbas, A.M., Hussein, F.H. Synthesis of few-wall carbon nanotubes using methanol/propanol mixture by chemical vapour deposition. *Front. Nanosci. Nanotech.*, 3(3), 1, 2017.

2

Synthesis and Characterization of Phosphorene: A Novel 2D Material

Sima Umrao[1], Narsingh R. Nirala[2], Gaurav Khandelwal[3] and Vinod Kumar[4]*

[1]School of Electronics and Electric Engineering, Sungkyunkwan University (SKKU), Suwon, Korea
[2]School of Materials Science and Technology, IIT (BHU), Varanasi, India
[3]Indian Institute of Technology Delhi, Hauzkhas, New Delhi, India
[4]Department of Materials Engineering, Ben Gurion University of the Negev, Beer-Sheva, Israel

Abstract
Phosphorene, a single or few-layered form of black phosphorus, has been discovered as a promising 2-D layered materials for applications in electronics and optoelectronics. The outstanding physicochemical properties of Phosphorene bridges gap between graphene and transition metal dichalcogenides. Fabrication of large-area and environmentally stable Phosphorene are main challenges in Phosphorene research. Few well known methods *viz.* mechanical, liquid exfoliation and pulsed laser deposition have been tried for getting good quality of Phosphorene but each of these methods have their own merit and demerits. In order to transfer the Phosphorene from research laboratories to the industries, large-area synthesis of Phosphorene remains a major challenges along with its environment stability. Current chapter describes various existing synthesis approaches and characterization tools of Phosphorene extending to the passivation methodologies.

Keywords: Black phosphorus, 2-D materials, phosphorene, stability, band gap

2.1 Introduction

In the last decade, two-dimensional (2D) materials are the focus of an intense research effort on nanomaterials because of their unique properties

**Corresponding author*: mail2vinod2@gmail.com, vinod@post.bgu.ac.il

Suvardhan Kanchi, Shakeel Ahmed, Myalowenkosi I. Sabela and Chaudhery Mustansar Hussain (eds.) Nanomaterials: Biomedical, Environmental, and Engineering Applications, (61–92)

and their potential for revealing fascinating new phenomena. Graphene is the most studied zero band gap 2D material because of its exceptional electronic, optoelectronic, electrochemical, and biomedical applications. Beyond graphene, a very wide spectrum of 2D materials is existing and possess seminal properties with additive a finite band gap to avoid the absence of a natural band gap in graphene [1]. Succeeding graphene, a theoretical study predicted that 2D hexagonal boron nitride (*h*BN) can induce a bandgap in graphene when graphene was deposited on top of a *h*BN sheet [2]. This result led in a significant experimental research on *h*BN, and ultimately found that *h*BN may be an ideal substrate for graphene electronics [6]. The success of graphene and *h*BN inspired the researcher to explore other 2D materials including transition metal dichalcogenides (MoS_2, $WeSe_2$ etc.) [3, 4], silicone [5], germanene [5, 6], stanine [7], and other 2D materials [8, 9]. The quest for a variety of high-performance devices in various fields including enviormental and biomedical applications has demanded the search for alternative 2D materials that possess a broad operating range in their key properties, such as carrier mobility and the electronic band gap. Recently, semiconducting phosphorene, a single layer of black phosphorous (BP), a layered material with phosphorus atoms forming 2D puckered sheets has captured great attention as a 2D family member because of its outstanding chemical, physical, and optoelectronic properties [10].

In this chapter, we cover briefly the synthesis methods and characterization techniques to explore phosphorene properties, which are beneficial for further future applications.

2.1.1 History of Phosphorene

In order to detail the path that phosphorene has taken, it is important to start with its bulk counterpart. In 1669, elemental phosphorus was discovered by Hennig Brand. Phosphorus has been extensively used in industrial level for matchsticks, fireworks, chemical fertilizers, and the napalm bomb. Since black phosphorus discovery in 2014, a layered allotrope of phosphorus synthesized for the first time by Bridgman [11] has not attracted any special attention by physicists and chemists due to its structural instability and strong toxicity [12]. In the American Physical Society March meeting in 2013, a talk on "Electronic Properties of Few-Layer Black Phosphorus" given by Yuanbo Zhang and co-workers, they dethroned graphene as the only elemental two-dimensional material isolated by mechanical exfoliation [13]. According to Zhang *et al.*, atomically thin layers (and eventually one-atom thick layers) of phosphorus can be prepared by mechanical exfoliation of bulk BP, termed as phosphorene, which have recently gained much attention. In the last 2 years, there have been exciting demonstrations of the material's applications in various fields such as transistors [14, 15, 16], photovoltaics [17, 18], photodetectors [19, 20], and batteries [21, 22].

Phosphorene has high and variable hole mobility ranging from 1000 cm^2/Vs down to 14 cm^2/Vs [83–91]. It has free standing capabilities like that of graphene and can be synthesized using many of the same techniques such as mechanical exfoliation [44], chemical vapor deposition [45], and liquid exfoliation [46]. An important thing is that the band gap of phosphorene covers a broad range according to the number of layer, and the band gap of single layer phosphorene, 2 eV [47, 48], lies above the zero-gap of graphene and 1.9 eV of MoS_2. The electronic and mechanical properties of phosphorene have been shown in Table 7.1 with a comparison of graphene and MoS_2 properties.

2.1.2 Crystal Structure

As phosphorene is a single layer of BP, graphene is a single layer of graphite. BP atoms are strongly bonded in-plane similar to graphite and form layers, which weakly interact through van der Waals forces. In BP, the

Table 2.1 Comparative summary of electronic and mechanical properties of monolayer phosphorene with graphene and MoS_2. The value in the bracket corresponding to the zigzag direction in contrast to the value in armchair direction.

	Phosphorene	**Graphene**	**MoS_2**
Band gap (eV)	0.3–2 [15]	0 [23]	1.2–1.8 [24]
Carrier mobility ($cm^2.V^{-1}.s^{-1}$)	~1000 [15]	200,000 [25]	200 [26]
On/Off ratio	10^3–10^5 [14, 15]	~5.5–44 [27]	10^6–10^8 [26]
Effective mass (m_e)	0.146 (1.246) [28]	~0 [23]	0.47–0.6 [29]
Thermal conductance (W/m-K)	36 (110) [30]	2000–5000 [31]	52 [32]
ZT	1–2.5 [33]	~0 [34]	0.4 [35]
Critical strain (%)	27 (30) [36]	19.4–34 [37]	19.5–36 [38]
Young's modulus (GPa)	44 (166) [39]	1 [40]	270±100 [41]
Poisson's ratio	0.4 (0.93) [42]	0.186 [40]	0.21–0.27 [43]

phosphorus atoms have five valence electrons available on 3p orbitals for bonding. Therefore, each phosphorus atom bonds covalently at 2.18 Å to three neighboring phosphorus atoms through sp^3 hybridized orbitals, resulting in a puckered honeycomb lattice structure (orthorhombic) of phosphorene with space group *Cmca*.

Figure 2.1 shows a schematic diagram of the phosphorene crystal structure. Two phosphorus atoms are in the plane of the layer from each other, and the third phosphorus atom is between the layers. The atomic arrangement yields two directions within the phosphorene lattice; the zigzag (x-axis, parallel to the atomic ridges) and the armchair (z-axis, perpendicular to the ridges). Recently, researchers have found that the lattice constants along the two perpendicular directions are different and depending on the number of layers, at $a_1 = 4.52 \pm 0.05$ Å and $a_2 = 3.31 \pm 0.03$ Å, respectively [14, 49, 50]. The layer number also has slight influence on the dihedral angle ($\theta 1 = 102.42°$ for bulk BP and $\theta 1 = 103.51°$ for single-layer phosphorene) and the hinge angle ($\theta 2 = 96.16°$ for bulk BP and $\theta 2 = 96.00°$ for single-layer phosphorene) [50]. Therefore, it is clear that the number of layer can be a function to tune the geometric properties of phosphorene. However, the number of layers has no significant influence on the adjacent P–P bond length (R2) and the connecting bond length (R1) unlike other parameters. The R1 value of single-layer phosphorene is very close to that of the R2 ~ 2.224 Å, which can be ascribed to the covalent bonds derived from phosphorus 3p orbitals [51]. BP is a highly reactive material [52] because

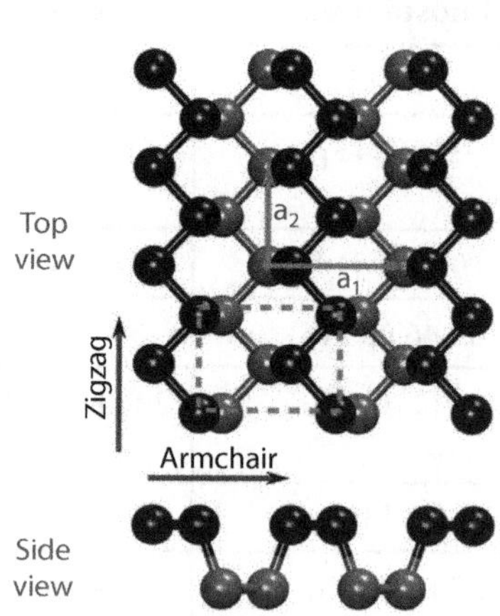

Figure 2.1 Crystal structure of phosphorene; top view of single-layer phosphorene; the puckered structure of three-layer phosphorene. The x and z axis are along the zigzag and armchair directions, respectively [30]. Reproduced with permission Copyright 2015, Nature Publishing Group.

of a lone pair of electrons on the phosphorus atom, which contribute to bonding with other elements, in particular water and oxygen. Phosphorene degrades to PO_x species [53] and phosphoric acid H_3O_4P [54] under ambient environmental conditions within a few hours. Recently, much effort has been made to stop degradation in phosphorene. Particulary, capping layers and advanced synthesis routes seem to be very promising [55, 56].

2.1.3 Band Structure

Density functional theory (DFT) is the most appropriate and used method to calculate band structure of phosphorene because of an exact formulation [57–59]. However, the exchange-correlation energy functional [60] in DFT is usually approximated such as include GGA generalized gradient approximations [61], LDA local-density approximations [62], and hybrids [63] among others. In phosphorene, sp^3 hybridization increases the interlayer spacing between layers unlike the sp^2 hybridization in graphene. More importantly, each layer of phosphorene has an influence with other adjacent layers like self-alignment, which supports the anisotropic behavior of phosphorene even in the bulk form [14]. The band gap of phosphorene is layer dependent like the TMDs materials. Phosphorene has puckered a hexagonal crystal structure as shown in Figure 2.1 and of our atom in one unit cell [64]. The armchair direction lines up with the *x*-axis (horizontal) and the zigzag direction lines up with the *y*-axis. The buckling parameter R1 is ~0.25 nm calculated from hybrid exchange-correlation functional HSE06 calculations [65, 66]. Buckling parameters are the vertical distance that separates the covalently bonded P atoms in the structure along the *z*-axis [15, 67]. DFT calculation results demonstrated that phosphorene has a direct band gap ranging from 1 to 2 eV at gama point, which fully supported the band gap value calculated by experiemntl results [14, 47, 48, 68].

2.2 Synthesis of Phosphorene

2.2.1 Mechanical Exfoliation

The mechanical exfoliation method has proved to be effective to cleave bulk layered materials into single and few layer materials [69, 70]. The structure of BP is layered and interconnected together by weak van der Wall interlayer forces, which submits that few-layer or even monolayer phosphorene can be obtained by the exfoliation method.

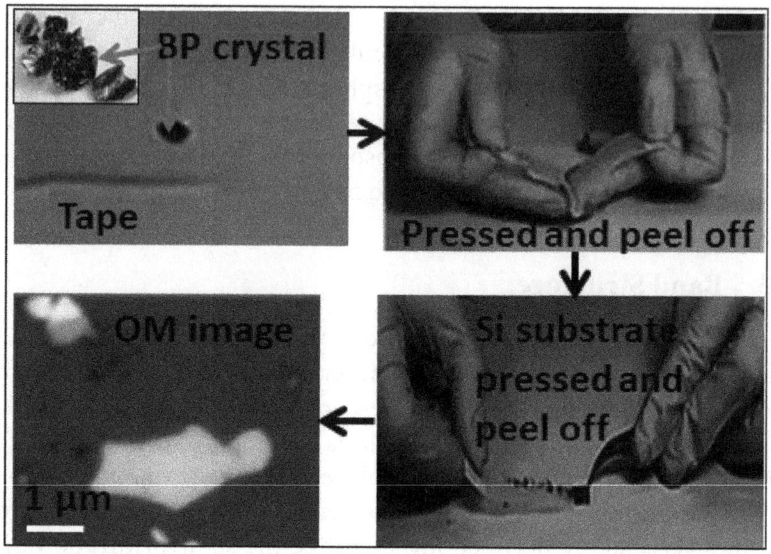

Figure 2.2 Mechanical exfoliation method to produce phosphorene from bulk BP by tape exfoliation.

The single-layer phosphorene was obtained by a combination of mechanical exfoliation and plasma thinning [44, 71]. Briefly, a thick phosphorene flake was mechanically exfoliated using a blue nitto tape to a 275-nm SiO_2/Si substrate and then the sample was treated under O_2 plasma etching by the ICP-RIE system under proper optimize conditions [44, 72]. Yuerui Lu group [44] used 400 W ICP generator power, 30 W RF bias power, with 30 sccm O_2 flow at 10 mTorr pressure conditions to get few to single layer phosphorene plasma etching. The controllable production of few- and monolayer phosphorene samples by O_2 plasma thinning is shown in Figure 2.2. Although high quality phosphorene can be produced by mechanical exfoliation but the main problem is the scalable production as well as a lack of systematic control of flake thickness and size. This is limited to be used in the laboratory. In addition, structural and chemical stability of phosphorene is low because of lone pair on each phosphorus atom and as a result, exfoliated phosphorene degrades at ambient environment conditions [48, 52].

2.2.2 Plasma-Assisted Method

Another promising alternative is the improved fabrication method that is faster and more controllable to get single- and few-layer phosphorene by the plasma-assisted process as also used for graphene and MoS_2

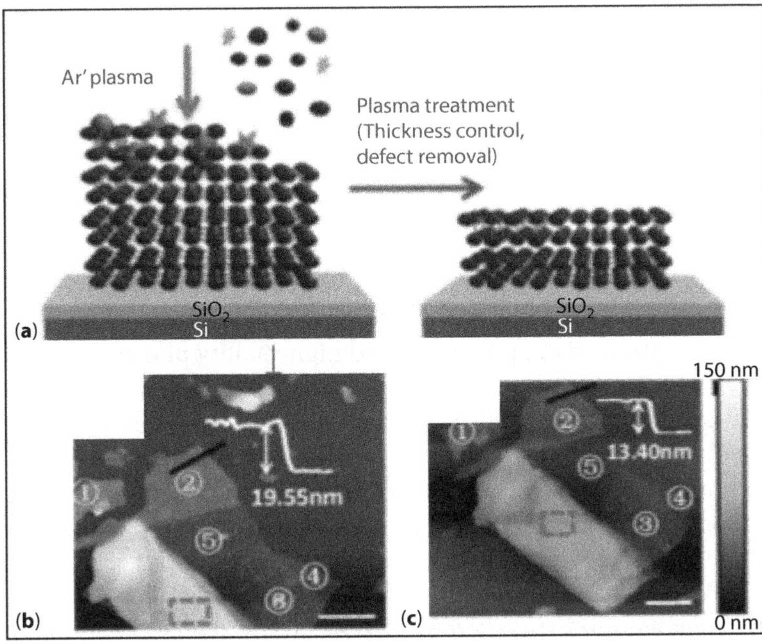

Figure 2.3 (a) Schmatic representation for plasma etching of phosphorene. (b, c) AFM image of multilayered pristine phosphorene after and before Ar+ plasma thinning, respectively. Reprinted (adapted) with permission from [75]. Copyright 2015, American Chemical Society.

[48, 73–75]. In this method, first few-layer BP was exfoliated by the tape exfoliation method on the SiO_2/Si substrate, after which it was treated with plasma under optimized conditions to get single-layer phosphorene via layer-by-layer etching as shown in Figure 2.3. Lu *et al.*, [73] used a focused Ar+ plasma (commercial 13.56 MHz RF source with a power of 30 W and a pressure of 30 Pa) to get single-layer phosphorene by thinning few-layer phosphorene flakes. Jia *et al.*, [75] used inductive coupled plasma (ICP) at 30 mTorr, 350 W rf power at 13.56 MHz to treat tape-exfoliated few-layer BP flakes on the SiO_2/Si substrate. Obviously, this method is combined with exfoliation but it provides an improved way to control the thickness of phosphorene as well as removed the chemical degradation of the oxidized phosphorene surface [75]. This method can be an alternative approach such as a modified exfoliation, which employs a silicone-based transfer layer to optimize high-quality atomically thin phosphorene. However, this method does not fill the requirements for the scale-up applications because of small-scale production for fundamental research.

2.2.3 Liquid-Phase Exfoliation

Two obtain large scale and size phosphorene nanosheets, liquid phase exfoliation methods are very promising. The most promising large scale production of 2D layered thin nanosheets from a direct conversion of bulk layered crystals by electrostatic repulsion in aqueous solvents and surface energy matching in organic solvent-based systems is known as liquid phase exfoliation [76]. In fact, liquid exfoliation [77] is just a general concept followed by different mechanisms for different approaches including ion intercalation, ion exchange, and sonication-assisted exfoliation as shown in Figure 2.4. Brent *et al.*, [78] produced high-quality phosphorene atomic layer by the sonication liquid exfoliation methods. Briefly, they sonicated bulk BP crystal with *N*-Methyl-2-pyrrolidone (NMP) solvent (5 mg/ml) at 820 W across four horns operating at 37 kHz frequency and 30% power for 24 hours and the temperature of bath was maintained below 30 °C throughout the sonication period using a water-cooling coil. The final turbid dispersions were centrifuged to remove larger flaks and get pale yellow/brown color stable dispersions of phosphorene.

After that, according to further applications needed, a thin film of phosphorene was made on the SiO_2 (300nm)/Si substrate by spin coating. Approximate in the same period, Yasaei *et al.*, [79] tried several organic solvents covering a wide range of polar interaction parameters (2.98–9.3 $MPa^{1/2}$) and surface tensions (21.7–42.78 dyne/cm) to exfoliate bulk BP into few-layer phosphorene. They practically found that the aprotic and polar solvents such as dimethylformamide (DMF) and dimethyl sulfoxide

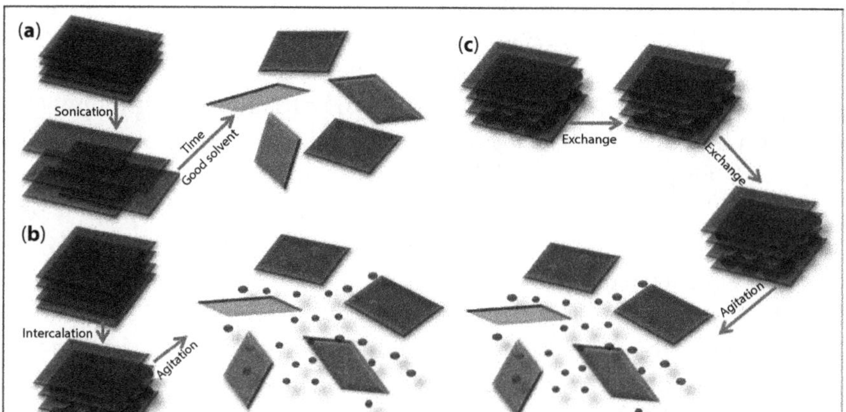

Figure 2.4 Schematic description of the liquid exfoliation method. (a) Sonication-assisted exfoliation, (b) ion intercalation, and (c) ion exchange.

(DMSO) were best candidates to exfoliate bulk BP after 6 h sonication at 130 W for 0.2 mg per 10 ml solvent. Further, AFM, SEM, RAMAN, optical absorption, and TEM were used to characterize the synthesized few-layer phosphorene as shown in Figure 2.5. The average phosphorene flake size in the DMF case was about 190 nm with thickness ~5 nm, while in the DMSO solution the average flake size was 532 nm with a thickness range of 15–20 nm. Raman bands with maxima at 361 cm^{-1}, 438 cm^{-1}, and 465 cm^{-1}, corresponding to the A_{1g}, $B_{2g,}$ and A_{2g} modes of few-layer phosphorene and for single layer only, 465 cm^{-1} band will be present corresponding to the A_{2g} mode. The brief characterization result explanation will be given in the coming characterization techniques. This method opens up new important

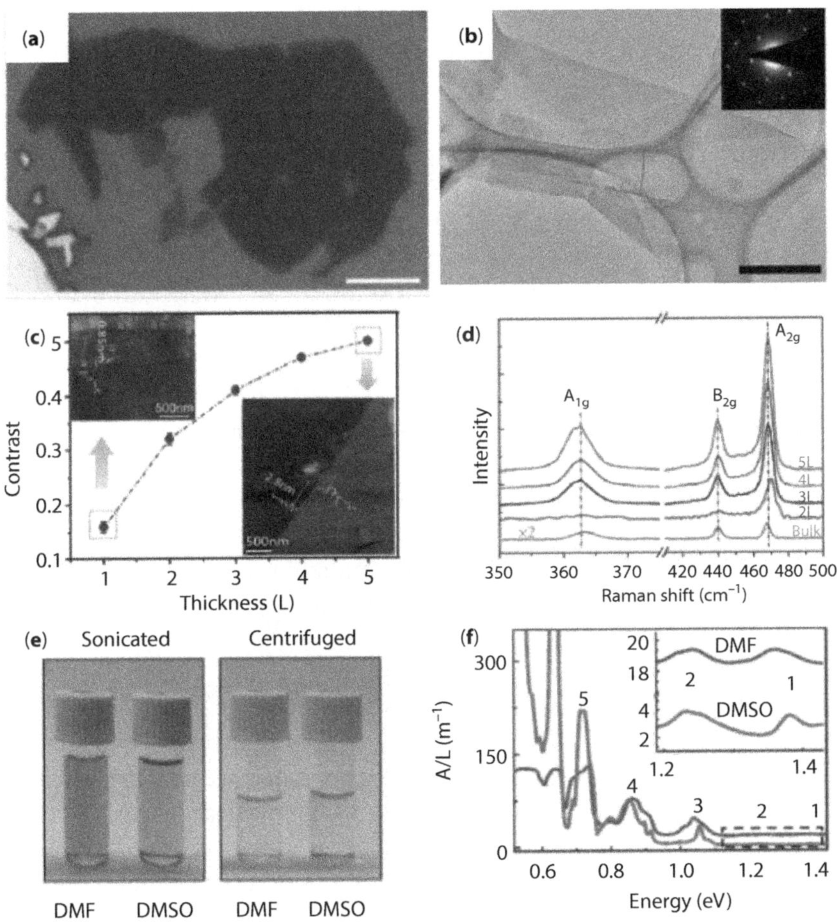

Figure 2.5 Photograph of the few-layer phosphorene dispersions in the solvents DMF and DMSO.

possibilities to get the atomically thin phosphorene thin films and its composites on large scales with a wide range of applications importantly in the sensing, flexible electronics, and optoelectronics.

2.2.4 Chemical Vapor Deposition

From the last decade, the chemical vapor deposition (CVD) method has been a well famous and high quality production method to grow 2D layered materials such as graphene, TMDs, etc. [26, 80, 81]. Unfortunately, phosphorene synthesis is not fully explored by CVD due to the complicated chemistry of phosphorus. The material science and chemistry specialists have put in combined efforts to the development of large-scale phosphorene synthesis methods in thin film form at the wafer scale, so that more application opportunities emerge like other 2D materials, such as graphene, TMDs, etc. [82–85]. Moreover, it is also important to develop a large-area single-crystal thin film in which the anisotropic properties of phosphorene may be explored at a larger scale [86].

Recently, Li *et al.*, developed a BP thin film of 4 nm thickness on a flexible substrate by depositing a red phosphorus thin film on a flexible polyester substrate [87]. The red phosphorus film converted into BP under high pressure in a multi-anvil cell at room temperature. Additionally, the poorly crystallized BP film was successfully grown with a thickness ranging from several nanometers to tens of nanometers on Si/SiO_2 or graphene/Cu substrates via pulsed laser deposition using BP crystal as precursor [88]. However, these processes need further improvement by optimizing the processing conditions to get a thin film of BP in one step. More importantly, the development of wafer-scale CVD on metal substrates [89] and epitaxial growth on insulating substrates [90] have facilitated a large-scale device fabrication based on graphene and TMDCs but still this approach has not yet been fully developed for high-quality phosphorene like other 2D materials.

2.3 Characterization of Phosphorene

The analysis of phosphorene possesses several issues because of its instability due to each phosphorous atom having a lone electron pair, which have a bonding tendency with the other atoms. Various characterization techniques have been used for the better understanding of phosphorene such as absorption spectroscopy, X-ray diffraction (XRD), neutron diffraction, scanning electron microscopy (SEM), transmission electron microscopy (TEM) and aberration-corrected TEM, Raman spectroscopy, scanning tunneling microscopy (STM), atomic force microscopy (AFM), and many other qualitative and quantitative techniques to understand fundamental properties of phosphorene in nanoscale and bulk scale BP. In this section, we present structural, morphological, and spectroscopic analyses of phosphorene.

2.3.1 Structural Charcterizations

In order to examine the structure and morphology of phosphorene, we can use SEM, TEM, STEM, and AFM. Under normal conditions, phosphorene is a layered structure consisting of puckered hexagonal rings in an orthorhombic crystal structure, whereas individual layers of phosphorene are stacked together by the van der Walls force. This structure is reversible and can be transformed into a semi-metallic rhombohedral phase and metallic simple cubic under ~5 GPa and ~10 GPa pressure, respectively [91].

In the atomic structure of BP, each phosphorous atom is bonded with three neighboring phosphorous atoms by sp3 hybridization. Side and top view of a single-layer phosphorene is shown in Figure 2.6 (a and b) and

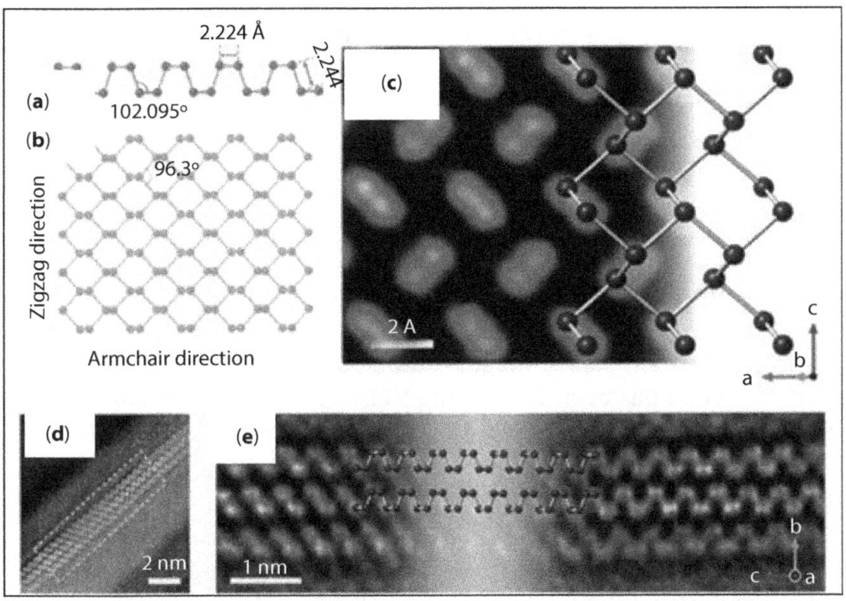

Figure 2.6 Structural view of phosphorene. (a) Side view and (b) top view of monolayer phosphorene. Reproduced with permission from [92]. Copyright 2015, Royal Society of Chemistry. (c) ADF-STEM image viewed along the [101] direction. (d) ADF-STEM image captured at an edge of a BP flake along the [100] direction showing multiple layers stacked together. (e) Magnified image of the region highlighted in (d). (c–f) Reproduced with permission from [93]. Copyright 2015, AIP Publishing.

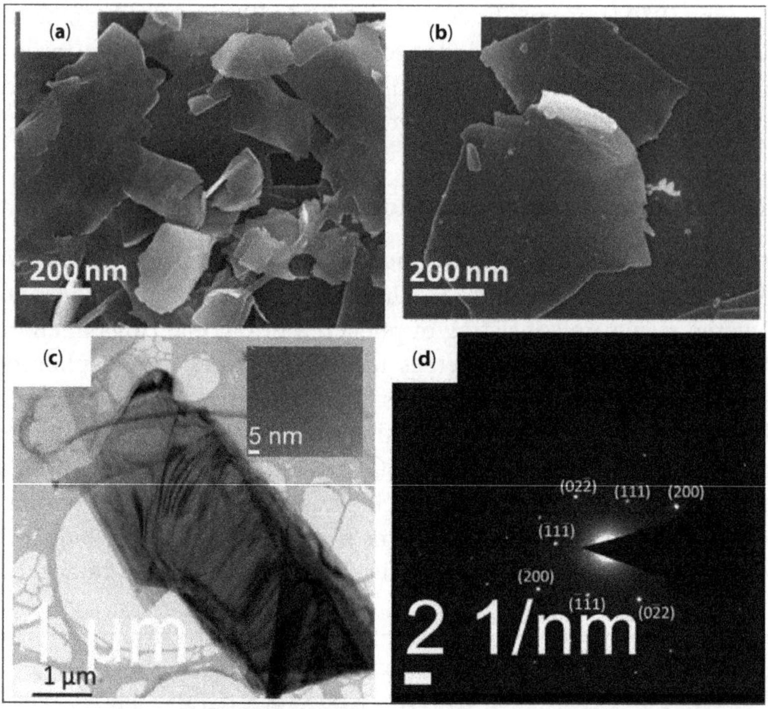

Figure 2.7 (a) and (b) SEM image of phosphorene nanoflakes. Reproduced with permission from [95]. Copyright 2015, IOP Publishing. (c) TEM and HRTEM image (in inset) of phosphorene flake. (d) Electron diffraction. Reproduced with permission from [96].

it clearly divulges the corrugated structure of each BP layer. The x and y directions are corresponding to the AM and ZZ directions and strong in-plane anisotropy exists along these two directions. Recently, the investigation on the atomic structure and individual atomic appearance visually by experimental has been done using STEM imaging along different crystallographic directions [94]. An annular dark field-scanning TEM (ADF-STEM) image along the [101] direction of an exfoliated BP flake from the bulk sample viewed is shown in Figure 2.6(c). Here the individual atomic columns are clearly visible because of the increased spacing between atomic columns. To see a clear cross-sectional view of 2D BP, the low- and high-magnification ADF-STEM images (Figure 6d and e) captured at the edge of the BP flake aligned along the [100] crystallographic direction. This imaging method can even disclose doping of any other atoms into phosphorene lattice.

However, topological (morphological) studies of as-synthesized phosphorene can be done using SEM. For SEM measurements, phosphorene flakes were transferred to the SiO_2/Si substrate. For example, a sample of phosphorene synthesized by liquid exfoliation spin coated on a substrate and recorded SEM images as shown in Figure 2.7a. A non-uniform distribution of phosphorene flakes across the substrate has been found, looks like flakes grouped together in close proximity at the solvent-drying time. There are areas on the substrate that have higher concentrations of phosphorene, while others have no visible flakes. Figure 2.7b shows that multiple phosphorene flakes seem to overlap with one another. This agrees with PL studies in the coming sections, where multiple PL peaks demonstrated corresponding to several different layering amounts in the same location. Therefore, SEM is a good tool to characterize the phosphorene sample as we can distinguish single flake in the whole substrate. Another morphological and crystal structure characterization tool is TEM. Once the phosphorene sample is transferred successfully in the TEM grid from the SiO_2/Si substrate, we can proceed TEM measurements. George Anderson *et al.*, [96] captured the TEM image of phosphorene (Figure 2.7c), which clearly reveals that the phosphorene flake has free-standing capabilities and the lateral dimensions of the flake is ~ 2 × 6 μm. The high resolution (HR)-TEM image of a few-layer sample is shown in the inset of Figure 2.7c, which confirmed the beam-induced breakdown of the structure of phosphorene atoms. As previously, the Gomez group found that few-layer phosphorene is beam sensitive for HR-TEM [48]. Further, the electron diffraction result of the same sample shows that the material is single crystal (Figure2. 7d), as no spreading of the diffraction pattern because of multiple orientated crystals. The d-spacing measured experimentally are approximately 0.261 nm, 0.161 nm, and 0.174 nm corresponding to planes (111), (200), and (022), respectively [97].

Further, the surface analysis and thickness of the phosphorene can be done using AFM. AFM is an extremely well-suited technique for the analysis of 2D materials. AFM results reveal that the single-layer phosphorene has a step height of ~0.85 nm [14] as shown in Figure 2.8(a). Therefore, according to the contrast of AFM image (Figure 2.8b), we can calculate the number of layers by thickness measurements. Additionally, we can also study about the surface impurity in the phosphorene flake by calculating surface roughness from AFM topography images.

2.3.2 Spectroscopic Characterizations

BP is characterized by various spectroscopic techniques such as Raman spectroscopy, infrared spectroscopy, polarization-dependent spectroscopy, and X-ray photoelectron spectroscopy to study the characteristic

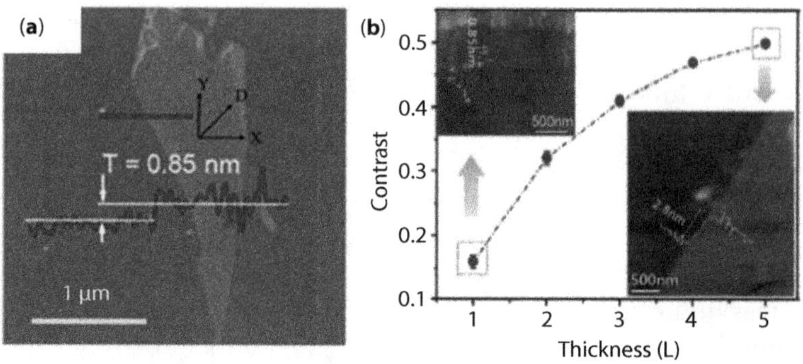

Figure 2.8 (a) and (b) AFM image of an exfoliated few-layered phosphorene crystal with a sectional profile displaying 0.85 nm. Reproduced with permission from [14]. Copyright 2014, American Chemical Society.

vibrational modes, intrinsic bonding energies, and crystallinity. The vibrational properties of phosphorene nanosheets with external stimuli such as strain, pressure, and temperature can study to unravel the intrinsic anisotropic physical properties because of the unique puckered structure of BP. The main vibrational modes of phosphorene are A_{1g}, B_{2g}, and A_{2g} modes. Raman spectral features of phosphorene are sensitive to the number of layers [71]. The intensity ratio of A2g to A1g modes increases monotonic with the decrease of thickness down to a monolayer [71]. Therefore, the Raman analysis can be an indirect way of finding the number of layers in phosphorene flakes. But Raman measurements have to be done carefully, for example, choice of substrate and crystalline orientation to the polarization of incident laser. Most importantly, the accuracy of the calculation of number of layers depends on the resolution of the spectrometer under Raman measurements. The typical Raman spectra of bulk BP (Figure 2.9b) consist of main features at 362 cm^{-1}, 439 cm^{-1}, 467 cm^{-1} corresponding to A_{g1}, B_{2g}, and A_{g2} phonon modes, respectively [48]. The intensity of the A1g peak in relation to the Si peak can also be demonstrated by the number of layers of phosphorene [48] according to the thickness as shown in Figure 2.9(a). The B_{2g} and A_{g2} modes correspond to in-plane vibrational modes of the atoms, and the A_{g1} mode corresponds to the out-of-plane vibration of the phosphorous atom.

Additionally, polarization-resolved Raman spectroscopy has been studied in order to address the anisotropic behavior of phosphorene and layer dependency in different crystalline orientations by Xia *et al.*, [100]. The Raman scattering results show that the standard peaks of BP have been appeared in all *x*, *y* and *D* (diagonal) directions for laser excitation

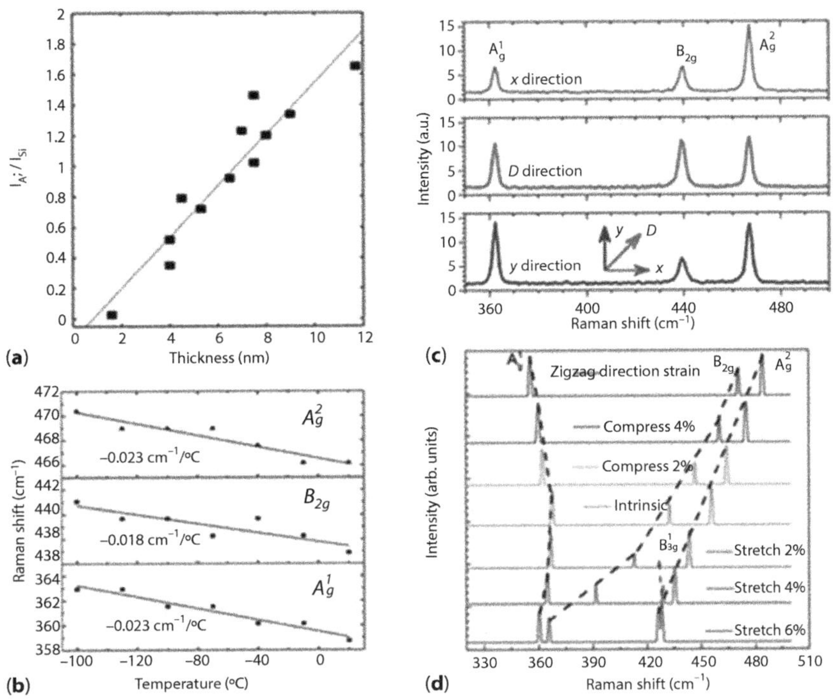

Figure 2.9 (a) Thickness dependence of the intensity ratio between the Ag1 and Si peaks [48]. Copyright 2014, IOP publishing. (b) Temperature dependence of A_{g1}, B_{2g}, and A_{g2} Raman peak positions. (c) Polarization-resolved Raman spectra of a BP layered thin film with 532-nm linearly polarized laser excitation incident in the *z* direction. The D direction is along the 45° angle relative to the *x*- and *y*-directions, as shown in the bottom panel. Reproduced with permission from [98] Copyright 2014, Nature Publishing Group. (d) Raman spectra of phosphorene under uniaxial strain along the ZZ direction. Reproduced with permission from [99]. Copyright 2014, AIP publishing.

(Figure 2.9b) regardless of the polarization. For all three different polarizations, there is no shift in the position of Raman peaks, but there is a relative significant change in the intensities of characteristic peaks corresponding to of A_{g1}, B_{2g} and A_{g2} phonon modes with polarization direction and the reasons need to be explained in future. The angle-resolved polarized Raman spectroscopy studies discovered that Raman modes of phosphorene not only depends on the polarization angle (the angle between the polarization vectors of incident laser and scattered light) but also relies on the sample rotation angle (the angle between the AM direction of BP and the polarization vector of scattered light) [101–103].

Because of the puckered structure of phosphorene, spatial inhomogeneity is of particular interest in phosphorene, and strain can modify a wide range of its properties such as electrical and mechanical properties. The higher resolutions in spatial strain distribution can be found by confocal Raman or near-field Raman scattering. The mechanical strain is an effective external stimulus on phosphorene, which can be moderate to the electronic band structure. This effect can be studied by Raman spectroscopy. Fei *et al.,* [104] studied theoretically the strain effect in phosphorene and they monitored the shift in the position of original strain-free Raman peaks to strained phosphorene with the relative frequency shifts between the different peaks (Figure 2.9d). According to this study, a considerable shift in the vibrational modes has been found corresponding to the type and amount of applied strain in monolayer phosphorene. Both B_{2g} and A_{g2} modes exhibit monotonic red shifts when stretched and blue shifted when compressed along the zig-zag direction, while the magnitude of frequency shifts along the zig-zag direction is much larger in comparison to the armchair strain [105]. Similarly, temperature can also give substantial shifts in Raman spectra of phosphorene [106, 107]. It is calculated by a linear equation $\omega = \omega_0 + \chi T$, where ω_0 is mode frequency at zero K, χ is the first-order temperature coefficient, and χ values for different modes within a low temperature range from 20 °C to 160 °C represented in Figure2 9(b). It is remarkable to mention that these coefficient values for phosporene are larger than other 2D materials such as graphene, MoS_2, $MoSe_2$, and WSe_2 [108–110] but less than that of TiS_3 nanosheets [111]. Therefore, BP is very much sensitive to the applied temperature because of its corrugated structure and good mechanical flexibility.

2.3.3 Optical Band Gap Characterization

Photoluminesecnce attributed the nature of excitons, which represent the fundamental band gap values of the material. The extreme variation in the band structure corresponding to flake thickness of phosphorene has provoked intense interest and debate. Nevertheless, the theory consistently predicts that the band gap of phosphorene is direct for all thicknesses, which has ambitious further interest in various application fields because most of other 2D semiconductors possess indirect band gaps.

PL is an especially useful tool to study phosphorene properties as the band gap of phosphorene increases with the decrease in number of layers [107]. PL spectra of few-layer BP exfoliated on the silicon substrate demonstrated strongly dependent PL results with the number of phosphorene layer (2 layers to 5 layers) by Zhang and his co-workers [107]. PL peaks with strong intensity are noticed at 961 nm, 1268 nm, 1413 nm, and 1558 nm corresponding to 2, 3, 4, and 5-layered phosphorene flakes,

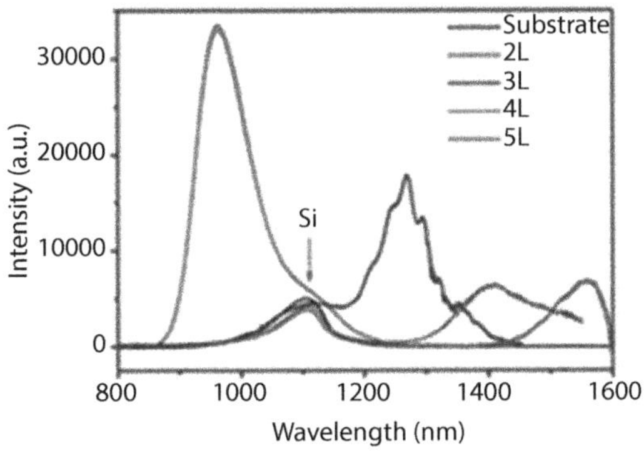

Figure 2.10 PL spectra of 2L, 3L, 4L, and 5L phosphorene flakes. Reproduced with permission from [112]. Copyright, American Chemical Society.

respectively. The corresponding energy peak values are 1.29 eV, 0.98 eV, 0.88 eV, and 0.80 eV, respectively (Figure 2.10). The PL emission process in phosphorene is due to electron–hole interactions. The mechanism for the PL emission from the phosphorene structure is shown briefly in Figure 2.11. Incident photons with energy $E = h\nu_i$ excite electrons from the ground electronic state of phosphorene, where h is Plank's constant and ν is the frequency of the photon. If the photon has a certain energy at least the same energy as the band gap of the material, it can excite electrons to move to higher energy levels. When the electron has been excited, there are several processes that take place such as non-radiative relaxation. However, once the electron reaches the conduction band minimum, the radiative relaxation process occurs by excitonic decay. Energy is released from this process in the form of a photon with energy equal to the lower bound of the energy band gap of the phosphorene. Therefore, PL results in the emission peak, which will be strongly dependent on the number of phosphorene layers because of the band gap variation corresponding to the number of layers. PL results support these quantitative predictions, such as the varying exciton binding energy from 0.01 to 0.9 eV in phosphorene [14, 48], which also depends on the static dielectric constant of the surrounding medium. However, surface defects, contamination, and oxidation of samples may introduce experimental uncertainty. In fact, the results so far are quite varied as in one study trilayer photoluminesce was at 1.60 eV [48], while in another, the measured value was 0.97 eV [113]. Electrical measurements have also been exposed such that mobility gaps were smaller than the band gap calculated by PL results [114]. This result is surprising because, generally, the mobility gap should be larger than the optical gap in a semiconductor with few inter-band states [115, 116].

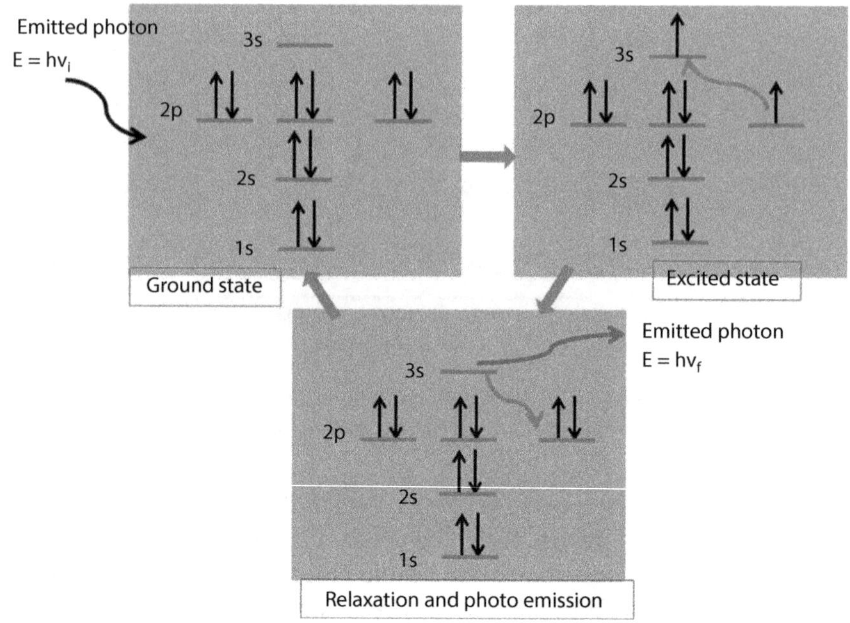

Figure 2.11 Schematic representation of the PL process in phosphorene.

Further optical absorbance of phosphorene and the corresponding calculated band gap can be measured using UV-vis-NIR spectroscopy and Tauc analysis. The Woomer group reported a detailed study of optical absoption of phosphorene using a single exfoliated phosphorene flake with a KBr pallete and liquid suspension with a varying fraction of phosphorene [117]. A high optical density had been found in polycrystalline bulk BP, which allowed us to measure light absorption near the threshold band gap value ~0.4 eV as shown in Figure 2.12(a). However, in case of exfoliated BP with thickness ~20–40 nm, it represented low optical density with an additional absorption edge at about 1.95 eV. In the case of liquid suspension with varying fraction, the optical absorbance spectra shows a blue shift (Figure 2.12b) corresponding to lowering thickness of the phosphorene flake. The two noticeable features have been recognized in this absorption spectrum: slowly increasing absorption in the near IR region as well as sharply rising absorption within the visible region. These spectral features may be attributed to the same high- and low-energy transitions in the bulk material [118].

Using these absorption features, Tauc analysis represented that the high-energy transition achieved an excellent fit with the Tauc model when $n = 2$ corresponding to direct and allowed transition (Figure 2.12c and d).

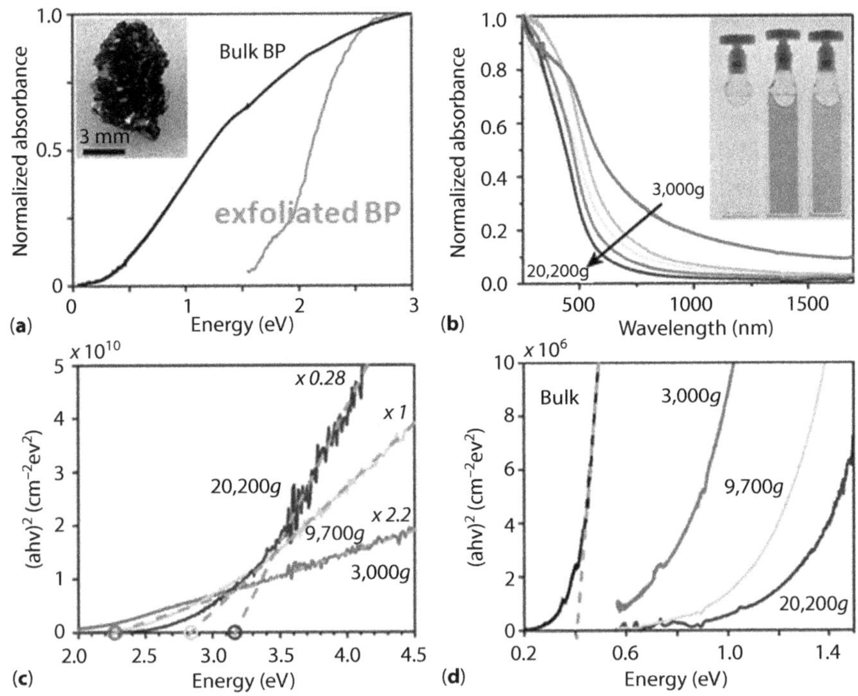

Figure 2.12 UV-vs-NIR spectroscopy of black phosphorus and its liquid-exfoliated few-layer flakes. (a) Optical absorbance of bulk phosphorus and exfoliated few layer BP. (b) Absorbance of phosporene suspensions with varying fraction. (c) Representative direct Tauc plots used to determine the high-energy band-to-band transition. (d) Representative direct Tauc plots of the low-energy optical transition. Reproduced with permission from [118]. Copyright 2014, AIP publishing.

But the value of high-energy transition energies is ~1.95 eV in bulk BP and 3.14 eV in a monolayer phosphorene suspension. The Tauc models fitted within this data and may suggest that the five experimental challenges such as light scattering, high exciton binding energy, Urbach tail, anisotropic optical properties, show the variation in the band gap assigned a negligible effect on this Tauc studies of the high-energy transition. Moreover, in the direct application of the Tauc model on bulk BP, the low energy transition is 0.40 eV. Most of the experimental results are evident that the band gap and the high-energy transitions are extremely dependent and change according to the flakes thickness lowering to the monolayer thickness [118]. The band gap of bulk phosphorene is 0.33 ± 0.02 eV and 1.88 ± 0.24 eV for bilayer and the higher energy transition can be modulated from 1.95 ± 0.06 eV in bulk to 3.23 ± 0.39 eV in bilayers [118]. These ranges exceed all known 2D materials and are as large as the most tunable quantum dots. Looking toward future applications of phosphorene, the surprising range of band gaps of 2D phosphorene, with tunable absorption threshold values from the visible to the IR, will provide a new material platform for the design and development of photonic, optoelectronic, and biomedical field applications.

2.4 Environment Stability Issue of Phosphorene

Even though phosphorene provides high mobility as well as tunable direct bandgap, it suffers from its instability in ambient conditions, which degrades the performance of phosphorene-based devices with time. Droplets containing impurities appear on the surface of phosphorus due to oxygen and water absorption from the environment when exfoliated to nanoscale dimensions [48, 52, 53], which act as carrier scattering centers and charge trapping centers. The rapid oxidation over a short period of time considerably degrades the charge carrier mobility and threshold voltage shifts of phosphorene-based transistors. Consequently, a theoretical study has also supported that the surface of phosphorene is hydrophilic due to its strong out-of-the plane dipole moment [119]. DFT calculations indicate a large distortion of the phosphorene lattice structure, which shrinks by around 25% because of strong dipole–dipole interactions [120]. The degradation in the phosphorene surface can be seen by a simple OM image as well as sheet resistance measurements with an atomic force microscopy-based microwave impedance microscope [121] as a function of time and electrical performance measurements of transistors [52, 53] as shown in Figure 2.13.

However, a study of the degradation mechanism in phosphorene can be done by Raman and transmission electron spectroscopies, which allow for better understanding the most plausible mechanism behind aging of phosphorene in ambient conditions, as photoassisted oxidation reaction with oxygen dissolved on the absorbed surface. Importantly, to protect phosphorene degradation, people started to fabricate devices in vacuum conditions to ensure their reliability. But, this is a very expensive method to develop a phosphorene-based device. Some researchers proposed a way to passivate or protect phosphorene-based devices by avoiding direct contact with ambient atmosphere at an early stage during the fabrication [53, 122, 123]. An effective encapsulation of phosphorene by other materials such as 2D materials (graphene, *h*-BN, etc.) [124, 125], Al_2O_3 [53], and PMMA [19, 126] can prevent its degradation under ambient conditions.

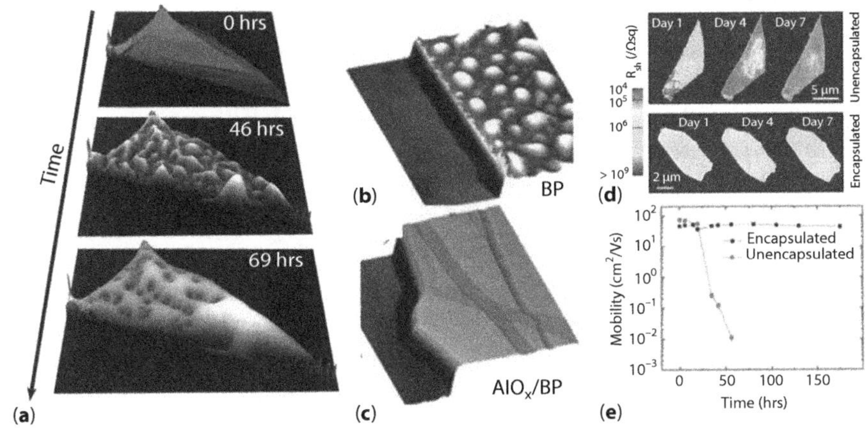

Figure 2.13 Time dependent degradation of unprotected and protected phosphorene.

The encapsulation technology may resolve the environmental instability of phosphorene, which is essential for modern electronics devices. This passivation technology may lead to a better performed device reliability. For example, BP was encapsulated by alumina to minimize the material degradation from air/moisture [53]. In this work, the workers examined how exfoliated BP crystals degrade to oxygenated phosphorus compounds in ambient conditions. Figure 2.13(a) shows clearly how to increase bubbles on the surface of the BP flake during the oxidation after a time interval. They reported that the deposition of an AlO_x layer by atomic layer deposition (ALD) is an effective, scalable strategy to passivate BP flakes and FETs from ambient deterioration [53]. Figure 2.13c shows the BP flake with and without encapsulation, where an exfoliated BP flake exposed to air for 3 days shows large topographic protrusions ("bubbles") above the surface of the unprotected BP flake (Figure 2.13b). Figure 2.13d and e shows that the sheet resistance of the BP flake was increasing with time, but after encapsulation the sheet resistance maintains its reliablity. Most importantly, the electrical performance of the BP device was improved by a considerable amount for Hall measurements over time after encapsulation (Figure 2.13d). It was found that the transfer curve shifts significantly by the off-current increasing about 7 times and threshold voltage increasing by 22 V. After 1 week of ambient exposure (~ 175 h), AlOx encapsulated BP FET was working without significant degradation more than 1 week under ambient environment. After that, a new approach was used to prevent degradation of monolayer phosphorene under ambient atmosphere by oxygen plasma dry etching [44]. The thick-exfoliated phosphorene flakes etched layer by layer using oxygen plasma to make thin phosphorene. In this process, the top layers of phosphorene flakes were oxidized and changed into the PxOy layer, which acts as a protective layer like the Al_2O_3 passivation layer deposited by ALD for the remaining below phosphorene layer.

On the other hand, the study is going on transport properties of phosphorene with van der walls passivation such as graphene and *h*BN under ambient conditions [125, 127, 128]. AFM and Raman spectroscopy measurements were performed to see the effect of capping BP by graphene and BN exposed to the ambient atmosphere. AFM height images have been obtained for BP film over time. It is evident from AFM height images that the unprotected surface of the BP film developed significant roughness after air exposure, while the regions covered with graphene showed no noticeable surface roughness change. Phosphorene capping with graphene and h-BN seems a promising way to make high performance BP electrical devices. Sandwiched structures of BN/BP/BN have been demonstrated by the Chen *et al.,* [127] and they found high mobility (~400 $cm^2 V{-}^1 s{-}^1$) and on/off ratio (10^5) with high stability. Graphene-capped BP transistors are showing negligible effect with ambient environment and almost eliminated hysteresis with stable transport properties [125]. The efficient, effective, and ultrathin BP nonlinear characteristic devices can be developed by encapsulation of suitable 2D thin materials. However, in scalable quantity electronic-grade, BP dispersions can be produced by a sealed tip-ultra sonication of BP flakes with anhydrous organic solvents, which avoids BP degradation that would otherwise occur via solvated O_2 or H_2O [129]. NMP is the most appropriate organic solvent among conventional solvents, which provide stable, highly concentrated (~0.4 mg $mL{-}^1$) BP dispersions. The structure and chemistry of NMP solvent-exfoliated BP nanosheets are comparable to mechanically exfoliated BP flakes and this method will avoid the direct contact of air with BP. This organic solvent BP showed significant high hole mobility and on/off ratio in spite of slight degradation of BP not more than 15% in organic solvents.

2.5 Summary and Future Prospective

In the last decade, two-dimensional (2D) layered nanomaterials, such as graphene and the transition-metal dichalcongenide (TMDC) family have received tremendous interest in the field of nanotechnology. However, the quest for a variety of high-performance 2D material based electronic devices or nanosensors has dictated to search the additional layered 2D materials with comparatively superior properties. In this continuation, recently, Phosphorene, the single- or few-layered form of black phosphorus, has been discovered as a promising 2-D layerd materials for applications in electronics and optoelectronics. The outstanding phyico-chemical properties of phosphorene bridges the gap between graphene (zeroband gap semiconductor) and transition metal dichalcogenides (wide band gap semiconductors).

In phosphorene research, the fabrication of large-area samples and the environmental stability of black phosphorus are two main challenges. Mechanical exfoliation method is the most appropriate synthesis method, but it is not scalable in industrial applications. Cheap and scalable production production of phosphorene by liquid exfoliation have good prospects for making electronic device with extending applications range. But, the quality of liquid exfoliated phosphorene might be not good enough for some applications because of defects and doping during exfoliation process. Very recently, the pulsed laser deposition method (PVD) has been used to produce thin films of Phosphorene, however, the PVD synthesized phosphorene layers lacks crystallinity, and their electrical properties are much poorer than pristine phosphorene. Therefore, in order to transfer the phosphorene from research laboratories to the industries, developing a large-area synthesis method for crystalline Phosphorene is still a major challenges. On the other hand, the stability of BP in the environment is a big issue in the research community, as phosphorene is hygroscopic and highly reactive with moisture from the air. Considering, the out standing wide range application potential of phosphoerene, the current chapter we have described the various realted extising synthesis technologies as well as effective characterization tools of phosphorene. A comprehensive characterization techniques such XRD, XPS, SEM, TEM and aberration corrected TEM, Raman spectroscopy, STM have been presented. Stbaility issue of phosphorene have been further discussed to realize the real practical applications of this novel 2-D material in both technological purposes and in biomedicine.

References

1. Jariwala, D., Srivastava, A., Ajayan, P.M. Graphene synthesis and band gap opening. *J. Nanosci. Nanotechnol.*, 11, 6621, 2011.
2. Chang, C.K., Kataria, S., Kuo, C.C., Ganguly, A., Wang, B.Y., Hwang, J.Y., Huang, K.J., Yang, W.H., Wang, S.B., Chuang, C.H., Chen, M., Huang, C.I., Pong, W.F., Song, K.J., Chang, S.J., Guo, J.H., Tai, Y., Tsujimoto, M., Isoda, S., Chen, C.W., Chen, L.C., Chen, K.H. Band gap engineering of chemical vapor deposited graphene by *in situ* BN doping. *ACS Nano.*, 7, 1333, 2013.

3. Radisavljevic, B., Radenovic, A., Brivio, J., Giacometti, V., Kis, A. Single-layer MoS2 transistors. *Nat. Nanotechnol.*, 6, 147, 2011.
4. Coehoorn, R., Haas, C., Dijkstra, J., Flipse, C.J.F., De Groot, R.A., Wold, A.. Electronic structure of MoSe 2, MoS 2, and WSe 2: I. Band-structure calculations and photoelectron spectroscopy. *Phys. Rev. B.*, 35, 6195, 1987.
5. Dimoulas, A., Silicene and germanene: Silicon and germanium in the flatland. *Microelectron. Eng.*, 131, 68, 2015.
6. Dávila, M.E., Xian, L., Cahangirov, S., Rubio, A., Le Lay, G. Germanene: a novel two-dimensional germanium allotrope akin to graphene and silicene. *New J. Phys.*, 16, 95002, 2014.
7. Zhu, F., Chen, W., Xu, Y., Gao, C., Guan, D., Liu, C., Qian, D., Zhang, S.C., Jia, J. Epitaxial growth of two-dimensional stanene. *Nat Mater.*, 14, 1020, 2015.
8. Bhimanapati, G.R., Lin, Z., Meunier, V., Jung, Y., Cha, J., Das, S., Xiao, D., Son, Y., Strano, M.S., Cooper, V.R., Liang, L., Louie, S.G., Ringe, E., Zhou, W., Kim, S.S., Naik, R.R., Sumpter, B.G., Terrones, H., Xia, F., Wang, Y., Zhu, J., Akinwande, D., Alem, N., Schuller, J.A., Schaak, R.E., Terrones, M., Robinson, J.A. Recent advances in two-dimensional materials beyond graphene. *ACS Nano.*, 9, 11509, 2015.
9. Zou, X., Yakobson, B.I. An open canvas—2D materials with defects, disorder, and functionality. *Acc. Chem. Res.*, 48, 73, 2015.
10. Eswaraiah, V., Zeng, Q., Long, Y., Liu, Z. Black phosphorus nanosheets: Synthesis, characterization and applications. *Small.*, 12, 3480, 2016.
11. Bridgman, P.W. Two new modifications of phosphorus. *J. Am. Chem. Soc.*, 36, 1344, 1914.
12. Chou, T.D., Lee, T.W., Chen, S.L., Tung, Y.M., Dai, N.T., Chen, S.G., Lee, C.H., Chen, T.M., Wang, H.J. The management of white phosphorus burns. *Burns.*, 27, 492, 2017.
13. Likai Li, Y.Z., Yu, Y., Ye, G.J., Chen, X.H. Electronic properties of few-layer black phosphorus. *APS March Meet.* College Park, MD: American Physical Society. Abstract I (2013). Available at http://meetings.aps.org/Meeting/MAR13/ Session/J6.
14. Liu, H., Neal, A.T., Zhu, Z., Luo, Z., Xu, X., Tománek, D., Ye, P.D. Phosphorene: An unexplored 2D semiconductor with a high hole mobility. *ACS Nano.*, 8, 4033, 2014.
15. Li, L., Yu, Y., Ye, G.J., Ge, Q., Ou, X., Wu, H., Feng, D., Chen, X.H., Zhang, Y. Black phosphorus field-effect transistors. *Nat Nano.*, 9, 372, 2014.
16. Koenig, S. P., Doganov, R. A., Schmidt, H., Castro Neto, A.H., Özyilmaz, B., Electric field effect in ultrathin black phosphorus. *Appl. Phys. Lett.*, 104, 103106, 2014.
17. Buscema, M., Groenendijk, D.J., Steele, G.A., van der Zant, H.S.J., Castellanos-Gomez, A. Photovoltaic effect in few-layer black phosphorus PN junctions defined by local electrostatic gating. *Nat. Commun.*, 5, 4651, 2014.

18. Deng, Y., Luo, Z., Conrad, N.J., Liu, H., Gong, Y., Najmaei, S., Ajayan, P.M., Lou, J., Xu, X., Ye, P.D. Black phosphorus–monolayer MoS2 van der Waals heterojunction p–n diode. *ACS Nano.*, 8, 8292, 2014.
19. Engel, M., Steiner, M., Avouris, P. Black phosphorus photodetector for multispectral, high-resolution imaging. *Nano Lett.*, 14, 6414, 2014.
20. Low, T., Engel, M., Steiner, M., Avouris, P. Origin of photoresponse in black phosphorus phototransistors. *Phys. Rev. B.*, 90, 81408, 2014.
21. Park, C.M., Sohn, H.J. Black phosphorus and its composite for lithium rechargeable batteries. *Adv. Mater.*, 19, 2465, 2007.
22. Dahbi, M., Yabuuchi, N., Fukunishi, M., Kubota, K., Chihara, K., Tokiwa, K., Yu, X., Ushiyama, H., Yamashita, K., Son, J.Y., Cui, Y.T., Oji, H., Komaba, S. Black phosphorus as a high-capacity, high-capability negative electrode for sodium-ion batteries: Investigation of the electrode/electrolyte interface. *Chem. Mater.* 28, 1625, 2016.
23. Geim, A.K., Novoselov, K.S. The rise of graphene. *Nat. Mater.*, 6, 183, 2007.
24. Song, J.G., Ryu, G.H., Lee, S.J., Sim, S., Lee, C.W., Choi, T., Jung, H., Kim, Y., Lee, Z., Myoung, J.M., Dussarrat, C., Lansalot-Matras, C., Park, J., Choi, H., Kim, H. Controllable synthesis of molybdenum tungsten disulfide alloy for vertically composition-controlled multilayer. *Nat Commun.*, 6, 1, 2015.
25. Bolotin, K.I., Sikes, K.J., Jiang, Z., Klima, M., Fudenberg, G., Hone, J., Kim, P., Stormer, H.L. Ultrahigh electron mobility in suspended graphene. *Solid State Commun.*, 146, 351, 2008.
26. Jeon, J., Jang, S.K., Jeon, S.M., Yoo, G., Jang, Y.H., Park, J.H., Lee, S. Layer-controlled CVD growth of large-area two-dimensional MoS2 films. *Nanoscale.*, 7, 1688, 2015.
27. Das, A., Pisana, S., Chakraborty, B., Piscanec, S., Saha, S.K., Waghmare, U.V., Novoselov, K.S., Krishnamurthy, H.R., Geim, A.K., Ferrari, A.C., Sood, A.K. Monitoring dopants by Raman scattering in an electrochemically top-gated graphene transistor. *Nat. Nanotechnol.,* 3, 210, 2008.
28. Fei, R., Yang, L. Strain-engineering the anisotropic electrical conductance of few-layer black phosphorus. *Nano Lett.*, 14, 2884, 2014.
29. Peelaers, H., de Walle, C.G. Effects of strain on band structure and effective masses in MoS2. *Phys. Rev. B.*, 86, 241401, 2012.
30. Jain, A., McGaughey, A.J.H. Strongly anisotropic in-plane thermal transport in single-layer black phosphorene. *Sci. Rep.*, 5, 8501, 2015.
31. Balandin, A.A. Thermal properties of graphene and nanostructured carbon materials. *Nat Mater.*, 10, 569, 2011.
32. Sahoo, S., Gaur, A.P.S., Ahmadi, M., Guinel, M.J.F., Katiyar, R.S. Temperature-dependent Raman studies and thermal conductivity of few-layer MoS2. *J. Phys. Chem. C.*, 117, 9042, 2013.
33. Fei, R., Faghaninia, A., Soklaski, R., Yan, J.A., Lo, C., Yang, L. Enhanced thermoelectric efficiency via orthogonal electrical and thermal conductances in phosphorene. *Nano Lett.*, 14, 6393, 2014.

34. Balandin, A.A. Thermal properties of graphene and nanostructured carbon materials. *Nat Mater.*, 10, 569, 2011.
35. Huang, W., Da, H., Liang, G. Thermoelectric performance of MX2 (M = Mo,W; X-S,Se) monolayers. *J. Appl. Phys.*, 113, 104304, 2013.
36. Wei, Q., Peng, X. Superior mechanical flexibility of phosphorene and few-layer black phosphorus. *Appl. Phys. Lett.*, 104, 251915, 2014.
37. Liu, F., Ming, P., Li, J. Ab initio calculation of ideal strength and phonon instability of graphene under tension. *Phys. Rev. B.*, 76, 64120, 2007.
38. Bertolazzi, S., Brivio, J., Kis, A. Stretching and breaking of ultrathin MoS2. *ACS Nano.*, 5, 9703, 2011.
39. Wei, Q., Peng, X. Superior mechanical flexibility of phosphorene and few-layer black phosphorus. *Appl. Phys. Lett.*, 104, 251915, 2014.
40. Liu, F., Ming, P., Li, J. Ab initio calculation of ideal strength and phonon instability of graphene under tension. *Phys. Rev. B.*, 76, 64120, 2007.
41. Li, T. Ideal strength and phonon instability in single-layer MoS2. *Phys. Rev. B.*, 85, 235407, 2012.
42. Jiang, J.W., Park, H.S. Negative poisson's ratio in single-layer black phosphorus. *Nat. Commun.*, 5, 4727, 2014.
43. Bertolazzi, S., Brivio, J., Kis, A. Stretching and breaking of ultrathin MoS2. *ACS Nano.*, 5, 9703, 2011.
44. Pei, J., Gai, X., Yang, J., Wang, X., Yu, Z., Choi, D.Y., Luther-Davies, B., Lu, Y. Producing air-stable monolayers of phosphorene and their defect engineering. *Nat. Commun.*, 7, 10450, 2016.
45. Smith, J.B., Hagaman, D., Ji, H.F. Growth of 2D black phosphorus film from chemical vapor deposition. *Nanotechnology.*, 27, 215602, 2016.
46. Hanlon, D., Backes, C., Doherty, E., Cucinotta, C.S., Berner, N.C., Boland, C., Lee, K., Harvey, A., Lynch, P., Gholamvand, Z., Zhang, S., Wang, K., Moynihan, G., Pokle, A., Ramasse, Q.M., McEvoy, N., Blau, W.J., Wang, J., Abellan, G., Hauke, F., Hirsch, A., Sanvito, S., Regan, D.D.O., Duesberg, G.S., Nicolosi, V., Coleman, J.N. Liquid exfoliation of solvent-stabilized few-layer black phosphorus for applications beyond electronics. *Nat. Commun.*, 6, 8563, 2015.
47. Castellanos-Gomez, A. Black phosphorus: Narrow gap, wide applications. *J. Phys. Chem. Lett.*, 6, 4280, 2015.
48. Castellanos-Gomez, A., Vicarelli, L., Prada, E., Island, J.O., Narasimha-Acharya, K.L., Blanter, S.I., Groenendijk, D.J., Buscema, M., Steele, G.A., Alvarez, J.V., Zandbergen, H.W., Palacios, J.J., van der Zant, H.S.J. Isolation and characterization of few-layer black phosphorus. *2D Mater.*, 1, 25001, 2014.
49. Kou, L., Chen, C., Smith, S.C. Phosphorene: Fabrication, properties, and applications. *J. Phys. Chem. Lett.*, 6, 2794, 2015.
50. Qiao, J., Kong, X., Hu, Z.X., Yang, F., Ji, W. High-mobility transport anisotropy and linear dichroism in few-layer black phosphorus. *Nat. Commun.*, 5, 4475, 2014.

51. Asahina, H., Morita, A. Band structure and optical properties of black phosphorus. *J. Phys. C: Solid State Phys.*, 17, 1839, 1984.
52. Island, J.O., Steele, G.A., van der Zant, H.S.J., Castellanos-Gomez, A. Environmental instability of few-layer black phosphorus. *2D Mater.*, 2, 11002, 2015.
53. Wood, J.D., Wells, S.A., Jariwala, D., Chen, K.S., Cho, E., Sangwan, V.K., Liu, X., Lauhon, L.J., Marks, T.J., Hersam, M.C. Effective passivation of exfoliated black phosphorus transistors against ambient degradation. *Nano Lett.*, 14, 6964, 2014.
54. Favron, A., Gaufres, E., Fossard, F., Phaneuf-L[rsquor]Heureux, A.L., Tang, N.Y.W., Levesque, P.L., Loiseau, A., Leonelli, R., Francoeur, S., Martel, R. Photooxidation and quantum confinement effects in exfoliated black phosphorus. *Nat Mater.*, 14, 826, 2015.
55. Guo, Z., Zhang, H., Lu, S., Wang, Z., Tang, S., Shao, J., Sun, Z., Xie, H., Wang, H., Yu, X.F., Chu, P.K. From black phosphorus to phosphorene: Basic solvent exfoliation, evolution of Raman scattering, and applications to ultrafast photonics. *Adv. Funct. Mater.*, 25, 6996, 2015.
56. Das, S., Demarteau, M., Roelofs, A. Ambipolar phosphorene field effect transistor. *ACS Nano.*, 8, 11730, 2014.
57. Kresse, G., Furthmüller, J. Efficient iterative schemes for ab initio total-energy calculations using a plane-wave basis set. *Phys. Rev. B.*, 54, 11169, 1996.
58. Kohn, W., Becke, A.D., Parr, R.G. Density functional theory of electronic structure. *J. Phys. Chem.*, 100, 12974, 1996.
59. Kohn, W., Sham, L.J. Self-consistent equations including exchange and correlation effects. *Phys. Rev.*, 140, A1133, 1965.
60. Kohn, W., Sham, L.J. Self-consistent equations including exchange and correlation effects. *Phys. Rev.*, 140, A1133, 1965.
61. Perdew, J.P., Burke, K., Ernzerhof, M. Generalized gradient approximation made simple. *Phys. Rev. Lett.*, 77, 3865, 1996.
62. Jones, R.O., Gunnarsson, O. The density functional formalism, its applications and prospects. *Rev. Mod. Phys.*, 61, 689, 1989.
63. Kim, K., Jordan, K.D. Comparison of density functional and MP2 calculations on the water monomer and dimer. *J. Phys. Chem.*, 98, 10089, 1994.
64. Jain, A., McGaughey, A.J.H. Strongly anisotropic in-plane thermal transport in single-layer black phosphorene. *Sci. Rep.*, 5, 8501, 2015.
65. Balendhran, S., Walia, S., Nili, H., Sriram, S., Bhaskaran, M. Elemental analogues of graphene: Silicene, germanene, stanene, and phosphorene. *Small.*, 11, 640, 2015.
66. Heyd, J., Scuseria, G.E., Ernzerhof, M. Hybrid functionals based on a screened Coulomb potential. *J. Chem. Phys.*, 118, 8207, 2003.
67. Balendhran, S., Walia, S., Nili, H., Sriram, S., Bhaskaran, M. Elemental analogues of graphene: Silicene, germanene, stanene, and phosphorene. *Small.*, 11, 640, 2015.

68. Cai, Y., Zhang, G., Zhang, Y.W. Layer-dependent band alignment and work function of few-layer phosphorene. *Sci. Rep.*, 4, 6677, 2014.
69. Li, H., Wu, J., Yin, Z., Zhang, H. Preparation and applications of mechanically exfoliated single-layer and multilayer MoS2 and WSe2 nanosheets. *Acc. Chem. Res.*, 47, 1067, 2014.
70. Yi, M., Shen, Z. A review on mechanical exfoliation for the scalable production of graphene. *J. Mater. Chem. A.*, 3, 11700, 2015.
71. Lu, W., Nan, H., Hong, J., Chen, Y., Zhu, C., Liang, Z., Ma, X., Ni, Z., Jin, C., Zhang, Z. Plasma-assisted fabrication of monolayer phosphorene and its Raman characterization. *Nano Res.*, 7, 853, 2014.
72. Li, L., Kim, J., Jin, C., Ye, G.J., Qiu, D.Y., da Jornada, F.H., Shi, Z., Chen, L., Zhang, Z., Yang, F., Watanabe, K., Taniguchi, T., Ren, W., Louie, S.G., Chen, X.H., Zhang, Y., Wang, F. Direct observation of the layer-dependent electronic structure in phosphorene. *Nat Nano.*, 12, 21, 2017.
73. Lu, W., Nan, H., Hong, J., Chen, Y., Zhu, C., Liang, Z., Ma, X., Ni, Z., Jin, C., Zhang, Z. Plasma-assisted fabrication of monolayer phosphorene and its Raman characterization. *Nano Res.*, 7, 853, 2014.
74. Liu, Y., Nan, H., Wu, X., Pan, W., Wang, W., Bai, J., Zhao, W., Sun, L., Wang, X., Ni, Z. Layer-by-Layer thinning of MoS2 by plasma. *ACS Nano.*, 7, 4202, 2013.
75. Jia, J., Jang, S.K., Lai, S., Xu, J., Choi, Y.J., Park, J.H., Lee, S. Plasma-treated thickness-controlled two-dimensional black phosphorus and its electronic transport properties. *ACS Nano.*, 9, 8729, 2015.
76. Coleman, J.N., Lotya, M., Neill, A.O., Bergin, S.D., King, P.J., Khan, U., Young, K., Gaucher, A., De, S., Smith, R.J., Shvets, I.V., Arora, S.K., Stanton, G., Kim, H.Y., Lee, K., Kim, G.T., Duesberg, G.S., Hallam, T., Boland, J.J., Wang, J.J., Donegan, J.F., Grunlan, J.C., Moriarty, G., Shmeliov, A., Nicholls, R.J., Perkins, J.M., Grieveson, E.M., Theuwissen, K., McComb, D.W., Nellist, P.D., Nicolosi, V. Two-dimensional nanosheets produced by liquid exfoliation of layered materials. *Science.*, 331, 568, 2011.
77. Nicolosi, V., Chhowalla, M., Kanatzidis, M.G., Strano, M.S., Coleman, J.N. Liquid exfoliation of layered materials. *Science.* 340(6139), 1226419, 2013.
78. Brent, J.R., Savjani, N., Lewis, E.A., Haigh, S.J., Lewis, D.J., Brien, P.O. Production of few-layer phosphorene by liquid exfoliation of black phosphorus. *Chem. Commun.*, 50, 13338, 2014.
79. Yasaei, P., Kumar, B., Foroozan, T., Wang, C., Asadi, M., Tuschel, D., Indacochea, J.E., Klie, R.F., Salehi-Khojin, A. High-quality black phosphorus atomic layers by liquid-phase exfoliation. *Adv. Mater.* 27, 1887, 2015.
80. Suk, J.W., Kitt, A., Magnuson, C.W., Hao, Y., Ahmed, S., An, J., Swan, A.K., Goldberg, B.B., Ruoff, R.S. Transfer of CVD-grown monolayer graphene onto arbitrary substrates. *ACS Nano.*, 5, 6916, 2011.
81. Li, Z., Wu, P., Wang, C., Fan, X., Zhang, W., Zhai, X., Zeng, C., Li, Z., Yang, J., Hou, J. Low-temperature growth of graphene by chemical vapor deposition using solid and liquid carbon sources. *ACS Nano.*, 5, 3385, 2011.

82. Berke, K., Tongay, S., McCarthy, M.A., Rinzler, A.G., Appleton, B.R., Hebard, A.F. Current transport across the pentacene/CVD-grown graphene interface for diode applications. *J. Phys. Condens. Matter.*, 24, 255802, 2012.
83. Wang, Y., Zheng, Y., Xu, X., Dubuisson, E., Bao, Q., Lu, J., Loh, K.P. Electrochemical delamination of CVD-grown graphene film: Toward the recyclable use of copper catalyst. *ACS Nano.*, 5, 9927, 2011.
84. Kim, K.S., Zhao, Y., Jang, H., Lee, S.Y., Kim, J.M., Kim, K.S., Ahn, J.H., Kim, P., Choi, J.Y., Hong, B.H. Large-scale pattern growth of graphene films for stretchable transparent electrodes. *Nature.*, 457, 706, 2009.
85. Huang, Y., Dong, X., Shi, Y., Li, C.M., Li, L.J., Chen, P. Nanoelectronic biosensors based on CVD grown graphene. *Nanoscale.*, 2, 1485, 2010.
86. Ling, X., Wang, H., Huang, S., Xia, F., Dresselhaus, M.S. The renaissance of black phosphorus. *Proc. Natl. Acad. Sci.*, 112, 4523, 2015.
87. Li, X., Deng, B., Wang, X., Chen, S., Vaisman, M., Karato, S., Pan, G., Lee, M.L., Cha, J., Wang, H., Xia, F. Synthesis of thin-film black phosphorus on a flexible substrate. *2D Mater.*, 2, 31002, 2015.
88. Yang, Z., Hao, J., Yuan, S., Lin, S., Yau, H.M., Dai, J., Lau, S.P. Field-effect transistors based on amorphous black phosphorus ultrathin films by pulsed laser deposition. *Adv. Mater.*, 27, 3748, 2015.
89. Lee, Y., Bae, S., Jang, H., Jang, S., Zhu, S.E., Sim, S.H., Il Song, Y., Hong, B.H., Ahn, J.H. Wafer-scale synthesis and transfer of graphene films. *Nano Lett.*, 10, 490, 2010.
90. Su, C.Y., Lu, A.Y., Wu, C.Y., Li, Y.T., Liu, K.K., Zhang, W., Lin, S.Y., Juang, Z.Y., Zhong, Y.L., Chen, F.R., Li, L.J. Direct formation of wafer scale graphene thin layers on insulating substrates by chemical vapor deposition. *Nano Lett.*, 11, 3612, 2011.
91. Morita, A. Semiconducting black phosphorus. *Appl. Phys. A.*, 39, 227, 1986.
92. Du, H., Lin, X., Xu, Z., Chu, D. Recent developments in black phosphorus transistors. *J. Mater. Chem. C.*, 3, 8760, 2015.
93. Wu, R.J., Topsakal, M., Low, T., Robbins, M.C., Haratipour, N., Jeong, J.S., Wentzcovitch, R.M., Koester, S.J., Mkhoyan, K.A. Atomic and electronic structure of exfoliated black phosphorus. *J. Vac. Sci. Technol. A: Vacuum, Surfaces, Film.*, 33, 60604, 2015.
94. Wu, R.J., Topsakal, M., Low, T., Robbins, M.C., Haratipour, N., Jeong, J.S., Wentzcovitch, R.M., Koester, S.J., Mkhoyan, K.A. Atomic and electronic structure of exfoliated black phosphorus. *J. Vac. Sci. Technol. A: Vacuum, Surfaces, Film.*, 33, 60604, 2015.
95. Xu, F., Ge, B., Chen, J., Nathan, A., Xin, L.l., Ma, H., Min, H., Zhu, C., Xia, W., Li, Z., Li, S., Yu, K., Wu, L., Cui, Y., Sun, L., Zhu, Y. Scalable shear-exfoliation of high-quality phosphorene nanoflakes with reliable electrochemical cycleability in nano batteries. *2D Mater.*, 3, 25005, 2016.
96. Anderson, G. Synthesis , characterization , and electronic properties of novel 2D materials : transition metal dichalcogenides and phosphorene. 2016. *Electronic Theses and Dissertations.* Paper 2428.

97. Monaco, G., Falconi, S., Crichton, W.A., Mezouar, M. Phosphorus: New *in situ* powder data from large-volume apparatus. *Powder Diffr.*, 18, 155, 2003.
98. Xia, F., Wang, H., Jia, Y. Rediscovering black phosphorus as an anisotropic layered material for optoelectronics and electronics. *Nat. Commun.*, 5, 4458, 2014.
99. Tokár, K Derian, R., Brndiar, J., Štich, I. Strain control of vibrational properties of few layer phosphorene. *J. Appl. Phys.*, 120, 194305, 2016.
100. Xia, F., Wang, H., Jia, Y. Rediscovering black phosphorus as an anisotropic layered material for optoelectronics and electronics. *Nat. Commun.*, 5, 4458, 2014.
101. Kim, J., Lee, J.U., Lee, J., Park, H.J., Lee, Z., Lee, C., Cheong, H. Anomalous polarization dependence of Raman scattering and crystallographic orientation of black phosphorus. *Nanoscale.*, 7, 18708, 2015.
102. Ribeiro, H.B., Pimenta, M.A., de Matos, C.J.S., Moreira, R.L., Rodin, A.S., Zapata, J.D., de Souza, E.A.T., Castro Neto, A.H. Unusual angular dependence of the Raman response in black phosphorus. *ACS Nano.*, 9, 4270, 2015.
103. Zhang, S., Yang, J., Xu, R., Wang, F., Li, W., Ghufran, M., Zhang, Y.W., Yu, Z., Zhang, G., Qin, Q., Lu, Y. Extraordinary photoluminescence and strong temperature/angle-dependent Raman responses in few-layer phosphorene. *ACS Nano.*, 8, 9590, 2014.
104. Fei, R., Yang, L. Lattice vibrational modes and Raman scattering spectra of strained phosphorene. *Appl. Phys. Lett.*, 105, 83120, 2014.
105. Fei, R., Yang, L. Lattice vibrational modes and Raman scattering spectra of strained phosphorene. *Appl. Phys. Lett.*, 105, 83120, 2014.
106. Late, D.J. Temperature-dependent phonon shifts in few-layer black phosphorus. *ACS Appl. Mater. Interfaces.*, 7, 5857, 2015.
107. Zhang, S., Yang, J., Xu, R., Wang, F., Li, W., Ghufran, M., Zhang, Y.W., Yu, Z., Zhang, G., Qin, Q., Lu, Y. Extraordinary photoluminescence and strong temperature/angle-dependent Raman responses in few-layer phosphorene. *ACS Nano.*, 8, 9590, 2014.
108. Calizo, I., Balandin, A.A., Bao, W., Miao, F., Lau, C.N. Temperature dependence of the Raman spectra of graphene and graphene multilayers. *Nano Lett.*, 7, 2645, 2007.
109. Late, D.J., Shirodkar, S.N., Waghmare, U.V., Dravid, V.P., Rao, C.N.R. Thermal expansion, anharmonicity and temperature-dependent Raman spectra of single- and few-layer MoSe2 and WSe2. *ChemPhysChem.*, 15, 1592, 2014.
110. Sahoo, S., Gaur, A.P.S., Ahmadi, M., Guinel, M.J.F., Katiyar, R.S. Temperature-dependent Raman studies and thermal conductivity of few-layer MoS2. *J. Phys. Chem. C.*, 117, 9042, 2013.
111. Pawbake, A.S., Island, J.O., Flores, E., Ares, J.R., Sanchez, C., Ferrer, I.J., Jadkar, S.R., van der Zant, H.S.J., Castellanos-Gomez, A., Late, D.J. Temperature-dependent Raman spectroscopy of titanium trisulfide (TiS3) nanoribbons and nanosheets. *ACS Appl. Mater. Interfaces*, 7, 24185, 2015.

112. McLintock, A., Cunha-Matos, C.A., Zagnoni, M., Millington, O.R., Wark, A.W. Universal surface-enhanced Raman tags: Individual nanorods for measurements from the visible to the infrared (514–1064 nm). *ACS Nano.*, 8, 8600, 2014.
113. Yang, J., Xu, R., Pei, J., Myint, Y.W., Wang, F., Wang, Z., Zhang, S., Yu, Z., Lu, Y. Optical tuning of exciton and trion emissions in monolayer phosphorene. *Light Sci. Appl.*, 4, e312, 2015.
114. Das, S., Zhang, W., Demarteau, M., Hoffmann, A., Dubey, M., Roelofs, A. Tunable transport gap in phosphorene. *Nano Lett.*, 14, 5733, 2014.
115. Jackson, W.B., Kelso, S.M., Tsai, C.C., Allen, J.W., Oh, S.J. Energy dependence of the optical matrix element in hydrogenated amorphous and crystalline silicon. *Phys. Rev. B.*, 31, 5187, 1985.
116. Lösche, A., Mott, A.N.F., Davis, E.A. Electronic Processes in Non-Crystalline Materials. Oxford: Clarendon-Press, 1971, pp 437 .
117. Woomer, A.H., Farnsworth, T.W., Hu, J., Wells, R.A., Donley, C.L., Warren, S.C. Phosphorene: Synthesis, scale-up, and quantitative optical spectroscopy. *ACS Nano.*, 9, 8869, 2015.
118. Woomer, A.H., Farnsworth, T.W., Hu, J., Wells, R.A., Donley, C.L., Warren, S.C. Phosphorene: Synthesis, scale-up, and quantitative optical spectroscopy. *ACS Nano.*, 9, 8869, 2015.
119. Du, Y., Ouyang, C., Shi, S., Lei, M. Ab initio studies on atomic and electronic structures of black phosphorus. *J. Appl. Phys.*, 107, 93718, 2010.
120. Du, Y., Ouyang, C., Shi, S., Lei, M. Ab initio studies on atomic and electronic structures of black phosphorus. *J. Appl. Phys.*, 107, 93718, 2010.
121. Kim, J.S., Liu, Y., Zhu, W., Kim, S., Wu, D., Tao, L., Dodabalapur, A., Lai, K., Akinwande, D. Toward air-stable multilayer phosphorene thin-films and transistors. *Sci. Rep.*, 5, 8989, 2015.
122. Avsar, A., Vera-Marun, I.J., Tan, J.Y., Watanabe, K., Taniguchi, T., Castro Neto, A.H., Özyilmaz, B. Air-stable transport in graphene-contacted, fully encapsulated ultrathin black phosphorus-based field-effect transistors. *ACS Nano.*, 9, 4138, 2015.
123. Tayari, V., Hemsworth, N., Fakih, I., Favron, A., Gaufrès, E., Gervais, G., Martel, R., Szkopek, T. Two-dimensional magnetotransport in a black phosphorus naked quantum well. *Nat. Commun.*, 6, 1, 2015.
124. Gillgren, N., Wickramaratne, D., Shi, Y., Espiritu, T., Yang, J., Hu, J., Wei, J., Liu, X., Mao, Z., Watanabe, K., Taniguchi, T., Bockrath, M., Barlas, Y., Lake, R.K., Lau, C.N. Gate tunable quantum oscillations in air-stable and high mobility few-layer phosphorene heterostructures. *2D Mater.*, 2, 11001, 2015.
125. Avsar, A., Vera-Marun, I.J., Tan, J.Y., Watanabe, K., Taniguchi, T., Castro Neto, A.H., Özyilmaz, B. Air-stable transport in graphene-contacted, fully encapsulated ultrathin black phosphorus-based field-effect transistors. *ACS Nano.*, 9, 4138, 2015.

126. Tayari, V., Hemsworth, N., Fakih, I., Favron, A., Gaufrès, E., Gervais, G., Martel, R., Szkopek, T. Two-dimensional magnetotransport in a black phosphorus naked quantum well. *Nat. Commun.*, 6, 1, 2015.
127. Chen, X., Wu, Y., Wu, Z., Han, Y., Xu, S., Wang, L., Ye, W., Han, T., He, Y., Cai, Y., Wang, N. High-quality sandwiched black phosphorus heterostructure and its quantum oscillations. *Nat Commun.*, 6, 1, 2015.
128. Gillgren, N., Wickramaratne, D., Shi, Y., Espiritu, T., Yang, J., Hu, J., Wei, J., Liu, X., Mao, Z., Watanabe, K., Taniguchi, T., Bockrath, M., Barlas, Y., Lake, R.K., Lau, C.N. Gate tunable quantum oscillations in air-stable and high mobility few-layer phosphorene heterostructures. *2D Mater.*, 2, 11001, 2015.
129. Kang, J., Wood, J.D., Wells, S.A., Lee, J.H., Liu, X., Chen, K.S., Hersam, M.C. Solvent exfoliation of electronic-grade, two-dimensional black phosphorus. *ACS Nano.*, 9, 3596, 2015.

3

Graphene for Advanced Organic Photovoltaics

Tanvir Arfin* **and Shoeb Athar**

Environmental Materials Division, CSIR-National Environmental Engineering Research Institute, Nehru Marg, Nagpur India

Abstract
Graphene is a promising one-atom-thick 2D material of nanoscale dimensions with sp^2-hybridized hexagonal carbon network having unusual properties such as excellent transparency, exception charge transport characteristics, high mechanical strength, and thermal stability, which has rendered it an ideal material for countless applications, specifically energy conversion and energy storage applications including super-capacitors, photovoltaic (PV) cells, fuel cells, etc. Out of these myriad applications, the development of advanced PV cells that can efficiently convert sunrays into electricity has particularly warranted great attention of research fraternity as it entails the solution of a very challenging prospective energy and global warming problems. This chapter summarizes and briefly discusses, with selected examples and findings, the recent progress in graphene applications as transparent electrodes, acceptor material, interfacial layer, etc. in organic photovoltaic devices.

Keywords: Graphene, organic photovoltaics, transparent electrode, acceptor material, interfacial layer

3.1 Introduction

Material science plays a critical role in our life as it provides the scope for designing and developing new materials via synthesis process or by

**Corresponding author*: tanvirarfin@ymail.com

Suvardhan Kanchi, Shakeel Ahmed, Myalowenkosi I. Sabela and Chaudhery Mustansar Hussain (eds.) Nanomaterials: Biomedical, Environmental, and Engineering Applications, (93–104)

artificial means. Life styles of human beings have an advanced way back due to the innovation of new materials.

A large sign in the development of our society is fully related with the material from the beginning of initial life right from the Stone Age to present era of telecom revolution. Materials are a part of our life without which survival is difficult if not impossible. The life in modern age is totally dependent on the various types of syntheses and man-made materials, which help us to improve the quality of life in the society and exist effortlessly in the civilization of the country.

3.2 History of Graphene

The innovation of carbon-based materials such as graphene and the successive growth of a graphene-based polymer composite plays a significant role in the field of nanoscience. Compared to the carbon nanotubes with minimum density and maximum aspect ratio, graphene has a great consideration due to its excellent mechanical and electrical properties and outstanding electronic features. The outcome shows that it is a promising excellent material for growth and functionalized development of material *via* synthesis and man-made process along with its derivatives.

3.3 Structure of Graphene

Graphene has the ability to show a 2D structure and it is atomically thick with sp^2 hybridization arranged in a honeycomb type of compact structure [1]. The structure of graphene is shown in Figure 3.1. Novoselov *et al.*, [2] has proved that graphene is the thinnest material when compared to other materials in this world and his group received a Noble Prize in the field of Physics in 2004 for graphene.

3.4 Graphene Family Nanomaterials

GFN are of several types in accordance with a variety of layers in the modification of sheet or in a chemically enhanced form. The various forms of GFNs are single-layer graphene (SLG), bi-layer graphene (BLG), multilayer graphene (MLG), graphene oxide (GO), and reduced graphene oxide (rGO). They vary from each other possessing properties such as amount of layers, composition, surface chemistry, horizontal dimensions, and purity.

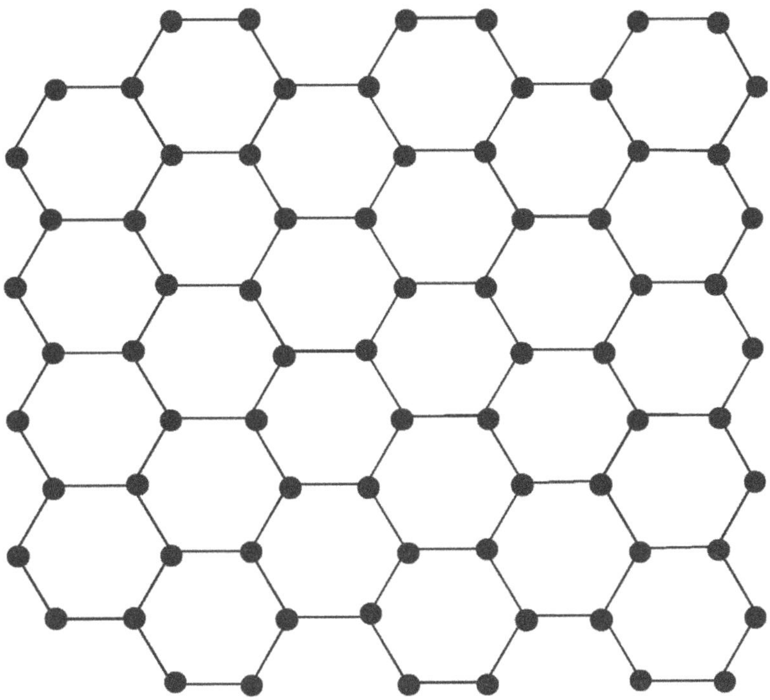

Figure 3.1 Basic structure of graphene.

3.5 Properties of Graphene

Graphene possesses varieties of mechanical properties and underlying physical and chemical properties such as thermal conductivity, large surface area, and high charge carrier mobility.

3.5.1 Physicochemical Properties

The graphene lattice structure shows a honeycomb-patterned one atom thick layer. It can be divided into two sub-lattices attached through σ bonds and π electrons where σ bonds connect with a single carbon atom molecule and free π electrons contribute to the delocalized electron system. These π electrons contribute for the maximum electron density up and down of the two-dimensional structure. These electrons can easily interact with FMO of various types of organic compounds, which renders the electrophilic substitution reaction easier in comparison to nucleophilic substitution.

3.5.2 Thermal and Electrical Properties

The excellent features of graphene molecules and the strong single bond between C-C molecules show outstanding electrical and thermal conductivity with a minimum thermal expansion coefficient. In the case of single-layer graphene (SLG), it shows excellent electrical and thermal conductivity because of minimum defect in crystal lattice. The extraordinary features of graphene in terms of thermal and electrical conductivity are further used in making electronic devices, biomedical devices, and electrochemical and biosensors.

3.5.3 Optical Properties

Graphene has become a curiosity in the research field because of outstanding optical features and electrical charge transport properties. SLG has proved that it can transmit nearly 97.7% of the overall incident light at large extent of wavelengths. It can be further stated that optical image contrast and light absorption increases with an increase in the amount of layer in the structure of graphene molecules.

3.5.4 Mechanical Properties

The breaking strength of graphene is around 200 times greater than steel, making it one of the best and strongest materials. Pure graphene has a higher mechanical feature than GO.

3.5.5 Biological Properties

Graphene has the ability to show a high surface area where it stimulates interaction with cells though particular uptake mechanisms are still unresolved. Graphene due to its biocompatibility, flexibility, and electrical conductivity can be used in neural interface electrode without gliosis and diminishing of signal strength over long time usage. Graphene and graphene-based materials are ideal candidates in the field of pharmaceutical as well as biomedical industries for a number of applications such as biosensors, tissue engineering, drug delivery, cancer treatment, etc.

3.6 Graphene for Advanced Organic Photovoltaics

3.6.1 Transparent Electrodes of OPVs

Thin film photovoltaic cells pose as a promising substitute for conventional silicon photovoltaic cells. A crucial feature of these organic cells is the conduction of current through the electrode of the cell within the transparent conductor, i.e., the electrode must be transparent with adequate conductance. Fluorine tin oxide (FTO) as well as indium tin oxide (ITO) caters to these requisites. Although, ITO is more efficient than its fluorine counterpart, it has its own disadvantages, such as limited indium resource, diffusion of ions into polymeric layers in case of organic photovoltaic cells (thus reducing efficiency), low transparency for the near-infrared (NIR) region (thereby rendering the cell unable to absorb a wider spectrum of solar radiation), instability at acidic or basic conditions, and high cost and brittle nature of ITO that limits its use for flexible photovoltaic cells [3].

The search for low cost and high performance novel window electrodes has brought the focus on carbon-based materials. The following unique properties of graphene make it an ideal 2-D material for application as electrodes in solar cells:

1. The ease of assembly into the film-electrode with an ultra-smooth surface
2. The ideal atomic thickness to facilitate high transparency in visible as well as NIR regions
3. Frugal production method

Yin *et al.*, [4] used a transparent electrode in the form of a transferred reduced GO film (rGO)-poly(ethylene terephthalate) (PET) composite to fabricate flexible OPV cells. An increase in photocurrent density (J_{sc}) and, by extension, power conversion efficiency (PCE) was observed when the resistance of the rGO film was reduced by decreasing the film thickness. The maximum PCE obtained was 0.78% when the transparency and resistance of the transparent electrode was 55% and 1.6 kΩ/sq., respectively. The devices were highly stable when tension was induced by bending and could perform consistently even upon bending a 1000 times.

Similarly, Choi *et al.*, [5] produced an indium-free organic photovoltaic cell using a multi-layered graphene electrode (MLG). The transparency of MLG-based electrodes, developed upon glass substrates via chemical vapor deposition and multi-transfer method at ambient temperature, was as high as 84.2% with minimal sheet resistance. The resulting OPV exhibiting a PCE of 1.17% was proposed as a cost-effective substitute for conventional ITO electrodes.

To overcome limitations of use of MLG films in OPVs arising out of high surface roughness, costly fabrication of transparent electrodes, low work-function, etc., Du *et al.*, [6] developed single-layer graphene films-based transparent anode for OPV cells comprised of light-absorbing films containing evaporable organic molecular semiconductor materials, namely zinc phthalocyanine (ZnPC)/fullerene (C60) along with an interfacial layer of molybdenum oxide (MoO). Besides increasing the optical transmittance, the single-layered electrode showed lesser surface roughness with respect to two- and four-layered graphene anodes obtained by multi-transfer and stacking of a single-layered graphene anode. The addition of an interfacial layer of MoO resulted in the reduction of energy barrier between the anode and active layer as well as caused an almost ten times decrease in the resistance of the SLG. The OPV cells fabricated in this work showed a PCE of nearly 0.84% which is merely 17.6% lesser than the OPV cells having an equivalent structure based on ITO anodes. Moreover, an increase in efficiency by 50% and 86.7% compared to two-layered graphene and four-layered graphene anodes was observed. The work proved the feasibility of SLG electrodes for flexible as well as wearable OPV cells.

Similarly, Lima *et al.,* [7] proposed an easy and commercially viable process to obtain a flexibly transparent and conductive GO-based composite by mixing GO and the conducting poly(3,4–ethylenedioxythiophene):poly(sty renesulfonate) (PEDOT:PSS) polymer in an aqueous solution without using surfactants. The exceptionally flexible composite thin film gave good transmittance as well as resistivity values and, after application as transparent electrodes in a double-layered structured OPV cells, yielded a PCE of 1.10%.

Although graphene is more stable, both chemically and mechanically, compared to ITO-based photovoltaic cells, their low PCE still remains a big challenge. Park *et al.,* [8] demonstrated the application of graphene anode and cathode in polymer photovoltaic (PPV) cells to get the highest PCEs ever achieved, i.e., 6.1% and 7.1%, correspondingly. The record-high efficiencies were gained by thermally treating the electron-blocking layer of the MoO_3 layer and directly depositing the electron-transporting layer of ZnO on graphene. The work also entailed the fabrication of graphene/PET-based PPV cells that were found to be stable under various bending conditions. The work paved the way to fabricate graphene-based efficient PV cells using a simply reproducible procedure.

3.6.2 Acceptor Material in OPVs

In conventional inorganic semiconductors, free holes and free electrons are simply generated upon solar illumination; however, in organic solar cells, the electrons and holes generated are strongly bound. Therefore, the separation of these electron–hole pairs (excitons) requires a strong driving force in OPV cells. This is achieved by forming a heterojunction with an acceptor material having an electron affinity (EA) greater than the donor polymer but still lesser than the ionization potential (IP). The difference between the EA and IP of these two materials in the heterojunction results in a driving force that dissociates the firmly bound pairs of electrons and holes into separate charges [9]. Two commonly used heterojunctions are: bilayer or planar heterojunction structure and an inter-mixed bulk heterojunction (BHJ) structure. In planar heterojunction devices, limited diffusion length (the travelling distance of exciton to reach exciton restricts their overall efficiency charge-transport channels) restricts their overall efficiency. This drawback can be overcome by employing the BHJ structure where all electron–hole pairs are expectedly generated within the limits of diffusion length of excitons in an inter-penetrating network of acceptor and donor materials. Presently, the best performing OPV devices are developed applying the BHJ structure using polymers having lower band gap polymers as donor and graphene-based materials as acceptor.

Liu *et al.*, [10] fabricated and comprehensively studied the BHJ structured photovoltaic cells using solution-processable functionalized graphene (S-PFG) in the form of acceptor material and P_3OT as a donor polymer. The functionalization of GO was carried out using phenyl isocyanate to convert hydrophilic character of GO nano-sheets into hydrophobic. The P_3OT/S-PFG composite film had nearly same absorption as the pristine P_3OT film within 400–650 nm of the wavelength range. A major observation was the remarkable quenching in the strong photoluminescence of P_3OT after the deposition of S-PFG, indicating the effective energy transfer along the P_3OT/S-PFG interface.

Hill *et al.*, [11] studied the electrochemical properties of GO nano-sheets and showed the fluorescence and electro-generated chemiluminescence quenching ability of GO nano-sheets deposited onto chloroform from aqueous media employing an innovative, surfactant-driven technique. The study revealed the feasible reduction of GO using charge injection. Fluorescence quenching of P_3HT was carried out to prove the potential application of GO as an electron acceptor material in a bulk hetero-junction OPV cell. Moreover, OPV devices with ITO/PEDOT:PSS/P_3HT-GO/Al architecture were developed. GO-consisting OPV devices showed a rise in short-circuit current as well as conductivity; however, a drop in open-circuit voltage was observed. The findings, specifically efficient quenching of photoluminescence, prove the potential use of non-organically modified GO as an electron acceptor material in OPV devices.

Gupta *et al.*, [12] used a hydrothermal method to functionalize graphene quantum-dots (GQ-Ds) (obtained from graphene sheets) with aniline for application as an acceptor material in OPV cells. P_3HT/An-GQ-Ds-based hybrid photovoltaic cells were developed having a device structure of ITO/PEDOT:PSS/P_3HT:An-GQ-Ds/LiF/Al. P_3HT/An-graphene sheets-based photovoltaic cells were also fabricated for comparison. The value of filling factor (FF) for P_3HT/An-GQ-Ds heterojunction OPV cells was 0.53 compared to 0.33 for graphene sheets-based heterojunction devices. Highest values of PCE, open circuit voltage (V_{oc}), photocurrent density (J_{sc}), and FF were found to be 1.14%, 0.61V, 3.51 mA/cm^2, and 0.53, respectively, for 1% w/w An-GQ-Ds in P_3HT, whereas for graphene sheets counterpart the corresponding maximum values were comparatively lower, i.e., 0.65%, 0.88 V, 2.65 mA/cm^2, and 0.28 at 10% w/w An-graphene sheets in P_3HT. Contrary to the large domains of P_3HT/An-graphene sheets, atomic force microscopy (AFM) images of P_3HT/An-GQ-Ds films showed uniformly fine features, indicating nano-scale phase separation that suggests a high potential of GQ-Ds as the acceptor material in OPV cells.

Recently, Tsai *et al.*, [13] configured a PV device with an Al/amorphous-Si/PEDOT:PSS-GQ-Ds/Ag structure by adding a layer of PEDOT:PSS and GQ-Ds to micro-structured Si heterojunctions.

The GQ-Ds were produced by the microwave method. The J_{sc} and FF had a positive correlation with GQ-Ds concentrations up to 0.5%; thereafter, a decrease in efficiency was observed because of more recombination reactions, possibly due to the formation of GQ-D aggregates. Thus, the best performance of nearly 13.22% was accomplished owing to the influence of GQ-Ds on light harvesting under 400 nm as well as on the enhancement in conductivity and consequently on efficiency of carrier collection.

3.6.3 Interfacial Layer in OPVs

The performance of organic electronic devices relies heavily on the "active layer-anode-cathode" interfaces. The interfacial material plays the following crucial functions [9]:

1. Adjustment of height of energetic barrier between active layer and electrodes
2. Formation of a selective and fine contact for typical carriers
3. Determination of the device polarity
4. Surface property modification to change the morphology of the active laver
5. Prohibition of any chemical/physical reaction that may occur between active layer and electrodes
6. Function as an optical-spacer

This section discusses the application of graphene as an interfacial layer in OPV devices.

Li *et al.* [14] demonstrated the application of GO thin-films as the hole-transport as well as electron-blocking layer in OPV cells. The introduction of GO between the photo-active P_3HT: phenyl C61-butyric acid methyl ester (PCBM) layer and the conducting as well as transparent ITO resulted in the reduction of electron–hole recombination along with the leakage currents. Consequently, a remarkable enhancement in the efficiencies of OPVs is obtained indicating the efficacy of solution-processable GO as the hole-transport and electron-blocking layer in OPVs.

Valentini *et al.* [15] reported a simplistic approach for using chemically synthesized few-layered graphene nano-sheets (FLGNS) as part of a transparent electrode for fabrication of PPV cells. GNS were chemically modified by covalently conjugating fluorine followed by the exposure of fluorinated GNS to aliphatic amine at ambient temperature. The PPV devices then developed having ITO/PEDOT:PSS/Butyl amine (BAM)-modified fluorinated-FLGNS/ Regioregular-P_3HT:PCBM/LiF/Al architecture performed superiorly with a PCE of 0.74%, against the corresponding values of 0.38% and 0.42% for the PPV cells with non-modified GNS, and 42% for PEDOT:PSS. The findings suggested that BAM-modified, low-cost, and simply prepared GNS can effectively improve the transport of charge carrier and decrease the recombination influence of the active layer, and can thereby be easily used as a hole acceptor material in PPV applications.

Feng *et al.* [16] introduced NH_3-modified GO (GO:NH_3) into perovskite-based photovoltaic cells having ITO/PEDOT:PSS-GO:NH3/ CH3NH3PbI3-xClx/phenyl C61-butyric acid methyl ester (PCBM)/solution Bphen (sBphen)/Ag structure, and found a significant improvement in the performance of cells and stability of a perovskite structure. The fabricated PV devices had an excellent PCE of 16.11% and performed superiorly with respect to all reference PV devices without the GO:NH_3 film. The enhanced performance were partially attributed to each enhanced crystallization and ideal alignment orderliness of perovskite structure, enhanced morphological characteristics with almost complete coverage, improved optical absorption owing to the PEDOT:PSS-GO:NH_3 sheet, and well-matched energy-level alignment on the interface of perovskite. Moreover, the PV device exhibited better stability under ambient conditions that evidently is the outcome of the better structural stability of perovskite due to the GO:NH_3 layer as also confirmed by synchrotron-based grazing incidence X-ray diffraction (GIXRD) results. Precisely, chemically modified GO can function as an effective interfacial layer in perovskite-based PV cells.

3.7 Conclusion

In this chapter, feasibility and myriad applications of graphene-based material in advanced OPV devices were discussed in brief. Graphene as transparent electrodes has shown great latent potential minus the negative features of its conventional analogs attributable to excellent conductivity and transparency in visible as well as NIR regions. Graphene offers several big advantages such as dispersibility, tunable band structure via regulation of dimension, and functionalization, rendering it a potential acceptor material for OPV devices, though their performance still needs improvement. Regarding the use of graphene as an interfacial layer, the work is still in infancy and requires cautious and rigorous optimization before a judgment can be made on their performance. Though performance of graphene-based OPV cells is still not comparable to conventional materials, such as ITO, exploiting exceptional electronic properties of graphene via tuning of its energy levels as well as band-gap, enhancing its wettability through flexible functionalization and employing the high chemical, thermal, and mechanical stabilities of low-cost graphene, must make graphene a promising and ideal material for advanced organic photovoltaic applications in the near future.

References

1. Arfin, T., Bushra, R., Mohammad, F. Electrochemical sensor for the sensitive detection of o-nitrophenol using graphene oxide-poly(ethyleneimine) dendrimer-modified glassy carbon electrode. *Graphene Technol.*, 1, 1, 2016.
2. Novoselov, K.S., Geim, A.K., Morozov, S.V., Jiang, D., Zhang, Y., Dubonos, S.V., Grigorieva, I.V., Firsov, A.A. Electric field effect in atomically thin carbon films. *Science*, 306, 666, 2004.
3. Hu Y.H., Wang H., Hu, B. Thinnest two-dimensional nanomaterial graphene for solar energy. *ChemSusChem*, 3, 782, 2010.
4. Yin, Z.Y., Sun, S.Y., Salim, T., Wu, S.X., Huang, X., He, Q.Y., Lam, Y.M., Zhang, H. Organic photovoltaic devices using highly flexible reduced graphene oxide films as transparent electrodes. *ACS Nano*, 4, 5263, 2010.
5. Choi, Y.-Y., Kang, S.J., Kim, H.-K., Choi, W.M., Na, S.-I. Multilayer graphene films as transparent electrodes for organic photovoltaic devices. *Sol. Energy Mater. Sol. Cells*, 96, 281, 2012.
6. Du, J.H., Jin, H., Zhang, Z.K., Zhang, D.D., Jia, S., Ma, L.P., Ren, W.C., Chenga, H.M., Burn, P.L. Efficient organic photovoltaic cells on a single layer graphene transparent conductive electrode using MoOx as an interfacial layer. *Nanoscale*, 9, 251, 2017.

7. Lima, L.F., Matos, C.F., Gonçalves, L.C., Salvatierra, R.V., Cava, C.E., Zarbin, A.J.G., Roman, L.S. Water based, solution-processable, transparent and flexible graphene oxide composite as electrodes in organic solar cell application. *J. Phys. D: Appl. Phys.*, 49, 1, 2016.
8. Park H., Chang, S., Zhou, X., Kong, J., Palacios, T., Silvija Gradecak, S. Flexible graphene electrode-based organic photovoltaics with record-high efficiency. *ACS Nano Lett.*, 14, 9, 5148.
9. Wan, X., Long, G., Huang, L., Chen, Y. Graphene – a promising material for organic photovoltaic cells. *Adv. Mater.*, 23, 5342, 2011.
10. Liu, Z., Liu, Q., Huang, Y., Ma, Y., Yin, S., Zhang, X., Sun, W., Chen, Y. Organic photovoltaic devices based on a novel acceptor material: graphene. *Adv. Mater.*, 20, 3924, 2008.
11. Hill, C.M., Zhu, Y., Pan, P. Fluorescence and electroluminescence quenching evidence of interfacial charge transfer in poly (3-hexylthiophene): graphene oxide bulk heterojunction photovoltaic devices. *ACS Nano*, 5, 942, 2011.
12. Gupta, V., Chaudhary, N., Srivastava, R., Sharma, G.D., Bhardwaj, R., S. Chand, S. Luminscent graphene quantum dots for organic photovoltaic devices. *J. Am. Chem. Soc.*, 133, 9960, 2011.
13. Tsai, M.-L., Wei, W.-R., Tang, L., Chang, H.-C., Tai, S.-H., Yang, P.-K., Lau, S.P., Chen, L.-J., He, J.-H. Si hybrid solar cells with 13% efficiency *via* concurrent improvement in optical and electrical properties by employing graphene quantum dots. *ACS Nano*, 10, 815, 2016.
14. Li, S.-S., Tu, K.H., Lin, C.-C., Chen, C.-H. Chhowalla, M., Solution-processable graphene oxide as an efficient hole transport layer in polymer solar cells. *ACS Nano*, 4, 3169, 2010.
15. Valentini, L., Cardinali, M., Bon, S.B., Bagnis, D., Verdejo, R., Lopez-Manchadob, M.A., Kenny, J.M. Use of butylamine modified graphene sheets in polymer solar cells. *J. Mater. Chem.*, 20, 995, 2010.
16. Feng, S., Yang, Y., Li, M., Wang, J., Cheng, Z., Li, J., Ji, G., Yin, G., Song, F., Wang, Z.-K., Li, J., Gao, X. High-performance perovskite solar cells engineered by an ammonia modified graphene oxide interfacial Layer. *ACS Appl. Mater. Interfaces*, 8, 23, 14503.

4

Synthesis of Carbon Nanotubes by Chemical Vapor Deposition

Falah H. Hussein[1,*] **and Firas H. Abdulrazzak**[2]

[1]*College of Pharmacy, Babylon University, Hilla, Iraq*
[2]*Chemistry Department, College of Education for Pure Sciences, Diyala University, Diyala, Iraq*

Abstract
Numerous literatures reported physiochemical properties, applications, characterization, and synthesis of different types of carbon nanotubes. In this review, we report our work with the synthesis of carbon nanotubes by chemical vapor deposition. The review includes the effect of many conditions that required synthesis of single wall carbon nanotubes (SWNTs), few-wall carbon nanotubes (FWNTs), and multiwall carbon nanotubes (MWNTs). The parameters were precursor as sources of carbon, catalyst, temperature, and the effect of the flow of transfer gas and precursor. In addition to the parameter, we reported the defect and deformation that accrued during the synthesis process while predicting effect on physiochemical properties of CNTs. Addition, the common methods for characterized carbon nanotubes such Raman spectroscopy, X-ray diffraction, thermal gravimetric analysis, transmittance TEM and scanning SEM spectroscopy are presented.

Keywords: CVD, temperature, Raman, tube furnace, CNT

4.1 Introduction

The real and active beginning that opened for treatments with carbon nanomaterials (CNM) should is to be refer to Iijima who synthesized the single wall carbon nanotubes (CNTs) with Ichihashi [1, 2]. CNTs consist of

**Corresponding author*: abohasan_hilla@yahoo.com

Suvardhan Kanchi, Shakeel Ahmed, Myalowenkosi I. Sabela and Chaudhery Mustansar Hussain (eds.) Nanomaterials: Biomedical, Environmental, and Engineering Applications, (105–132)

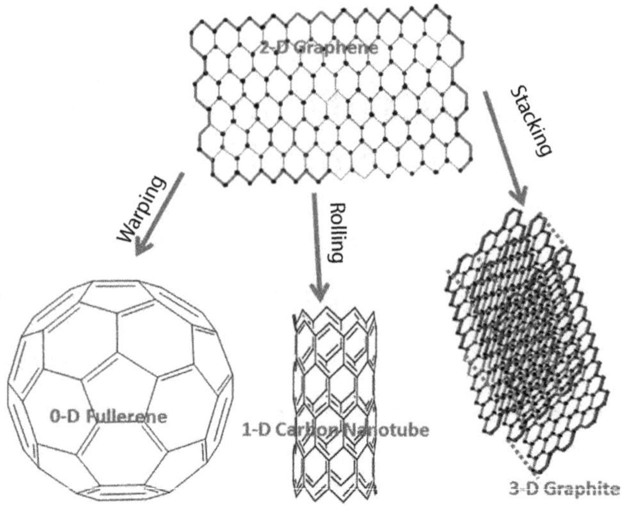

Figure 4.1 The structure of graphene in nature.

pristine carbon atoms linked together to forming a polymer in a hexagonal arrangement with a monolayer of carbon atoms [3] using specific connections that are represented by hybridization sp^2. Carbon atoms can form many different crystal structures, with a variety of properties. Figure 4.1 shows a typical examples of a sp^2-hybridized crystal structure representing one of the softest materials, a characteristic bonding π and antibonding π^* orbitals known as graphene. It consists of carbon atoms bonded with three neighboring atoms in a honeycomb lattice with a lattice constant or the distance of a = 0.142 nm between carbon atoms [4]. Graphene represents a two-dimensional (2-D) material with an edge energy that includes the position of armchair (A) to zig-zag (Z) and all the intermediate orientation chiral angles. The π-orbitals distributed over all the surfaces of the sheets enhance the formation of weak van der Waals forces resulting to distance of 0.34 nm between the layers [5]. When the graphene or graphite wrap around one of the axes, the structure will be convert from either 2D or 3D to 1D represented by tubular structure of carbon sheets. The direction of the sheets wrap will predict whether the tubes will be conductive or semi-conductive[6]. The CNTs structure got the attention of the scientists globally because of it physiochemical properties [7]. Saito *et al.*, [4] found that the inter-sheet distance in a multi-sheet nanotube is 0.344 nm, which is close to the distance of 0.335 nm between two sheets of graphene in graphite [8].

The common types of CNTs are single-walled carbon nanotubes (SWNTs) and multi-walled carbon nanotubes (MWNTs) (see Figure 4.2).

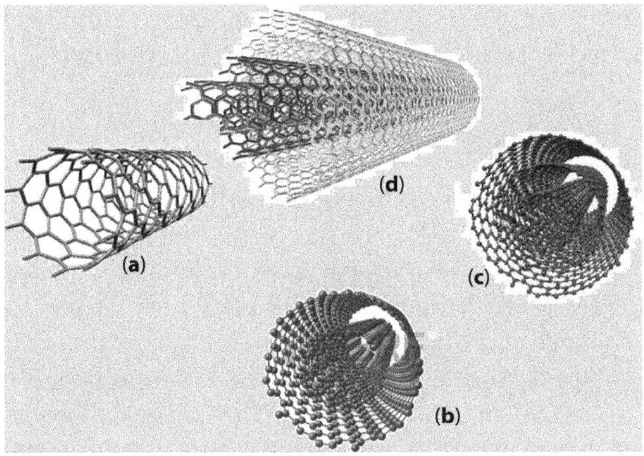

Figure 4.2 The classification of carbon nanotubes by the number of graphene layers: (a) SWNT, (b) DWNT, (c) FWNT, (d) MWNT.

Recently, a special kind of MWNT which can be considered as an intermediate structure between SWNTs and MWNTs has been reported. It is known as few-walled carbon nanotubes (FWNTs) and it consists of 2–6 layers of graphene sheets [9]. They have a diameter in the range of nanometers from 0.3 up to 100 nm [10], with a length that can reach to more than 2 cm [9]. The diameter of a typical SWNT is around 1 nm while for MWNTs can reach to more 10 nm [11].

In this review, we focus on the popular chemical vapor deposition CVD methods for synthesis of CNTs due to the possibility of producing nanotubes on a large commercial scale [12]. Generally, chemical vapor deposition (CVD) [13], arc-discharge [2], flame method [14], and laser ablation [15] represent the common methods for synthesized CNTs. The economic feasibility of the production of CNTs is seen in the CVD method, when hydrocarbon is dissociated in the presence of suitable metal catalysts or without a catalyst.

4.2 Synthesis Methods

The main methods reported commonly depend on the synthesis of carbon nanotubes including three types as we mentioned earlier. Many attempts were made to enhance the activity of methods such as varying the temperature, catalyst composition, and other process parameters. Consequently, the average diameter and length of the carbon nanotubes can be varied.

In the beginning, we will refer to the general information about the three methods before we go into the details of the CVD method.

4.2.1 Arc-Discharge

The arc-discharge method is used to produce fullerenes and CNTs [1] when an electric arc between two graphite rods is placed in an inert atmosphere or liquid of nitrogen. Carbon evaporation is initiated by a high-intensity electric current passing through the two rods, which are placed at 1 mm of distance to enhance and initiate the arc production as shown in Figure 4.3 (1), driven by approximately 20 V, creating a high temperature with low pressure (between 50 and 700 mbar) [2]. The high yield production of the carbon nanotubes depends on the homogeneity of the plasma arc and the temperature of the deposit on the two electrodes. MWNTs can be produced when the two electrodes include graphite without a catalyst while SWNTs and FWNTs are produced when the graphite rods was included catalytic materials such Molybdenum (Mo) [16].

The two carbon rods are different in size, the deposition will occur on the large rod and on the wall of precipitation chamber. The product usually short in length is with diameters ranging from 0.6 to 1.4 nm for single-walled and more than this value for multi-walled carbon nanotubes.

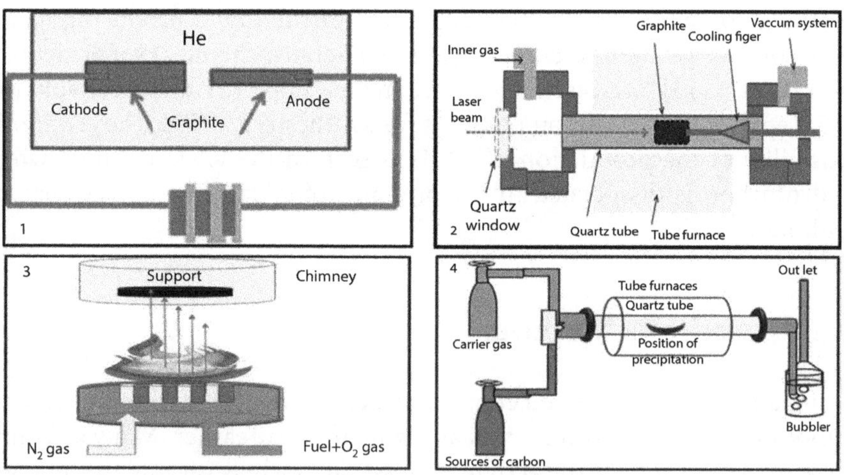

Figure 4.3 Methods for synthesis CNTs by Arc discharge, laser ablation, flame, and, chemical vapor deposition.

The most important parameter that influences the various activities involved in this method is the efficient cooling system [1] of the cathode, which has been shown to be essential in controlling the quality. Generally, the types and the quality of the product depend on many parameters such as the metal concentration, the inert gas pressure, current, and the system geometry. Possible disadvantage of this technique is the production of mixture of components.

4.2.2 Laser Ablation

The second way of producing high-quality CNTs from carbon plasma is by using a laser beam typically a YAG or CO_2 laser, where intense laser pulses ablate graphite as a source of carbon [15]. Figure 4.3 (2) shows graphite placed into a furnace heated to 1200 °C in the presence of an inert gas such as helium, and then it is directed toward a cold collector which causes the vapor to quickly condense into large clusters. The result of the process depends on the catalyst, which forms SWNTs, while the absence of a catalyst leads to the formation of MWNTs. This method was first discovered by Guo *et al.*, at Rive University in 1995 [17]. The tubes produced by this method are in the form of a mat of ropes 10–20 nm in diameter and up to 100 microns or more in length. The advantage of this method is high-quality SWNT, diameter control, the investigation of growth dynamics, and the production of new materials.

4.2.3 Flame Methods

Decomposition of hydrocarbon in gaseous phase with control conditions mostly causes growth CNT filaments which are called premixed flame. The most important difference between CVD and flame method, is the high concentrations of intermediate radicals formed in flame medium during the decomposition reaction.

Figure 4.3 (3) shows the typical reactor for decomposition of hydrocarbon with oxygen in atmospheric pressure. It is an exothermic reaction that produces high-heat with a rich carbon radical atmosphere that is suitable for CNT growth. The flame method uses the materials in gas or liquid (such as ethane, ethylene, acetylene, and propane) in a premixed or non-premixed reactor that is modified for this purpose [18]. The flame method can be classified depending on the nature of mixing the fuel and oxidizing into three types: premixed, non-premixed (diffusion), and partially premixed. The parameters that influence the nature and yield of carbon nanotubes [19] are gas flow rates, nature of catalyst, the fuel molecular constitution, the flame temperature, and growth times. Gulder reported that [20] the ratios of soot and carbon nanotube formation in laminar diffusion flames depend on the hydrocarbon molecular constitution and the temperature of decomposition. The fuel molecular constitution and the flame temperature govern soot and carbon nanotube formation in laminar diffusion flames [20]. Li Ming *et al.*, [21] used a stainless grid flame supplied by propane-air to synthesize CNTs on the surfaces that are covered with iron, chromium, and nickel oxide in a nitrogen atmosphere. The control in conditions of precipitation can form [22] SWNTs when particularly using the catalyst as mixes with the hydrocarbon fuel and oxygen at the burner surface or fixed on the support of precipitation. The growth of the SWNTs in the flame was related to catalyze by the presence of metals.

4.2.4 Chemical Vapor Deposition

The catalytic chemical vapor deposition of carbon was already reported in 1959 [23], however only in 1993 where carbon nanotubes were formed using this method [24]. The CVDs refer to the process of forming a thin film by reactions through chemical deposition to build high-quality layers of a designated material by using a special chamber that is a tube furnace containing one or more heated objects to be coated. The tube furnace uses a special container for precipitation made from quartzite or silica/quartzite in different lengths and diameters with a tubular stricture.

CVD seems the most promising method for possible industrial applications due to the relatively low growth temperature, high yields, and high purities with many specific properties that can be achieved during its production. The precursor mostly supplied in gases phase from gaseous containers or other sources are stored as liquids and their vapors are mixed with the carrier gases. Occasionally, solid sources could be used that undergo sublimation at low temperatures as compared with the process of precipitation [25].

In CVD, the synthesis of carbon nanotubes depends on the pyrolysis of hydrocarbons over the catalyst particle or without a catalyst, when deposition of carbon clouds at a specific site [13]. The catalyst material may be solid, liquid, or gas and can be placed inside the furnace or fed in continuously from outside. Figure 4.3 (4) shows the general structure of the CVD system. The carbon source is typically a hydrocarbon material, possibly a gas such as acetylene, ethylene, or a liquid such as different types of alcohol, which are usually supplied to the reactor by evaporation using a suitable method. The carrier gases are used to input the carbon clouds into the reactor. Sometimes a mixture of carrier gas (inert gas) and hydrogen are used as a reducing agent. The concentration of reactants in the mixture is determined by accurate flow meters. The operating temperature inside the quartz tube ranges from 500 °C to 1200 °C. Inside the tube, there are support materials that are covered with a suitable catalyst that behaves as an active site for the growth of carbon nanotubes.

The four main parameters that decided the type of CNTs, i.e., whether SWNTs or MWNTs, are the atmosphere of the reactor, the hydrocarbon source, the catalyst, and the growth temperature. Generally a low temperature in the range of 600–900 °C yields MWNTs, whereas a higher temperature of more than 900 °C during the reaction mostly yields SWNT growth. However, despite the many uses and applications of this technique, CVD also has a number of disadvantages, some of which could be removed or at least reduced while others cannot be prevented. The disadvantages are explained briefly as follows:

1. The typical process with a need for precursors should be volatile at near-room temperature. This is significant for a number of elements, although the use of metal-organic precursors have limited this situation.
2. The most important disadvantage is the health and safety aspect of this technique, which is represented by the precursors being highly toxic such as ($Ni(CO)_4$), or explosive (B_2H_6), or in many conditions causing the corrosion of the reactor ($SiCl_4$).
3. The byproducts of CVD reactions can also be hazardous (CO, or HF).
4. Some of these precursors, especially the metal-organic precursors, can also be quite costly.
5. The other major disadvantage is related to the process of synthesis, whereby the films are usually deposited at high temperatures.

This causes limitations on the kinds of substrates that can be used. In addition, the parameter which deals with the temperature of synthesis and thermal expansion coefficients can cause mechanical instabilities in the deposited films. Michael *et al.*, [26] developed a new modified method to produce high-purity SWNTs, at high pressures of ~30–50 atm and high temperatures of ~900–1100 °C, by flowing CO HiPco onto catalytic clusters of iron. Hernadi [27] used another modified CVD method named for the mixture of three catalysts: cobalt, molybdenum, and CoMoCat. The precursor of carbon in these methods was carbon monoxide, which decomposes within the temperature range of between 700 °C and 950 °C. The advantage of this method is represented by the lower ratios of the byproducts that form during the precipitation process as compared with the arc discharge and laser ablation methods.

4.3 The Parameters of CVD

The main parameters that influence the quality, purity, and quantities of carbon nanotubes are reported in this section, which are arranged according to the role of each type.

4.3.1 CNT Precursors

The most common sources for the synthesis of CNTs are methane [25], acetylene [28], benzene [29], and carbon monoxide [30] but the most popular CNT precursor in the CVD method worldwide is ethanol [31]. Ethanol is the most important due to no amorphous carbon produce, and the enhancement effect of the OH radical, which evolves from its dissociation [31–32]. The molecular structure of the precursor has a specific effect on the structure and skeletons of carbon nanotubes that are grown using this method. Linear hydrocarbons such as methane, ethylene, and acetylene thermally decompose into atomic carbon or linear dimmers and trimmers of carbon, and generally directly produce hollow CNTs. The precursors with the higher number of carbon atoms, more than seven atoms, produce branching CNTs, while cyclic hydrocarbons such as benzene, xylene, and cyclohexane relatively produce curved CNTs with curved tube walls, with many bridged. General experiments show that low temperatures under 900 °C yield MWNTs, while those over 900 °C yield SWNTs. This view is concerned with the important belief that SWNTs have a higher energy of formation [32], which may be related to the small diameters and high curvature having high strain energy. Most MWNTs can be synthesized in easier conditions and from most hydrocarbon sources, while SWNTs are produced under specific [9–11, 13, 15, 32] conditions and from selected hydrocarbons. Thus, to attain an ideal synthesis, the precursor of carbon represents a sensitive parameter in producing specific types and yields. These sources of carbon are mostly used as sources of energy and for many industrial purposes; a lot of these sources are at risk of depletion in the near future and the high costs compared with many other materials. The natural hydrocarbon precursors have generated a great deal of interest because of the possibility of synthesizing CNTs from the bank of hydrocarbon

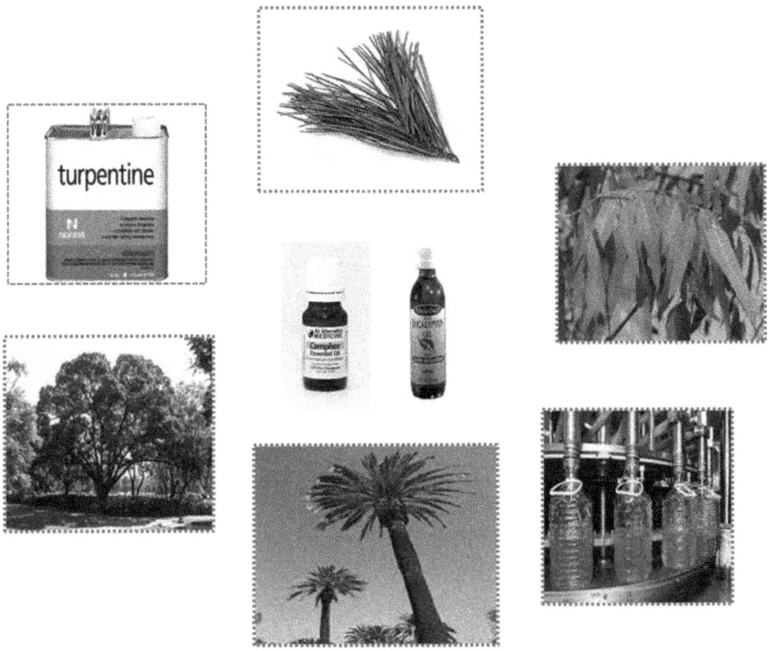

Figure 4.4 Different natural sources to synthesize CNTs.

compounds. The advantage is related to renewables produced by nature, and easily available and low in cost, such as essential oils. Figure 4.4 shows the commonly reported natural precursors are palm oil [33], camphor oil [34], maize [35], turpentine oil [36], castor oil [37], coconut oil, corn oil, sesame oil [38], and eucalyptus oil [39].

Most of these types mentioned above represent an important food for humans, or use in many food industries. Some research has, where appropriate, been directed away from the natural sources mentioned above by substituting these materials with animal and plant waste with a high carbon content. The wastes that were used in the literature were waste cooking oil [40], cellulosic materials [41], and chicken fat [42]. polyethylene has three types: high density polyethylene (HDPE), low density polyethylene (LDPE), and linear low density polyethylene (LLDPE) [43]. Tires for automobiles [44], fullerene waste soot, which are produced from the process of the synthesis of fullerene by arc-discharge [45], are also used for this purpose. The process of using waste as a source of carbon involves many drawbacks.

1. Before using this waste, a set of processes and treatments are carried out in order to make the waste suitable for the

reactor, such as washing, removal of intervening materials, and thermal treatments, in addition to a final configuration for the reaction, as well as other operations that depend on the type of waste.
2. A relatively high temperature is required for the use of these materials and for the liberation of the carbon content from this waste.
3. A special type of reactor is usually needed such as two-stage tube furnaces.
4. The major products of the combustion of the waste lead to the formation of byproducts that are harmful to the environment, which are mostly useless due to the high costs involved in reusing them.

4.3.2 Type of Catalyst

A critical parameter that influences the process of synthesizing CNTs is represented by the catalyst of precipitation. The catalyst plays critical influence in two ways: the first ideal size of metal particles required to build the tubular structure, and the second enhance the abilities of surface to decomposition hydrocarbon at a lower temperature. The catalyst particles serve as an active site to nucleate the growth of nanotubes. In order to be suitable the catalysts need to fulfill at least three important requirements, all supposed to be available. The first is represented by the high solubility of carbon [46] in these metals at high temperatures. The second does not prevent or reduce the diffusion rate of carbon on its surfaces. The third condition is the high melting point and low equilibrium-vapor pressure of these metals offering a wide temperature range of CVD for wide possibilities for the use of different types of carbon precursors. The Fe, Co, and Ni are widely used as transition metals for this purpose that is characterized by stronger adhesion and the ability to form a low dimension for synthesizing the product. These elements are often used and complete the reaction in two ways: the first is *in situ* by using organometallocene materials such as ferrocene [13, 46], cobaltocene, and nickelocene when evolving the catalyst particles in nano size. The second way is *out situ*, which is represented by preparing films of a few micrometers thickness, which is done by different methods on the surfaces of support. The diameter of CNTs is strongly dependent on the diameter of the catalyst particle; it is approximately the same size as the catalyst nanoparticles since the diameter also defines the number of walls of CNTs, and there is a strong connection between the catalyst particle diameter and the number of walls. The transition metals are proven to be efficient catalysts, not only in CVD but also in arc-discharge and laser-vaporization methods. Noble metals (Au, Ag, Pt, Pd, etc.) have a very low solubility for carbon, but they can dissolve carbon for CNT growth when their particle size is slightly less than 5 nm. Kondo *et al.*, [47] succeeded in the controlled growth of SWNTs by using nanoparticles of Au, which are distributed in the atomic phase with the support of Si.

4.3.3 Effect of Temperature

Heat represents the main factor for synthesizing carbon nanotubes, regardless of the techniques that are used for this purpose (arc-discharge, laser ablation, or chemical vapor deposition). One advantage of CVD compared to other methods that makes it the best method is lower operating costs due to the lower synthesis temperature [48]. The role of temperature is divided into two functions: the first is the conversion of the sources of carbon into vapor before going into the reactor, and the second causes decomposition of the vapor inside the precipitation reactor. To achieve this goal, special reactors are used; some are one stage and others two stages, which are used depending on the work requirements. The process of decomposition represents the most important step in the mechanism of forming tubular structures, which affects the length, diameter, deformation, type, and properties of the product [48]. The temperature of a decomposition precursor, will activates the catalyst, making it more effective towards increasing sensitivity. The synthesis of CNTs with a specific diameter is limited by converting the catalyst from a few micrometers to nanometers at high temperatures; thus, the activity of the catalysts decreases with lower temperatures [49]. The yield increases as the temperature also increases, which indicates that typical growth represented by catalysts and the best decomposition for the sources of carbon is more active at higher temperatures. A lot of the literatures propose that at higher temperatures the catalyst agglomerate converts into a large area for agricultural CNTs. The promotion of the sources of carbon decomposition leads to more wall formation [50], which in turn causes the growth of SWNTs with MWNTs. Thus, CNTs are produced very densely at high temperatures [51].

When increasing the growth temperature to a higher value, the ratios and thin lengths for producing CNTs are reduced. Aksak *et al.*, [52] postulated that increasing the growth temperature to 925 °C causes the production of very thin and long nanotubes with an average diameter of about 10.5 nm. Reducing the temperature below 925 °C decreases the average diameter compared to those at temperatures between 850 °C and 875 °C. Sivakumar *et al.*, found that [53] MWNTs form at low temperatures and

SWNTs at high temperatures. They also found that the number of CNTs decreases at high temperatures compared with the optimum range of temperature for both SWNTs and MWNTs. The SWNTs with a narrow diameter [51–53], distribution, and a higher yield were obtained at temperatures above 750 °C, whereas the best product with specific properties of MWNTs was observed at lower temperatures. Toussi *et al.*, [48] found that higher temperatures may cause a higher speed of decomposition, which prevents regular precipitation that occurs when the decomposition rate of precursor is higher than the carbon diffusion rate. However, this causes growth termination without producing CNTs or producing CNTs with higher ratios of amorphous carbon. Mitri *et al.*, [54] and Rajard *et al.*, [55] studied the effects of temperature on the synthesis of carbon nanotubes. The results reflects the importance of choosing the optimum temperature for growth in order to produce optimum crystalline. This estimates the product by finding the ratios I_D/I_G, as in Figure 4.5, where the Raman spectrum for synthesized CNTs at different temperatures is depicted.

4.3.4 Gas Flow Rates

This parameter mainly refers to the carrier gas and the precursor that are used as sources of carbon; therefore, in order to avoid confusion and to show the effect of each in the process of chemical vapor deposition. The carrier gas is one of the most fundamental requirements for the process; its role is limited to carry a cloud of the precursor stream into the deposition reactor only without causing any interference [52]. In the laboratory, the flow rate of the carrier gas directly influences the process of precipitation. When the flow rate of the carrier gas has slowed, very few CNTs are formed, because the flow rate cannot carry enough precursor vapors through the reactor to be deposited onto the catalysts [56–57]. It could decrease the CNT production due to a lack of a carbon source, and any further transformation may cause the polymerization of the precursor [58]. The high flow rate of the carrier gas and most of the precursor are carried out of the reactor with very slow or without any decomposition and in best cases incomplete decomposition, and thus no deposited occurs in the reactor in the presence and also in the absence of a catalyst [55]. It has been found both theoretically and practically [59] that the best flow rate for a carrier gas is one that provides the time required carrying out a complete decomposition of the carbon source. This allows for a full and regular precipitation while minimizing the less loss of the source. On the other hand, the impact of other precursors affects the vapor pressure. This represents the concentration of the precursor vapor in the reactor, which is influenced by

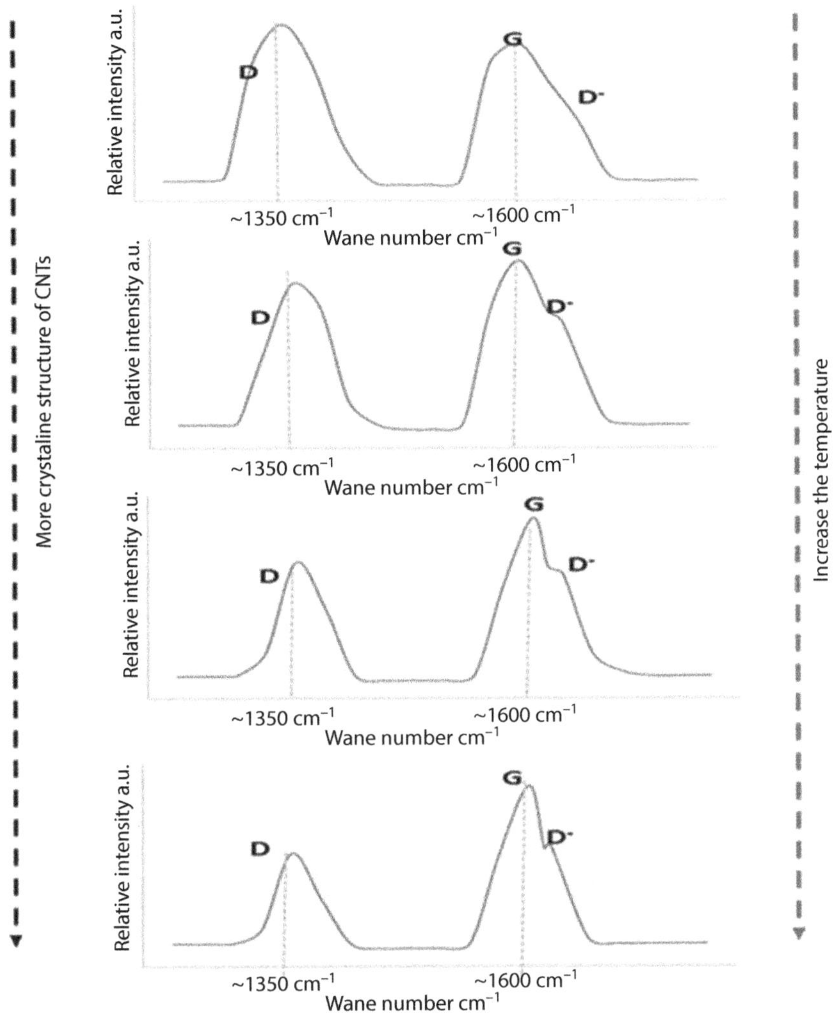

Figure 4.5 Raman spectra of purified carbon nanotubes grown at different temperature.

the rate of decomposition and the rate of diffusion. However, equilibrium is to be achieved between the two processes to allow for horizontal growth and the formation of a tubular structure while preventing the formation of a carbon layer on the surface. When excessive adsorption and decomposition happen, two cases arise. The first is when the decomposition rate of the precursor is higher than the carbon diffusion rate, thus causing a growth termination without producing any CNTs. The second case is when the decomposition rate of the precursor is lower than the carbon diffusion rate, which provides the appropriate time to allow for carbon atoms for building CNTs [57, 60]. Generally, the CNTs length decreases with the increasing flow rates of the carrier gas and a high vapor pressure within the range that causes growth [61–63]. At the same time, it can be deduced from Raman spectroscopy that the G and D bands are influenced directly by the flow rate of the carrier gas and the vapor pressure. When the flow rate and vapor pressure are at optimum conditions, this causes the growing CNTs to have a good crystalline graphitic structure. The best identification of ideal crystalline can be calculated by determining the ratio of I_G/I_D that gives a value more than 1 that indicates a good graphitization process for the product. Many experiments use H_2 to enhance the pyrolysis process of the precursor that represents its main job. Thus, at higher flow rates of hydrogen, the ratios of CNTs decrease, which may be attributed to a reduction in the optimum time of the reactant in the reactor. The last effect may be due to the high velocity of hydrogen gas in the mixture of gases, which remove the reactant at high speed from the reaction zone [63].

4.4 Deformations and Defects in Carbon Nanotubes

This section focuses on the distortion that may be accrued during growth of the tubular structure on the surface of precipitation. Mostly, the distortion happened when the condition of precipitation was not ideal or when some parameters were changed negatively. Sometimes the tubular structure in the hollow and the large aspect ratio of length to diameter, as well as the forces or interaction between the tubes, can cause deformations of bending, and the degree of deformation can be enhanced.

4.4.1 Deformations in Carbon Nanotubes

Figure 4.6 shows different schemes of deformations that can be observed in the tubular structures. CNT deformations under bending exhibit quite an interesting mode. A pure bending load acting on a CNT leads to real change in the cross-section; thus, the bending progresses, which is due to two instability deformation modes that are represented by kinking and rippling.

In order to find the actual influences of these forces, the radial deformation of a CNT is necessary to assess the van der Waals forces by taking the cantilever, tip, and sample geometry into account [64–65]. As shown in Figure 4.7, the CNTs have three macroscopic deformations, which are axial, radial, and torsional strains, in addition to two microscopic positions

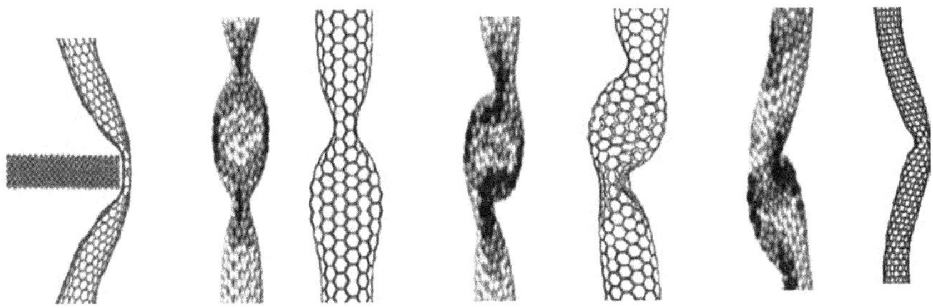

Figure 4.6 Different deformation in the skeleton of carbon nanotubes.

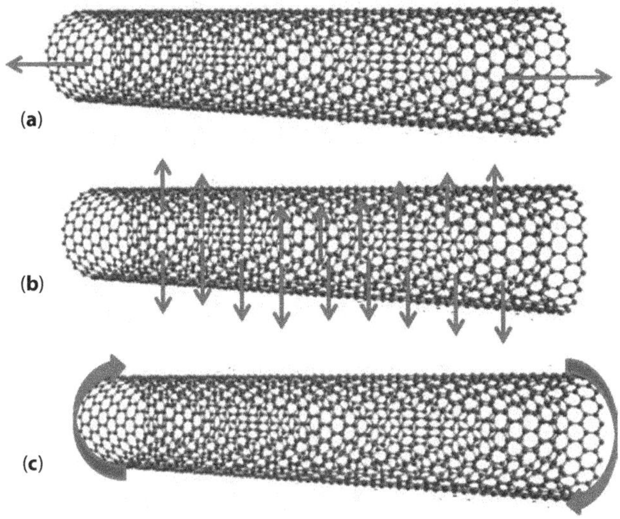

Figure 4.7 Deformation modes in a nanotube: (a) axial deformation, (b) radial deformation, and (c) twisting deformation.

of the carbon atoms within the unit cell deformation modes that do not break the symmetry of the underlying graphene lattice [65–66].

The radial deformation increases with the radius of single-walled carbon nanotubes and decreases with the number of layers. However, Figure 4.7 shows the radial deformation of SWNTs is the same as MWNTs when the radius of the first one is equal to the inner radius between the layers of graphene in a multi-walled structure. The radial deformations have an important effect on the electronic properties of CNTs. For example, the radial deformation of CNTs strongly affects their electrical properties [67]. The increasing in the number of walls directly affects the types and intensities of deformation, which can be explained as a result of the inner walls [68] of the double- and triple-wall tubes acquiring charges. In the triple-wall, the inner tube is always negatively charged, which indicates an increased electron affinity for small-diameter tubes. The screening effect of the outer tube is overestimated in full nonorthogonal tight-binding since on a minimal basis set, atoms cannot polarize. The magnitude of these values must thus be regarded as a lower limit.

One way to characterize radial deformation is to perform execute a nanoindentation test, as reported by Shen *et al.*, [69], by using contact mode AFM. The deformability (up to 46%) of a tube and it's ability to withstand a great compressive load of 20 μN were both reported. A similar experiment was done by Yu *et al.* [70], who used AFM in tapping-mode. The flexibility constant corresponding to the radial deformation was found to range from 0.3 GPa to 4 GPa based on a Hertzian contact model by Sato [68]. It has also been broadly accepted that the mechanical deformation of a carbon nanotube causes significant changes in its physical and chemical properties. A precise knowledge of its deformation mechanism and available geometry is, therefore, crucial for understanding the precise physics of CNT systems and in developing CNT-based applications.

4.4.2 Defects in Carbon Nanotubes

The defects in the structure of carbon nanotubes and the concentration of defects make it very sensitive for physiochemical properties such as chemical reactivity, mechanical strength, optical absorption, and electronic transport. Also, the defects may reduce the strength of CNTs by more than 85% CNTs representing an ideal material system for studying and probing the possible effects of defects, particularly in SWNTs. The most important [67] differences between graphite and CNTs have been found. First, the allowed categories of defects are restricted by the dimensionality of SWNTs; obviously, they cannot contain higher dimensional defects like line and screw imbalances. Isolated SWNTs also cannot support many of the common interstitial defects. In addition, the defects found in graphite are more complicated in CNTs due to their cylindrical nature. Experimental investigations have proven that the loss of mechanical strength, the change in optical activity, or the increase in electrical resistance can be attributed to point defects. The most typical type of defects in crystalline lattices is point vacancies, interstitials, and bound complex of the two. Figure 4.8 shows vacancy defects are common results in three dangling links that immediately rehybridize or react with neighboring molecules.

The metastable chemistry of a single vacancy also drives a tendency toward a vacancy merger. In graphite, a di-merger formed of two missing

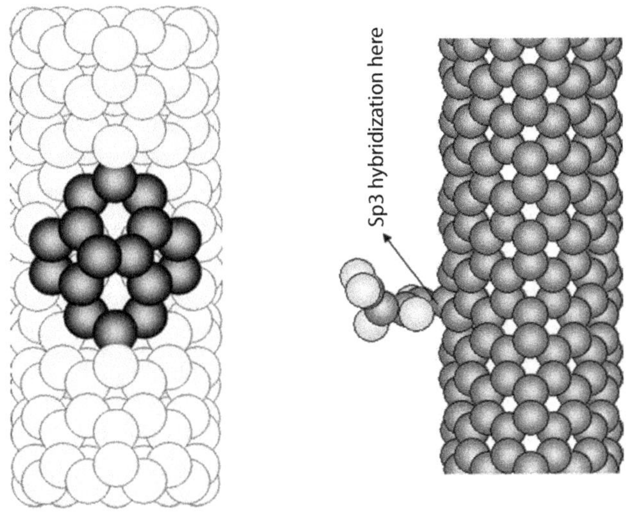

Figure 4.8 Post-synthesis defect on the outer surfaces of CNTs.

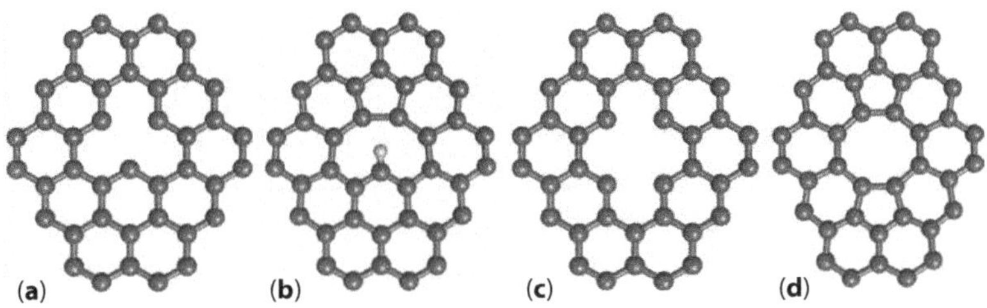

Figure 4.9 Small vacancy defects in the graphene system. Mono-vacancy (a) before and (b) after reconstruction and the H-termination of the remaining dangling bond. Di-vacancy (c) before and (d) after reconstruction.

atoms only costs ~1 eV more than a mono-merger, and nearly 6 eV less than two separated mono-mergers. Thus [71] particularly during annealing processes, single defects are observed to merge and grow into larger voids in graphene sheets. In SWNTs, the merger migration barrier is only 1 eV, suggesting mobility at temperatures as low as (100–200) °C. Figure 4.9 shows that the di-merger has a few notable properties, including the ability to reconstruct into a pentagon, octagon, and pentagon (5–8–5) structure that is free of dangling bonds. The additional strain of curvature and di-vacancies in SWNTs are believed to have smaller formation energies than mono-vacancies by nearly 1.5 eV.

The effects of defects appear in the properties of synthesized carbon nanotubes as follows:

1. Mechanical properties, which represent the changes in stiffness observed. The stiffness decreases with topological defects and increases with functionalization. The defect generation and growth are observed during plastic deformation and the fracture of nanotubes, which in addition to the synthesized composite will show improved properties with chemical bonding between the matrix and nanotubes.
2. Electrical properties, when the defect produces different types of shapes not only single-, few-, and multi-walled carbon nanotubes, but also branching carbon nanotubes which show a new behavior toward conductivity.

The most common results for the effects of deformation and defects are represented by the abilities for adsorption which can be explained by comparing graphite and carbon nanotubes. Graphite is many layers of graphene on a 2-D plane, while carbon nanotubes are represented by one or many layers of graphene that wrap to form a tubular structure in a 1-D plane. Generally, three differences between CNTs and graphite indicate that CNTs are even more sensitive to adsorbents than graphite surfaces: First, the CNT curvature results in partial sp3 hybridization, accentuated in small SWNTs, which enhances the π electron density on the cylinder's outer surface. This makes the adsorbed positive species such that Na^+ and H^+ dynamically interact with this surface of CNTs that include a high electron density, even in the absence of chemical bonding or static charge transfer [72]. Adsorbents in these voids can be better coordinated than on flat graphene surfaces. The voids readily contain a wide range of molecular shapes and sizes than do interlayer graphite interstices [71], which will be enhanced with the existence of defect and deformation, thus increasing the surface area. The graphite crystal is not changed by air at room temperature; the inter-cavities on the surfaces of tubular structures between the mono-filaments of SWNTs and bundles must be considered as filled with gases. Finally, every atom in a hollow SWNT is a surface atom, and the addition of adsorbents is a proportionally larger perturbation in SWNTs than in solid materials. The system can no longer be considered a simple carbon lattice if: (i) there is physical and chemical adsorption that occurs on a carbon lattice, (ii) there is interaction with the surfaces of many species such as H-bonded water dipoles, or chemisorbed oxygen as well as physisorbed hydrocarbons. All of these probabilities cause at least the breaking of the remaining rotational and translational symmetries of the tubular structure of SWNTs, however, they are physically extended from an idealized or the typical structure of a 1-D line.

The defect formation in metallic armchair-type tubes can cause the region surrounding that defect to become semiconducting. Furthermore, single monoatomic vacancies induce magnetic properties. Hertel *et al.,* [71] proposed adsorption on a substrate, where nanotubes are likely to face difficulties or defects; they will be subject to both radial and axial deformations. Depending on the tube diameter and the number of shells [72], the Van der Waals interaction between the nanotubes and a substrate result in high binding energies, which has been determined experimentally. Nanotubes may consequently experience radial and axial deformations, which significantly modify the idealized geometry of the free nanotubes. These findings have implications for electronic transport and the tribological properties of adsorbed nanotubes.

4.5 Characterization of CNTs

Many techniques were used to characterize CNTs. In this section, the common methods were explained briefly such as Raman spectroscopy and X-Ray diffraction. Raman spectroscopy is one of the most extensively employed methods for the characterization of carbon nanotubes, and which is a tool for the characterization of carbon nanotubes and functionalized carbon nanotubes [73], attracting a lot of attention in recent years. Theoretically, it is possible to predict morphological characteristics such as the diameter of the tubes and experimentally a powerful method for determining the degree of structural ordering or the presence of contaminants [74–76]. The variety of carbon materials arises from the strong dependence of their physical properties on the ratio of a sp2 such as graphite to a sp3 such as diamond [77]. There are many forms of sp2-bonded carbons with various degrees of graphitic ordering, ranging from single crystals of graphite, to nanocrystals, to glassy carbon [78].

As shown in Figure 4.10, the most distinguished Raman features in CNTs are the radial breathing modes (RBMs), caused by the higher frequency of disordered D, the G graphite network, and the G' (second-order Raman scattering from D-band variation) modes. The D, G, and G^- modes are found in graphite; and the RBM is specific to CNTs and is representative of the isotropic radial expansion of the tube. The RBM frequency is inversely proportional to the diameter of the tube, making it an important feature for determining the diameter distribution in a sample. The RBM bands are a useful diagnostic tool for confirming the presence of CNTs in a sample. The composite of CNTs with different materials has been evaluated by using Raman spectroscopy, which shows the state of dispersion

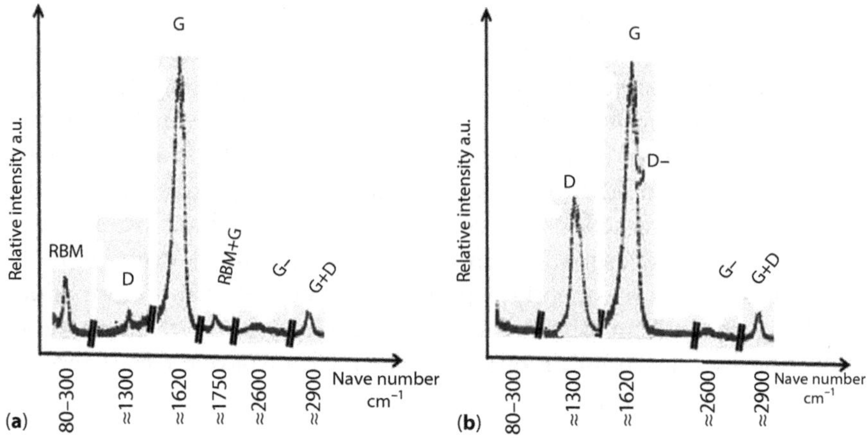

Figure 4.10 Typical Raman spectroscopy for (a) SWNT and (b) MWNT.

and the polymer–filler interactions reflected by shifts or width changes of the peaks. The sensitivity of some bands of CNTs to an application of mechanical distortion of the composite has also been used to quantify the load transferred from the matrix to the nanotubes and the interfacial adhesion [79].

The G band as shown in Figure 4.10 is a tangential shear mode of carbon atoms assigned to the in-plane vibration of the C–C bond that corresponds to the stretching mode in the graphite plane [80]. In simple graphite, a single mode is observed at 1580 cm^{-1} while in CNTs, this mode transforms into two modes as a result of the confinement of wave vectors along the circumference. The position of the G-band can be used to monitor the energy state change due to the environment. The frequency of the high-energy branch G^+ does not differ with diameter, while the lower energy peak G^- becomes more regular for smaller diameter CNTs.

The second peak is the D band, which is a longitudinal optical (LO) phonon and known as the disordered or defect style because a defect is required to scatter flexibly in order to maintain momentum. This property may relate to scattering from that defect and amorphous carbon impurities present in preparing CNTs. This style is usually located between 1250 and 1450 cm^{-1} and has a linear according to the laser excitation energy [80–81]. The D band is present in all carbon allotropes, including sp^2 and sp^3 amorphous carbon. This band is activated from the first-order scattering process of sp^2 carbons by the presence of in-plane substitution hetero-atoms, vacancies, grain boundaries, or other defects, and by finite-size effects. All of these characteristics reduce the crystal symmetry [82] of the lattice network. When observed in MWNTs, the D band is generally represented by a defect in the tubes. It can also be used to qualitatively characterize the chemical functionalization of the tube. Sidewall functionalization damages the tube, thus increasing the D band intensity to evaluate the quality using the D/G band intensities. For high-quality samples without defects and amorphous carbon, the D/G ratio is often less than 2%. The D-band width for CNTs is generally 10 to 20 cm^{-1}.

The D to G band intensity ratio (I_D/I_G) is the intensity of the disorder mode divided by the intensity of the graphite mode. This ratio is commonly used to evaluate the distortion on the surfaces of CNTs, and an increase in the ID/IG ratio indicates an increase in the number of defects on the sidewall of the G' band [83]. The G-band frequency is close to twice that of the D band and is found from 2500 to 2900 cm^{-1}. This is a second-order process from two-zone boundary LO phonons, or it may be attributed to the overtone of the D band. This band is commonly used to evaluate the load transfer between SWNTs and other types. The G^- band is an intrinsic property of the nanotube and graphite, and is present even in defect-free nanotubes for which the D band is completely absent.

The RBM used to characterize between graphene and carbon nanotubes does not exist in graphite. This mode is found between 75 and 300 cm^{-1} from the excitation line, and is associated with the symmetric transmission carbon atoms in the radial direction. The RBM [79–84] frequency (ωr) is used to find the inner and outer diameter when [$\omega_r = 224(cm^{-1})/d_t(nm)$]. Tube diameters between 0.8 and 1.3 nm give nearly identical results. Most single-grating Raman spectrometers have cutoff frequencies between 100 and 120 cm^{-1}, which limit the range of tube diameters to smaller than 2 to 2.5 nm. Larger tubes can be measured with high Rayleigh rejection multi-grating systems that allow frequencies of less than 100 cm^{-1}. The XRD pattern for CNTs generally shows two characteristic peaks at $2\theta \approx 26°$ which related to normal graphite for sp^2 (C=C) [85] and take the C(001) plane. The second peak at ≈43° can be attributed to the diffraction from the C(002) planes of the carbon nanotubes. The second peak is more intense in MWNTs than in SWNTs [86]. One of the most important uses of XRD is ascertaining the quality and crystalline nature of nanotubes as opposed to amorphous carbon materials, as well as the purities of synthesized CNTs.

Thermal-gravimetric analysis commonly used for evaluation of the purities of synthesized carbon nanotubes, the nature of the surfaces of the tubular structures, and the types of CNTs. A typical analysis using a TGA measurement of the as-produced nanotube material in air generally shows one peak in the value of change in weight loss as the temperature increases. An analysis of purified nanotube material in air may produce more than one peak that may relate to many causes: one reason for this is related to the deformation found on the surfaces of carbon nanotubes, in addition to various components in the nanotube material such as amorphous carbon, nanotubes, and graphitic particles. Transmission electron microscopy (TEM) and scanning electron microscopy (SEM) represent the two important analyses that are mostly used in nanomaterials. The importance of these two instruments can be due to abilities to find the size, inner and outer diameter, density, and nature of surfaces.

4.6 Conclusion

Many methods were used to synthesize carbon nanotubes. There are many disadvantages in using these methods. The main one is the cost of carbon source and the cost involved in processes of production of CNTs, which limited using them to produce carbon nanotubes. The cost and techniques represent the critical parameter that likely encourages quality over quantity account vice versa. Chemical vapor deposition is the common method for the synthesis of CNTs in all the world for technical and material considerations; thus, we focus on it to explain many details for CVD. The review confirms on choosing appropriate conditions in preparing CNTs, which certainly increases the sensitivity and efficiency both quantitative and qualitatively.

References

1. Iijima, S. Helical microtubules of graphitic carbon. *Nature.*, 354, 56, 1991.
2. Iijima, S., Ichihashi, T. Single-shell carbon nanotubes of 1-nm diameter. *Nature.*, 363, 603, 1993.
3. Dresselhaus, M., Jorio, A., Saito, R. Characterizing graphene, graphite, and carbon nanotubes by Raman spectroscopy. *Annu. Rev. Condens. Matter Phys.*,1, 89, 2010.
4. Saito, R., Dresselhaus, M., Dresselhaus, G. *Physical Properties of Carbon Nanotubes.* 1st edn. World Scientific, Imperial College Press London 259, 1998.
5. Bandow, S., Kokai, F., Takahashi, K., Yudasaka, M., Qin, L.C., Iijima, S. Interlayer spacing anomaly of single-wall carbon nanohorn aggregate. *Chem. Phys. Lett.*, 321, 514, 2000.
6. Wang, X., Li, Q., Xie, J., Jin, Z., Wang, J., Li, Y., Jiang, K., Fan, S. Fabrication of ultra long and electrically uniform single-walled carbon nanotubes on clean substrates. *Nano Lett.*, 9, 9, 3137, 2009.

7. Kenan, S., Yiying, Z., Jiangsha, M., Emily, C., Navid, T. Structural polymer-based carbon nanotube composite fibers: understanding the processing structure performance relationship. *Materials.*, 6, 2543, 2013
8. Kiselev, N., Hutchison, J., Ryabenko, A., Rakova, E., Chizhov, P., Zhigalina, O., Artemov, V., Grigoriev, V. Two structural types of carbon bi-filaments. *Carbon.*, 43, 1897, 2005.
9. Cheng, Q., Hang, Q., Bo, G., Yuan, C., Qi, Q., Lu, C., Otto, Z., Jie, L. Fabrication of small diameter few-walled carbon nanotubes with enhanced field emission property. *J. Nanosci. Nanotechnol.,* 6, 5, 1346, 2006.
10. Gruneis, A., Rummeli, M.H., Kramberger, C., Barreiro, A., Pichler, T., Pfeiffer, R., Kuzmany, H., Gemming, T., Buchner, B. High quality double wall carbon nanotubes with a defined diameter distribution by chemical vapor deposition from alcohol. *Carbon.,* 44, 15, 3177, 2006.
11. Gruneis, A., Rummeli, M.H., Kramberger, C., Barreiro, A., Pichler, T., Pfeiffer, R., Kuzmany, H., Gemming, T., Buchner, B. High quality double wall carbon nanotubes with a defined diameter distribution by chemical vapor deposition from alcohol. *Carbon.,* 44, 15, 3177, 2006.
12. Awasthi, K., Kumar, R., Raghubanshi, H., Awasthi, S., Pandey, R., Singh, D., Srivastava, O. Synthesis of nano-carbon (nanotubes, nanofibres, graphene) materials. *Bull. Mater. Sci.*, 34, 4, 607, 2011.
13. Kumar, M., Ando, Y. Chemical vapor deposition of carbon nanotubes: A review on growth mechanism and mass production. *J. Nanosci. Nanotechnol.*, 10, 6, 3739, 2010.
14. Howard, J.B., McKinnon, J.T., Johnson, M.E., Makarovsky, Y., Lafleur, A.L. Production of C-60 and C-70 fullerenes in benzene oxygen flames. *J. Phys. Chem. A.,* 96, 16, 6657, 1992.
15. Scott, C., Arepalli, S., Nikolaev, P., Smalley, R. Growth mechanisms for single-wall carbon nanotubes in a laser-ablation process. *Appl. Phys. A.,* 72, 5, 573, 2001.
16. Ando, Y., Zhao, X. Synthesis of carbon nanotubes by arc-discharge methods. *NDFCT*, 16, 3, 125, 2006.
17. Guo, T., Nikolaev, P., Thess, A., Colbert, D., Smalley, R.E. Catalytic growth of single-walled nanotubes by laser vaporization. *Chem Phys Lett.*, 243, 1, 49, 1995.
18. Vander, R.L., Hall, L.J., Berger, G.M. Optimization of flame synthesis for carbon nanotubes using supported catalyst. *J. Phys. Chem. B.,* 106, 13122, 2002.
19. Shaijumon, M.M., Ramaprabhu. S. Studies of yield and nature of carbon nanostructures synthesized by pyrolysis of ferrocene and hydrogen adsorption studies of carbon nanotubes. *Int. J. Hydrog. Energy* 30., 311, 2005.
20. Gulder, Q.L. Influence of hydrocarbon fuel structural constitution and flame temperature on soot formation in laminar diffusion flames. *Combust. Flame.*, 78, 179, 1989.
21. Yuan, L.M., Saito, K., Hu, W., Chen, Z. Ethylene flame synthesis of well-aligned multi-walled carbon nanotubes. *Chem. Phys. Lett.*, 346, 23, 2001.

22. Diener, M., Nichelson, N., Alford, J.M. Synthesis of single-walled carbon nanotubes in flames. *J. Phys. Chem. B.*, 104, 9615, 2000.
23. Walker, P., Rakszawski, J., Imperial, G. Carbon formation from carbon monoxide-hydrogen mixtures over iron catalysts: I. Properties of carbon formed. *J. Phys. Chem.*, 63, 2, 133, 1959.
24. Guo, T., Nikolaev, P., Thess, A., Colbert, D., Smalley, R.E. Catalytic growth of single-walled nanotubes by laser vaporization. *Chem. Phys. Lett.*, 243, 1, 49, 1995.
25. Satiskumar, B.C., Govindaraj, A., and Rao, C.N.R. Bundles of aligned carbon nanotubes obtained by the pyrolysis of ferrocene–hydrocarbon mixtures: role of the metal nanoparticles produced *in situ*. Chem. Phys. Lett., 307, 158, 1999.
26. Michael, J., Peter, A., Colbert, D., Smith, K., Smalley, R.E. Gas-phase production of carbon single-walled nanotubes from carbon monoxide via the HiPco process: A parametric study. *American Vacuum Society, J. Vac. Sci. Technol. A.*, 19, 4, 1800, 2001.
27. Hernadi, K., Fonseca, A., Nagy, J.B., Bernaerts, D., Lucas, A.A. Fe-catalyzed carbon nanotube formation. *Carbon.*, 34, 1249, 1996.
28. Li, W., Xie, S., Qian, L., Chang, B., Zou, B., Zhou, W., Zhao, R., and Wang, G. Large-scale synthesis of aligned carbon nanotubes. *Science.*, 274, 1701, 1996.
29. Sen, R., Govindaraj, A., Rao, C. Carbon nanotubes by the metallocene route. *Chem. Phys. Lett.*, 267, 276, 1997.
30. Nikolaev, P., Bronikowski, M., Bradley, R., Rohmund, F., Colbert, D., Smith, K., and Smalley, R. Gas-phase catalytic growth of single-walled carbon nanotubes from carbon monoxide. *Chem. Phys. Lett.*, 313, 91, 1999.
31. Li, N., Chen, X., Stoica, L., Xia, W., Qian, J., Abmann, J., Schuhmann, W., and Muhler, M. The catalytic synthesis of three-dimensional hierarchical carbon nanotube composites with high electrical conductivity based on electrochemical iron deposition. *Adv. Mater.*, 19, 19, 2957, 2007.
32. Okubo, S., Sekine, T., Suzuki, S., Achiba, Y., Tsukagoshi, K., Aoyagi, Y., and Kataura, H. Purification of single-wall carbon nanotubes synthesized from alcohol by catalytic chemical vapor deposition. *Jpn. J. Appl. Phys.*, 43, 3, 396, 2004.
33. Kumar, R., Tiwari, R.S., Srivastava, O. Scalable synthesis of aligned carbon nanotubes bundles using green natural precursor: neem oil. *Nanoscale Res. Lett.*, 6, 92, 2011.
34. Termeh Yousefi, A., Bagheri, S., Shinji, K., Rouhi, J., Mahmood, M., Ikeda, S. Fast synthesis of multilayer carbon nanotubes from camphor oil as an energy storage material. *BioMed. Res. Int.*, 2014.
35. Shukla, J., Maldar, N., Sharon, M., Tripathi, S., and Sharon, M. Synthesis of carbon nano material from different parts of maize using transition metal catalysts. *Der Chemi. Sin.*, 3, 5, 1058, 2012.
36. Bhattacharjee, C., Nath, A., Purkayasth, D., Mukherjee, B., Sharon, M., and Sharon, M. Synthesis and characterization of carbon nanotubes using a natural precursor: turpentine oil. *Sci. J. UBU.*, 2, 1, 36, 2011

37. Tripathi, S., Sharon, M., Maldar, N., Shukla, J., Sharon, M. Carbon nano spheres and nano tubes synthesized from castor oil as precursor: for removal of arsenic dissolved in water. *Appl. Sci. Res.*, 4, 4, 1788, 2012.
38. Azmina, M., Suriani, A., Salina, M., Azira, A., Dalila, A., Asli, N., Rosly, J., Nor, R.M., Rusop, M. Variety of bio-hydrocarbon precursors for the synthesis of carbon nanotubes. *Nano Hybrids.*, 2, 43, 2012.
39. Ghosh, P., Afre, R., Soga, T., Jimbo, T. A simple method of producing single-walled carbon nanotubes from a natural precursor: Eucalyptus oil. *Mater. Lett.*, 61, 17, 3768, 2007.
40. Suriani, A., Nor, R., Rusop, M. Vertically aligned carbon nanotubes synthesized from waste cooking palm oil. *J. Ceram. Soc. Jpn.*, 118, 10, 963, 2010.
41. Goodell, B., Xie, X., Qian, Y., Daniel, G., Peterson, M., Jellison, J. Carbon nanotubes produced from natural cellulosic materials. *J. Nanosci. Nanotechnol.*, 8, 5, 2472, 2008.
42. Suriani, A., Dalila, A., Mohamed, A., Mamat, M., Salina, M., Rosmi, M., Rosly, J., Nor, M., Rusop, M. Vertically aligned carbon nanotubes synthesized from waste chicken fat. *Mater Lett.*, 101, 1, 61, 2013.
43. Jagdale, P., Sharon, M., Kalita, G., Maldar, N., Sharon, M., Carbon nano material synthesis from polyethylene by chemical vapour deposition. *Adv. Mater. Phys. Chem.*, 2, 1, 1, 2012.
44. Oliveira, J., Zhuo, C., Angelo, Y., Alberto, J. Microstructural analysis of carbon nanomaterials produced from pyrolysis/combustion of styrene-butadiene-rubber (SBR). *Mater. Res.*, 14, 4, 499, 2011.
45. Qiu, J., Chen, G., Li, Z., Zhao, Z. Preparation of double-walled carbon nanotubes from fullerene waste soot by arc-discharge. *Carbon.*, 48, 4, 1312, 2010.
46. Yah, C., Simate, G., Moothi, K., Maphutha, K., Iyuke, S. Synthesis of large carbon nanotubes from ferrocene: the chemical vapour deposition technique. *Trends Appl. Sci. Res.*, 6, 11, 1270, 2011.
47. Kondo, D., Sato, S., Awano, Y. Low-temperature synthesis of single-walled carbon nanotubes with a narrow diameter distribution using size-classified catalyst nanoparticles. *Chem. Phys. Lett.*, 422, 481, 2006.
48. Toussi, S., Razi, A., Chuah, A., Suraya, A. Effect of synthesis condition on the growth of SWCNTs via catalytic chemical vapour deposition. *Sains Malays.*, 40, 3, 197, 2011.
49. Singh, C., Shaffer, M., Koziol, K., Kinloch, I., Windle, A. Towards the production of large-scale aligned carbon nanotubes. *Chem. Phys. Lett.*, 372, 860, 2003.
50. Yap, Y.K., Kayastha, V., Hackney, S., Dimovski, S., Gogotsi, Y. Effect of carrier gas on the growth rate, growth density, and structure of carbon nanotubes. *Mater. Res. Soc.*, 818, 1, 2004.
51. AMelezhyk, A.V., Rukhov, A.V., Tugolukov, E.N., Tkachev, A.G. Some aspects of carbon nanotubes technology. *Nanosystems.*, 4, 2, 247, 2013.

52. Aksak, M., Kir, S., Selamet, Y. Effect of the growth temperature on carbon nanotubes grown by thermal chemical vapor deposition method. *J. Optoelectron. Adv. M.,* 1, 3, 281, 2009.
53. Siva kumar, V., Rahman, M.A., Abdullah, A., Chai, S. Role of reaction and factors of carbon nanotubes growth in chemical vapour decomposition process using methane. *J. Nanomater.*, 2010.
54. Mitri, S., Sotrirchos, S. Production of carbon nanotubes using CVD: Study of the operating parameters. *J. Rev. Adv. Mater. Sci.,* 10, 314, 2005.
55. Rajarad, R., Ramachndra, B. Study of effect of temperature on the synthesis of carbon nanotubes by floating catalyst method. *J. Met. Mater. Min.*, 22, 2, 1, 2012.
56. Pigos, E., Tokune, T., Harutyunyan, R. Effect of Mo on the catalytic activity of Fe catalyst for the growth of carbon single-walled nanotubes. *Digest of American Chemical Society Meeting,* 2006.
57. Mendez, B., Campos, J., Gomez, M.S., Herrera, J., Rodrıguez, A., Navarro, H., Vidal, M., Terrones, H., Terrones, M. Controlling the dimensions, reactivity and crystallinity of multiwalled carbon nanotubes using low ethanol concentrations. *Chem. Phys. Lett.*, 453, 55, 2008.
58. Conover W. Chemistry: The Central Science, 8th Ed. student edition with media companion, *J. Chem. Educ.*, 77, 1126, 2000
59. Baker, R.M., Barber, M., Harris, P., Feates, S., Waite, R., Nucleation and growth of carbon deposits from the nickel catalyzed decomposition of acetylene. *J. Catal.*, 26, 51, 1972.
60. Terrones, M. Carbon nanotubes: Synthesis and properties, electronic devices and other emerging applications. *Int. Mater. Rev.*, 49, 325, 2004.
61. Dijon, J., Szkutnik, P., Fournier, A., Goislard, T.H., Quesnel, E., Muffato, V., E. DeVito, E., Bendiab, N., Bogner, A., Bernier, N. Growth of graphite spheres in liquid. *Carbon.*, 48, 3953, 2010.
62. Van der, R., Tichich, M., Curtis, V. Substrate-support interactions in metal-catalyzed carbon nanofiber growth. *Carbon.,* 39, 2277, 2001.
63. Reilly, P., Whitten, W. The role of free radical condensates in the production of carbon nanotubes during the hydrocarbon CVD process. *Carbon.*, 44, 1653, 2006.
64. Gartstein, Y., Zakhidov, A., Baughman, R. Mechanical and electromechanical coupling in carbon nanotube distortions. *Phys. Rev. B.*, 68, 115415, 2003.
65. Palaci, I., Fedrigo, S., Brune, H., Klinke, C., Chen, M., Riedo, E. Radial elasticity of multiwalled carbon nanotubes. *Phys. Rev. Let.*, 94, 175502, 2005.
66. Qian, D., Liu, W., Subramoney, S., Ruoff, R. Effect of interlayer interaction on the mechanical deformation of multiwalled carbon nanotube. *J. Nanosci. Nanotechnol.*, 3, 1, 185, 2003.
67. Collins, G. Defect and disorder in carbon nanotubes. *Oxford Handbook of Nanoscience and Technology, Frontiers and Advances.* A.V. Narlikar and Y.Y. Fu, Eds. Oxford: Oxford University Press, 2009.

68. Sato, M. Elastic and plastic deformation of carbon nanotubes. *Proc. Eng.*, 14 , 2366, 2001.
69. Shen, W., Jiang, B., Han, B., Xie, S. Investigation of the radial compression of carbon nanotubes with a scanning probe microscope. *Phys. Rev. Lett.*, 84, 16, 3634, 2006.
70. Yu, M., Kowalewski, T., Ruoff, R. Investigation of the radial deformability of individual carbon nanotubes under controlled indentation force. *Phys. Rev. Lett.*, 85, 7, 1456, 2000.
71. Hertel, T., Robert, E., Avouris, P. Deformation of carbon nanotubes by surface van der Waals forces. *The American Physical Society, Phys. Rev. B.,* 58, 20, 1998.
72. Plaksin, G.V., Rao, V., Stimming, U., Savinova, E.R., Simonov, P.A., Cherepanova, S.V., Kryukova, G.N. The influence of carbon support porosity on the activity of PtRu/Sib unit anode catalysts for methanol oxidation. *J. Power Sources,* 145, 178, 2005.
73. Tuinstra, F., Koenig, L. Raman spectrum of graphite *J. Chem. Phys.,* 53, 1126, 1970.
74. Hou P.-X., Liu, C., Cheng, H.M. Purification of carbon nanotubes. *Carbon.,* 46 2003–2025, 2008.
75. Thien-Nga, L., Hernadi, K., Ljubovic, E., Garaj, S., Forro, L. Mechanical purification of single-walled carbon nanotube bundles from catalytic particles. *Nano Lett.*, 2(12), 1349, 2002.
76. Yang, Y.L., Xie, L.M., Chen, Z., Liu, M.H., Zhu, T., Liu, Z.F. Purification and length separation of single-walled carbon nanotubes using chromatographic method. Synth. Met., 155, 455, 2005.
77. Saito, R., Kawarada, H. Optical properties and Raman spectroscopy of carbon nanotubes. In Carbon Nanotubes: Synthesis, Structure, Properties, and Applications, *Topics Appl. Phys.*, 80, 213, 2001.
78. Wang, Y., Alsmeyer, D.C., McCreer, R.L. Raman spectroscopy of carbon materials: Structural basis of observed spectra. *Chem. Mater.*, 2, 557, 1990.
79. Graupner, R. Raman spectroscopy of covalently functionalized single-wall carbon nanotubes. *J. Raman Spectrosc.*, 38, 673, 2007.
80. Brar, V., Samsonidze, G., Dresselhaus, G., Dresselhaus, M., Saito, R., Swan, K. Second-order harmonic and combination modes in graphite, single-wall carbon nanotube bundles, and isolated single-wall carbon nanotubes. *Phys Rev. B.*, 66, 155418, 2002.
81. Park, Y., Choi, Y., Kim, K., Chung, D., Bae, D., An, K. High yield purification of multiwalled carbon nanotubes by selective oxidation during thermal annealing. *Carbon.* 39, 655, 2001.
82. Ferrari, A., Robertson, J. Resonant Raman spectroscopy of disordered, amorphous, and diamond-like carbon. *Phys Rev. B.*, 64, 75414, 2001.
83. Ferrari, A., Robertson, J. Interpretation of Raman spectra of disordered and amorphous carbon. *Phys. Rev. B.*, 61, 14095, 2000.
84. Lei, X., Ni, Q., Shi, J., Natsuki, T. Radial breathing mode of carbon nanotubes subjected to axial pressure. *Topics Appl. Phys.,* 6, 492, 2011.

85. Abdulrazzak, F.H., Esmail, S.K., Dawod, H.A., Abbas, A.M., Almaliki, M.K.K. X-ray analysis for purification process of synthesized multi-walled carbon nanotubes by chemical vapor deposition. *Inter. J. Theor. Appl. Sci.*, 8, 37, 2016.
86. Abdulrazzak, F.H., Hussein, F.H., Alkaim, A.F., Ivanova, I., Emeline, A.V., Bahnemann, D.W. Sonochemical/hydration–dehydration synthesis of Pt–TiO_2 NPs/decorated carbon nanotubes with enhanced photocatalytic hydrogen production activity. *Photochem. Photobiol. Sci.*, 15, 1347, 2016.

Part II

ENVIRONMENTAL AND ENGINEERING APPLICATIONS

5

A Review of Pharmaceutical Wastewater Treatment with Nanostructured Titanium Dioxide

Lavanya Madhura and Shalini Singh*

Department of Operations and Quality Management, Durban University of Technology, Durban 4000, South Africa

Abstract

Wastewater contains a wide range of organic pollutants, which could have an adverse effect on human health. Nanotechnology has allowed researchers to develop efficient decontamination methods for the degradation of persistent organic pollutants, persistent organic pollutants from waste water. TiO_2 has shown to be a potential candidate for water purification based on the oxidation/photocatalytic degradation process. This chapter focusses on state-of-the-art advancements on TiO_2 photocatalytic degradation and its applications in pharmaceuticals wastewaters.

Keywords: Titanium dioxide, photocatalytic degradation, pharmaceuticals, wastewaters, nanotechnology

5.1 Introduction

Titanium dioxide is effectively and frequently used as a photocatalyst for the treatment of air and water due its easy availability and low price. Titanium dioxide is insoluble in water, is a non-hazardous material, and has a high resistance to acids, bases, and solvents. The photocatalytic activities depend on the size of the particles in which the surface area-to-volume ratio is large.

**Corresponding author*: shalinis@dut.ac.za

Suvardhan Kanchi, Shakeel Ahmed, Myalowenkosi I. Sabela and Chaudhery Mustansar Hussain (eds.) Nanomaterials: Biomedical, Environmental, and Engineering Applications, (135–152)

On the other hand, due to its semi-conducting nature, TiO_2 is regarded as a very good photocatalyst. In TiO_2, electron mobility can be observed under certain conditions. For example, the correct amount of energy is required for the electron mobility from ground to excited states to undergo electron transitions. This process takes place when TiO_2 is irradiated with UV-visible light, at 400 nm. The rapid growth in world population leads to major water concerns such as poor water quality and scarcity of water and climate change. On the other hand, it is very difficult to maintain a clean environment, due to waterborne diseases prevalent in the society. In recent years, personal care products, endocrine disruptors, surfactants, and pharmaceuticals are categorized as emerging intractable contaminants to water due to their poor systems, particularly less degradation capacity. Since the year 2000, there has been an increase in the treatment of pharmaceutical wastewaters [1–4]. Results obtained through studies [1–4] have raised the awareness on the impact of pharmaceutical compounds on the human and aquatic systems, in spite of observing in trace quantities ranging from ng L^{-1} to μg L^{-1} [5, 6]. A survey of the literature suggests that the existing sewage techniques are not sufficiently specific, selective, or sensitive to remove all micropollutants from the wastewaters, especially pharmaceutical compounds [7]. This suggests the urgency needed in the development of a promising and cost-effective technology for the treatment of pharmaceutical compounds from wastewaters [8, 9]. Based on the physical and chemical properties of organic compounds, some of these pollutants are non-degradable or poorly degradable. However, advanced oxidation processes (AOPs) are known to be suitable candidates for the degradation of organic pollutants especially for pesticides. Ozonation, photocatalysis, Fenton and photo-Fenton, electrochemical oxidation, sonolysis, wet air oxidation, and ultrasound radiation are some of AOPs used in the treatment of water and wastewaters. Dalrymple and co-workers studied the presence of reactive oxygen species which reacts with non-degradable pollutants in water and wastewaters and is one of the characterization methods for AOPs [10]. Reactive oxygen species or free radicals are oxidative in nature and therefore these species mineralize the pollutants into simple and harmless molecules. Free radicals are based on atoms or molecules with one or more unpaired electrons such as hydroperoxyl radical ($HO_2^\bullet$), hydroxyl radical ($HO^\bullet$), alkoxyl radical ($RO^\bullet$), or superoxide anion radical ($O2^{\bullet-}$). These species have gained more attention due to their strong oxidation capacity. Among all species mentioned above, $HO^\bullet$ exhibit a high potential of 2.8 V when compared to $HO_2^\bullet$, $RO^\bullet$, and $O2^{\bullet-}$. It has a fair interaction capability with an extensive variety of pollutants without adding any additives, and rate constant in the range of 10^6–10^9 mol L^{-1} s^{-1} [11]. Kanakaraju and co-workers have developed a semiconductor-based photocatalysis with TiO_2 and explained its distinctive properties over other AOPs for the removal of non-degradable pollutants from wastewaters [12].

5.2 Heterogeneous Photocatalysis

According to IUPAC (International Union of Pure and Applied Chemistry), photocatalysis is defined as an "initiation or change in the rate of the reaction in the presence of a substance, when it is exposed to ultraviolet, visible, or infrared radiation. The photocatalyst absorbs light quanta and undergoes chemical transformation [13]. Fujishima and co-workers [14] have invented a photochemical splitting of water in 1972. This process occurs in photochemical cell consisting of rutile TiO_2 as a photoanode and platinum as a counter electrode [14]. This invention has led to the novel applications such as anti-cancer therapy, organic synthesis, air purification, disinfection, and self-cleaning surfaces. The most interesting application of this invention is water treatment, by allowing organic molecules such as pesticides, dyes, and pharmaceuticals to undergo degradation in the presence of a photocatalyst. The significant features of an ideal photocatalyst should be photostable, cost-effective, chemically and biologically inactive, non-toxic, and should be excited with ultraviolet, visible, or infrared radiations. Although several oxides and sulfates of chalcogenide semiconductor photocatalyst such as Fe_2O_3, CeO_2, ZnS, CdS, ZnO, WO_3, TiO_2, and SnO_2 are available, these materials do not meet the characteristics of an ideal photocatalyst. The most known and frequently used photocatalyst is TiO_2 for the treatment of pharmaceuticals in wastewaters being photostable, non-toxic, cost-effective, and biologically and chemically inactive [15]. Based on the literature, several reports have reflected on the mechanistic aspects of TiO_2-induced photocatalytic degradation of organic pollutants [16–20]. Interfacial photocatalytic reactions and photogenerated holes have been observed in the photocatalytic degradation process due to the exposure of TiO_2 to ultraviolet, visible, or infrared radiation with sufficient energy [15]. In photocatalytic processes, TiO_2 is generally exposed to near-ultraviolet light in the range of wavelength from 300 to 400 nm light with artificial ultraviolet lamps or by a small section of the solar spectrum or by sunlight [21].

5.3 Pharmaceuticals in the Environment

The presence of pharmaceuticals and their metabolites show harmful effects on humans and other living systems and this is one of the foremost concerns ascribed in this chapter. So far there is no suitable documentation available in the literature on the pharmaceuticals effect to the environment. Due to their complex physicochemical properties TiO_2 can be used as a potential photocatalyst for the degradation of pharmaceuticals in various water systems [22–25].

Most of the pharmaceuticals are chemically synthesized and some of them exhibit endocrine-disrupting properties and therefore these are regarded as emerging environmental pollutants [26]. In general, the synthesized pharmaceuticals are highly stable for their anticipated function on humans and sooner or later undergo transformation into metabolites in the body due to a biochemical phenomenon. In later stages, these metabolites can be removed from the body either after being partially or completely changed to water-soluble metabolites or, in some cases, without being metabolized [27]. Generally, pharmaceuticals are classified into different groups based on their therapeutic applications and those of environmental alertness such as antihistamines, hormones, antiepileptics, non-steroidal anti-inflammatory drugs, lipid-lowering agents, beta-blockers, antidepressants, and antibiotics [28]. After verification of the reported literature, there is evidence of pharmaceuticals in ground and surface waters and sewage effluents [29–33]. The studies carried out by Daughton and co-workers and Ziylan and co-workers has proved that wastewater treatment plants are the major sources of pharmaceuticals in the environment. The removal efficiency of pharmaceuticals mainly depends on the various stages of reactor design, physio-chemical properties of pharmaceuticals together with seasonal conditions [34, 35]. Some of the literature also suggested the occurrence of pharmaceutical residues in tap and drinking waters [36, 37].

5.4 Role of TiO_2 in Photocatalysis for Degradation, Mineralization, and Transformation Process of Pharmaceuticals

To enhance the photocatalytic performance of TiO_2 in terms of degradation and mineralization, different experimental operational parameters have been optimized in various studies. The optimized parameters include initial concentration of analytes, pH, type, and nature of photocatalyst light intensity and wavelength. Other optimized parameters such as concentration of electron acceptors and co-oxidants also enhance the rate of the degradation process. The literature suggests that the kinetics of Active Pharmaceutical Ingredients (APIs) in the presence of UV/TiO_2 degradation is highly complex, due to the formation of different degradation products (hydroxyl radicals) that are non-selective in nature [26]. During this process, the transformation of parent-active pharmaceutical ingredients into new degradable products may also take place. Some studies confirmed that the design and geometry of the photoreactor will also affect the rate of degradation of APIs [38, 15]. Augugliaro and co-workers proposed a novel degradation route for several APIs using mass spectrometry for the identification of crucial intermediates [20]. Calza and co-workers projected photocatalysis as powerful for the identification and prediction of different metabolites in APIs' degradation pathway [39].

5.5 Applications

Li and co-workers developed a method based on the photodegradation and detoxification of antiviral pharmaceuticals using graphitic carbon nitride (g-C_3N_4)/TiO_2) and titanium dioxide hybrid as a potential photocatalyst under UV-visible light [40]. Their results suggested that the mineralization process of acyclovir is very difficult, but it takes 90 min to complete the process with a highly stable photocatalyst. Under UV-visible radiation, acyclovir was stable with pure TiO_2. However, very slight change in the concentration of acyclovir was observed within 300 min. Acyclovir undergoes photocatalytic degradation more efficiently with TiO_2 under visible light irradiation. The complete photocatalytic degradation can be achieved within 240 min with *g*-C_3N_4/TiO_2 as shown in Figure 5.1.

Further studies revealed that the three major intermediates that is (P1, P2, and P3) were formed during photocatalytic degradation due to low oxidation capacity of highest occupied molecular orbital (HOMO) of *g*-C_3N_4 as shown in Figure 5.2.

A sensitive and selective chemometric technique coupled to the photocatalytic ozonation system was developed for the simultaneous degradation of metronidazole (MET), ciprofloxacin (CIP), and acetaminophen (APAP) using TiO_2 nanoparticles immobilized onto montmorillonite support [41]. Then, the nanocomposite was irradiated with UV-visible light in the presence of ozone and characterized with a scanning electron microscope (SEM), transmission electron microscope (TEM), photoluminescence (PL), X-ray fluorescence spectrometry (XRF), and N_2 adsorption–desorption analysis. Figure 5.3 shows the photocatalytic ozonation reactor. This reactor was furnished with various parts such as a magnetic stirrer, a diffuser, an inlet for ozone, a sampling point, and an outlet for non-absorbed ozone gas. The walls of the reactor were initially covered with an aluminum

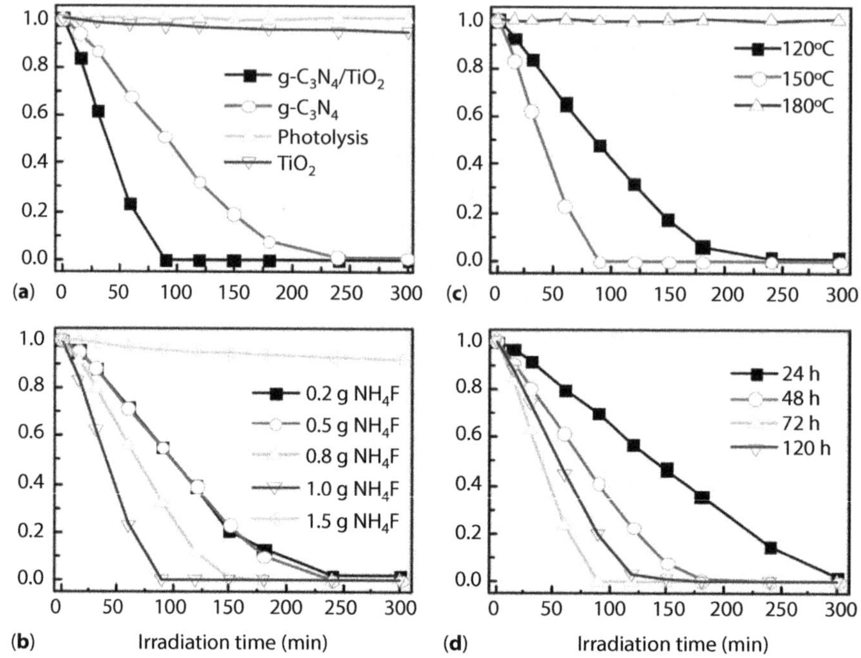

Figure 5.1 The photocatalytic degradation of acyclovir under visible light irradiation using (a) pure TiO_2, g-C_3N_4, and g-C_3N_4/TiO_2; (b) the photocatalysts prepared at 1.0 g NH_4F and treated for 72 h with different hydrothermal temperatures; (c) the photocatalysts prepared at hydrothermal temperature of 150°C treated for 72 h with different NH_4F concentrations; (d) the photocatalysts prepared at 1.0 g NH_4F and hydrothermal temperature of 150°C treated at different times (reproduced with permission from [40]).

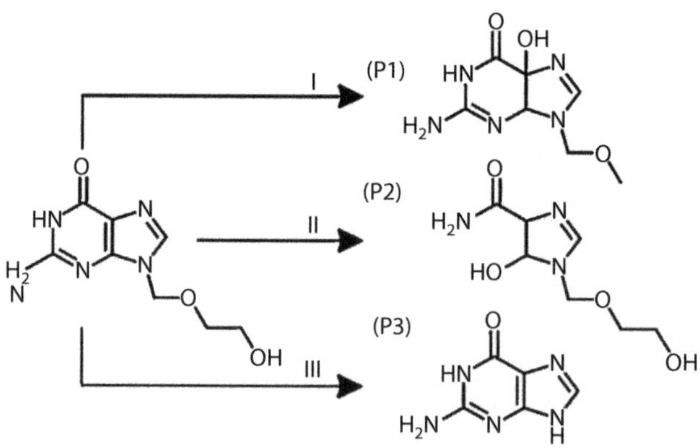

Figure 5.2 Proposed visible-light-driven photocatalytic degradation pathway of acyclovir in water by g-C_3N_4/TiO_2 hybrid photocatalyst (reproduced with permission from [40]).

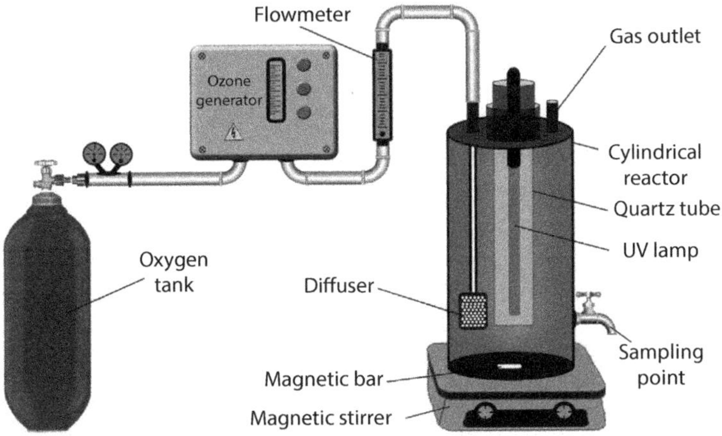

Figure 5.3 Schematic representation of the reactor used for photocatalytic ozonation process (reproduced with permission from [41]).

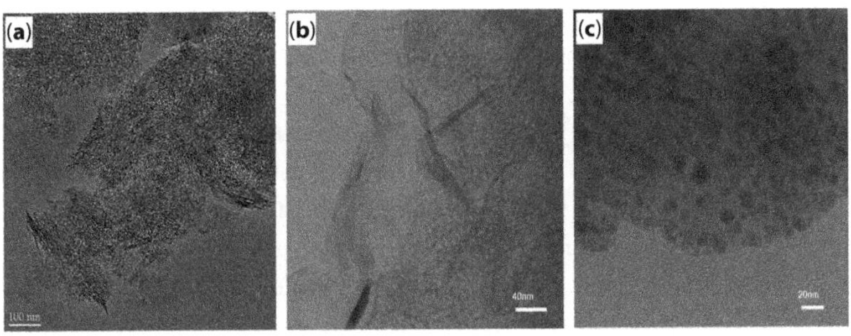

Figure 5.4 TEM images of (a) MMT and (b–c) TiO_2/MMT samples (reproduced with permission from [41]).

foil and then with the non-conducting materials to avoid radiations to the surroundings. Finally, ozone was prepared from pure oxygen by using an ozone generator (Triogen, Scotland).

Moreover, the morphology of the montmorillonite (MMT) and synthesized TiO_2 nanoparticles on the MMT was studied with TEM as illustrated in Figure 5.4.

The degradation of pharmaceuticals was monitored using a UV–vis spectrophotometer and the concentration of pharmaceutical molecules was measured using the partial least squares (PLS) method, due to the severe overlap of their spectra. In this study, a central composite design (CCD) was made to investigate the model and also optimize the effects of various experimental parameters on multiple responses for metronidazole (MET), ciprofloxacin (CIP), and acetaminophen (APAP) degradation. The results obtained suggest that 25 mg L^{-1} of MET, 5 mg L^{-1} CIP, and 5 mg L^{-1} APAP at 10 L h^{-1} ozone flow rate and a 15 min of reaction time were found to be the optimum conditions for the degradation of pharmaceuticals. The degradation percentages of MET, CIP, and APAP were found to be 64.60%, 80.58%, and 50.12%, respectively. Finally, the degraded products were analyzed using the GC–MS technique [41].

Chun-Te Lin and co-workers developed a method for the photodegradation of APAP with a $K_2S_2O_8$-doped TiO_2 [42]. In this method, various optimal parameters such as initial concentration of APAP (0.1 mM), pH (9.0), temperature (22 °C), and concentration of catalyst (1 g L^{-1}) with irradiation time of 9 h were used to enhance the degradation performance of acetaminophen. Additionally, three degradation kinetic models (i.e., zero, pseudo–first, and second order) were evaluated and it was found that the pseudo-first-order model fits well to the data obtained [42].

Salaeh and co-workers developed a novel pathway to investigate the efficiency of photocatalysis with solar/TiO_2-FeZ/H_2O_2 for the degradation, mineralization, and removal of diclofenac (DCF). This study was based on the conversion kinetics and optimization of experimental parameters to evaluate the quality of water. During the removal and mineralization of DCF, other parameters such as biodegradability, total organic content, toxicity to Vibrio fischeri, and dechlorination of DCF and its by-products were monitored. The data obtained from the experiments were in alignment with the HPLC-MS/MS analysis in the detection of by-products during degradation, mineralization, and removal of DCF [43].

The photocatalytic degradation of tetracycline was studied with the MWCNT/TiO_2 nanocomposite under UV-visible irradiation. Different experimental parameters such as photocatalyst dosage, analyte concentration, irradiation time, pH, and weight ratio of MWCNT to TiO_2 and tetracycline concentration were studied to enhance the removal percentage of tetracycline from wastewaters [44].

Figure 5.5(A–B) shows surface morphology and size distribution of MWCNTs and MWCNT/TiO_2 hybrid with field emission scanning electron microscopy (FE-SEM). The uniform distribution of TiO_2 nanoparticles was confirmed with a size ranging from 30 to 70 nm as shown in Figure 5.5(B). The well-dispersed TiO_2 nanoparticles on MWCNTs indicate the high reactivity and UV-visible adsorption of the photocatalyst. The energy dispersive X-ray (EDX) results showed that the nanocomposite (MWCNTs/TiO_2) comprised of 49.75% titanium, 22.33% carbon, and 27.91% oxygen. The EDX spectra showed peaks for Ti, C, and O, and no

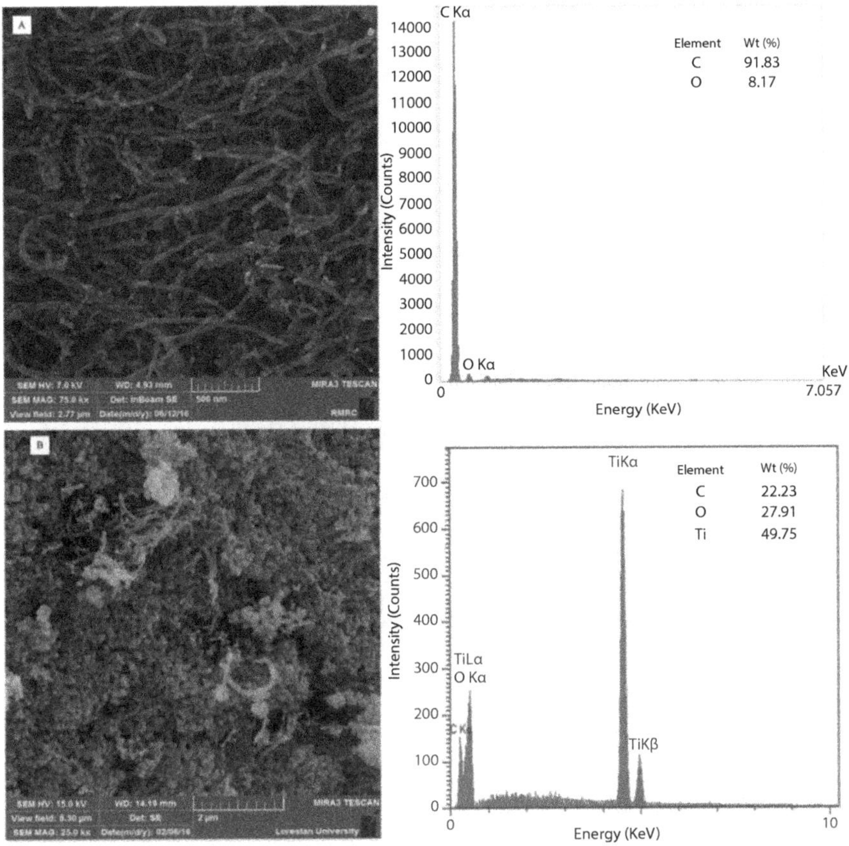

Figure 5.5 FE-SEM images of (A) MWCNT and (B) MWCNTs/TiO_2 nano-composites, along with corresponding EDX micrographs (reproduced with permission from [44]).

other peaks were found which indicates the highest purity of the nanocomposite. The MWCNTs/TiO_2 ratio of 1.5, pH 5, photocatalyst dosage of 0.2 g L^{-1} were fixed as optimum parameters to remove maximum concentration (10 mg L^{-1}) of tetracycline. In this study, the pseudo-first-order kinetic model fits well with experimental results [44].

The degradation studies of four different pharmaceutical molecules such as amoxicillin, ampicillin, diclofenac, and paracetamol were evaluated with bare TiO_2 and TiO_2 immobilized on activated carbon using solar irradiation. The temperature-impregnated method was adopted to prepare TiO_2/AC composite and it was characterized with scanning electron microscope (SEM), Brunauer–Emmett–Teller (BET) analysis, and Fourier transforms infrared spectroscopy (FTIR). Figure 5.6(A–B) illustrated the

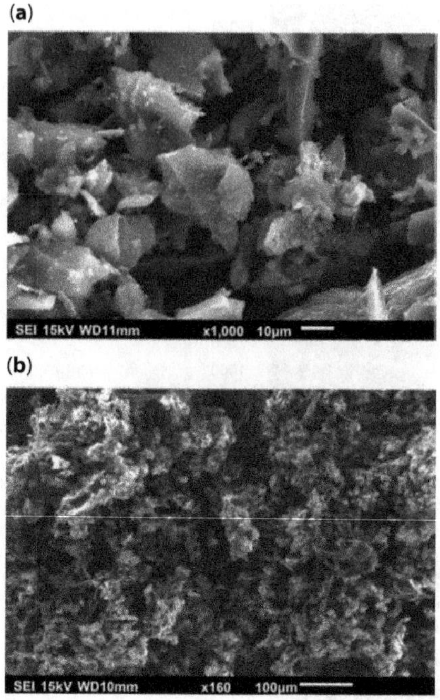

Figure 5.6 Scanning electronic micrographs (SEM) of (a) PAC and (b) TiO_2/AC (reproduced with permission from [46]).

SEM images of activated carbon and TiO_2-immobilized activated carbon. From Figure 5.6(A), the activated carbon surface appears to be rough with heterogeneous pores that indicate a chance of trapping TiO_2 on to the surface of activated carbon thus enhancing the surface area and photocatalytic activity. The SEM image (Figure 5.6B) shows the uniform immobilization of TiO_2 on to the surface area of activated carbon and some of TiO_2 could deposit in the mesopores and macrospores of activated carbon [45].

From this study, it was confirmed that amoxicillin and ampicillin were completely degraded with TiO_2/AC. In the presence of bare TiO_2, 89% and 83% of amoxicillin and ampicillin were removed from wastewaters, respectively, whereas in the case of diclofenac and paracetamol, the removal percentages were found be 85% and 70% with TiO_2/AC as compared with bare TiO_2 [46].

A hybrid of TiO_2 and montmorillonite (MMT) was prepared for the photocatalytic degradation of ciprofloxacin. The synthesized nanocomposite was characterized with Brunauer–Emmett–Teller (BET), scanning electron microscopy (SEM), X-Ray fluorescence (XRF), Fourier transform infrared spectroscopy (FTIR), energy-dispersive X-Ray spectroscopy

(EDX), transmission electron microscopy (TEM), and X-Ray diffraction (XRD) techniques. The TEM and XRD results showed that the average size of TiO_2 nanoparticles decreased from 60–80 nm to 40–60 nm after immobilization of MMT. Different experimental parameters, namely, reusability and dosage of catalyst (TiO_2/MMT), concentration of analyte, pH, UV light regions, and electrical energy were evaluated. The degradation process was studied in the presence of additional radical scavengers (sulfate, chloride, bicarbonate, and iodide) and enhancers (hydrogen peroxide, peroxydisulfate, and potassium iodate) were also studied on the efficiency of degradation. The artificial neural network model was designed to examine the photodegradation of ciprofloxacin and the results obtained were in agreement with the experimental data ($R^2 = 0.9864$) [47].

Magnetically separable flower-like TiO_2/Fe_2O_3 nanocomposite was synthesized for the photocatalytic degradation of paracetamol from the aqueous solutions. Various characterization techniques such as TEM, XRD, Raman spectroscopy, N_2 sorption (BET method), SEM, FTIR, and vibrating sample magnetometer (VSM) were used for the TiO_2/Fe_2O_3 nanocomposite. The results obtained showed that photomineralization and photodegradation of paracetamol enhances with an increase in the concentration of TiO_2 content in the TiO_2/Fe_2O_3. The important intermediate byproducts during paracetamol was determined with gas chromatography (GC) and gas chromatography coupled to mass spectroscopy (GC-MS). The results showed that 33% of TiO_2/Fe_2O_3 was found to be optimum for the stable and efficient photocatalytic degradation of paracetamol after four repeated cycles. In this study, pseudo-first-order reaction fits well into the photodegradation process of paracetamol [48].

A novel nanocomposite, namely, titanium-doped MCM-41 was synthesized with various ratios of Si/Ti at ambient temperature for the photodegradation of tetracycline antibiotics in an aqueous solution. The ratio of Si/Ti was optimized and found to be 25 (w/w%) to attain maximum (99%) removal of oxytetracycline in 150 min. The stability of Ti/MCM-41 was also studied with different cycles. It was found that after 5 reuses, 98% of oxytetracycline was removed. The products obtained from degradation of oxytetracycline, tetracycline, and chlortetracycline were detected by *Escherichia coli* DH5α and HPLC–MS/MS [49].

Vaiano and co-workers designed a novel photocatalyst, namely, N-doped TiO_2 as a potential material for the degradation of antibiotic, spiramycin. This study was conducted in a slurry photoreactor equipped with UV Black Light Tube and Blue LEDs as irradiation sources. This reaction system and method is proved to be rapid and sensitive for the removal of organic compounds from wastewaters. This heterogeneous photocatalytic system was effective in the removal of organic compounds present in a real pharmaceutical wastewater reaching high values of depollution in short times. It demonstrated the feasibility of photocatalytic visible treatment of streams containing Spiramycin with N-doped TiO_2, yielding a promising method for wastewater treatment [50].

Metoprolol tartrate (MET) was removed from municipal secondary effluent and ultrapure water by photocatalytic degradation using B-doped TiO_2 using a Xenon lamp (photon flux of 2.99×10^{-6} Einstein s^{-1}) as an irradiation source. Other parameters namely chemical oxygen demand, acute toxicity, biochemical oxygen demand, and total organic carbon were also analyzed. In this method, the concentration of photocatalyst and irradiation time were optimized. It was found that 44% and 70% of MET was obtained from municipal secondary effluent and ultrapure water using 0.4 g L^{-1} and 2.0 g L^{-1} of B/TiO_2 within 180 min, respectively. Various reaction intermediates produced during MET removal were determined using 5% (w/w %) B/TiO_2. Therefore, it can be concluded that B/TiO_2 acts as a potential photocatalyst in the presence of solar energy for the removal of organic molecules that also make the method cost effective [51].

Multiwalled carbon nanotubes integrated with TiO_2/SiO_2 was designed for the photocatalytic removal of carbamazepine and bisphenol A from water solution. A nanocomposite with the addition of 0.15–17.8% (w/w%) of MWCNTs was found to be an optimal photocatalyst for the maximum removal of both pollutants. In this study, photocatalytic degradation followed pseudo-first-order with the reaction constants of k_1 in the range of 0.0131–0.0743 min^{-1} and 0.0827–0.1751 min^{-1} for carbamazepine and bisphenol A, respectively [52].

TiO_2 impregnated coconut shell powder was developed for the photocatalytic degradation of three pharmaceutical and personal care products (PPCPs). In general, the rate of photodegradation of PPCPs increases with the increase in light intensity and concentration of dissolved oxygen, whereas the photodegradation reaction decreases with the increase in initial concentration of PPCPs. Under the UVC/TCNP combination, 99% removal was achieved compared to 30% for TiO_2 [53].

5.6 Conclusion

The surface and ground water systems with pharmaceuticals cause an adverse impact on both human and aquatic life. Treating wastewaters for persistence organic pollutants, especially pharmaceuticals, is a challenging environmental problem. Therefore, this chapter mainly focused on the heterogeneous semiconducting material, TiO_2, and many hybrid systems for the photocatalytic degradation of various classes of pharmaceutical compounds. Particularly in this area, many research studies have demonstrated the present challenges and analyte (drug compound) reaction kinetics after optimizing the experimental parameters. Several studies explained different experimental parameters such as initial concentration of analyte, solution pH, and water matrix to enhance the photodegradation process of the photocatalyst. However, very few studies focused on the determination of by-products produced during the reaction. Therefore, this area of research has a potential to improve the existing methodologies for water purification by focusing mainly on mineralization and advanced oxidation process. In conclusion, though several promising TiO_2-tailored materials have been synthesized and applied for the treatment of pharmaceutical wastewaters, still a few drawbacks such as variations in removal efficiency, incomplete mineralization, and photocatalytic activity of TiO_2 hybrid toward the complex drug molecules remain challenging. More information on optimizing the kinetics of degradation of mixtures of drug compounds in water of varying quality is thus needed, particularly at the pilot scale and for application to real wastewater treatment.

Acknowledgment

The authors are highly grateful to Durban University of Technology and National Research Foundation of South Africa for their financial support in the form of NRF-DST Innovation Doctoral Scholarship (UID: 107643) to carry out this work.

References

1. Heberer, T. Tracking persistent pharmaceutical residues from municipal sewage to drinking water. *J. Hydrol.*, 266(3–4), 175, 2002.
2. Tixier, C., Singer, H.P., Oellers, S., Müller, S.R. Occurrence and fate of carbamazepine, clofibric acid, diclofenac, ibuprofen, ketoprofen, and naproxen in surface waters. *Environ. Sci. Technol.*, 37(6), 1061, 2003.
3. Fent, K., Weston, A.A., Caminada, D. Ecotoxicology of human pharmaceuticals. *Aquat. Toxicol.*, 76(2), 122, 2006.
4. Mie`ge, C., Choubert, J.M., Ribeiro, L., Euse`be, M., Coquery, M. Fate of pharmaceuticals and personal care products in wastewater treatment plants—conception of a database and first results. *Environ. Poll.*, 157(5), 1721, 2009.

5. Kümmerer, K. The presence of pharmaceuticals in the environment due to human use-present knowledge and future challenges. *J. Environ. Manage.*, 90(8), 2354, 2009.
6. Mompelat, S., Le Bot, B., Thomas, O. Occurrence and fate of pharmaceutical products and by-products, from resource to drinking water. *Environ. Int.*, 35(5), 803, 2009.
7. Sua′rez, S., Carballa, M., Omil, F., Lema, J.M. How are pharmaceutical and personal care products (PPCPs) removed from urban wastewaters? *Rev. Environ. Sci. Biotechnol.*, 7, 125, 2008.
8. Ternes, T.A. Occurrence of drugs in German sewage treatment plants and rivers. *Water Res.*, 32(11), 3245, 1998.
9. Zhang, Y.J., Geissen, S.U., Gal, C. Carbamazepine and diclofenac: removal in wastewater treatment plants and occurrence in water bodies. *Chemosphere.*, 73(8), 1151, 2008.
10. Dalrymple, O.K., Yeh, D.H., Trotz, M.A. Removing pharmaceuticals and endocrine-disrupting compounds from wastewater by photocatalysis. *J. Chem. Technol. Biotechnol.*, 82(2), 121, 2007.
11. Andreozzi, R., Caprio, V., Insola, A., Marotta, R. Advanced oxidation processes (AOP) for water purification and recovery. *Catal. Today*, 53(1), 51, 1999.
12. Kanakaraju, D., Glass, B.D., Oelgemöller, M. Heterogeneous photocatalysis application in pharmaceutical wastewater remediation. In: Lichtfouse E, Schwarzbauer J, Robert D (eds) *Environmental Chemistry for a Sustainable World*, vol 3. Dordrecht: Springer, 2013.
13. Braslavsky, S.E. Glossary of terms used in photochemistry, 3rd edition. *Pure Appl. Chem.*, 79(3), 293, 2007.
14. Fujishima, A., Zhang, X.T., Tryk, D.A. TiO_2 photocatalysis and related surface phenomena. *Surf. Sci. Rep.*, 63(12), 515, 2008.
15. Friedmann, D., Mendive, C., Bahnemann, D. TiO_2 for water treatment: parameters affecting the kinetics and mechanisms of photocatalysis. *Appl. Catal. B: Environ.*, 99(3–4), 398, 2010.
16. Fox, M.A., Dulay, M.T. Heterogeneous photocatalysis. *Chem. Rev.*, 93(1), 341, 1993.
17. Legrini, O., Oliveros, E., Braun, A.M. Photochemical processes for water treatment. *Chem. Rev.*, 93(2), 671, 1993.
18. Hoffmann, M.R., Martin, S.T., Choi, W.Y., Bahnemann, D.W. Environmental applications of semiconductor photocatalysis. *Chem. Rev.*, 95(1), 69, 1995.
19. Chong, M.N., Jin, B., Chow, C.W.K., Saint, C. Recent developments in photocatalytic water treatment technology: a review. *Water Res.*, 44(10), 2997, 2010.
20. Augugliaro, V., Bellardita, M., Loddo, V., Palmisano, G., Plamisano, L., Yurdakal, S. Overview of oxidation mechanisms of organic compounds by TiO_2 in heterogeneous photocatalysis. *J. Photochem. Photobiol. C: Photochem. Rev.*, 13(3), 224, 2012.
21. Bahnemann, D. Photocatalytic water treatment: solar energy applications. *Sol. Energy*, 77(5), 445, 2004.

22. Abella´n, M.N., Bayarri, B., Gime´nez, J., Costa, J. Photocatalytic degradation of sulfamethoxazole in aqueous suspension of TiO_2. *Appl. Catal. B: Environ.*, 74(3–4), 233, 2007.
23. Yurdakal, S., Loddo, V., Augugliaro, V., Berber, H., Palmisano, G., Palmisano, L. Photodegradation of pharmaceutical drugs in aqueous TiO_2 suspensions: mechanism and kinetics. *Catal. Today* 129(1–2), 9, 2007.
24. Giraldo, A.L., Penuela, G.A., Torres-Palma, R.A., Pino, N.J., Palominos, R.A., Mansilla, H.D. Degradation of the antibiotic oxolinic acid by photocatalysis with TiO_2 in suspension. *Water Res.*, 44(18), 5158, 2010.
25. Tong, A.Y.C., Braund, R., Warren, D.S., Peake, B.M. TiO_2-assisted photodegradation of pharmaceuticals—a review. *Cent. Eur. J. Chem.*, 10(4), 989, 2012.
26. Oller, I., Malato, S., Sa´nchez-Pe´rez, J.A. Combination of advanced oxidation processes and biological treatments for wastewater decontamination—a review. *Sci. Total Environ.*, 409(20), 4141, 2011.
27. Khan, S.J., Ongerth, J.E. Modelling of pharmaceutical residues in Australian sewage by quantities of use and fugacity calculations. *Chemosphere.*, 54(3), 355, 2004.
28. Khetan, S.K., Collins, T.J. Human pharmaceuticals in the aquatic environment: a challenge to green chemistry. *Chem. Rev.*, 107(6), 2319, 2007.
29. Andreozzi, R., Marotta, R., Paxéus, N. Pharmaceuticals in STP effluents and their solar photodegradation in aquatic environment. *Chemosphere.*, 50(10), 1319, 2003.
30. Carballa, M., Omil, F., Lema, J.M., Llompart, M., García-Jares, C., Rodríguez, I., Gómez, M., Ternes, T. Behavior of pharmaceuticals, cosmetics and hormones in a sewage treatment plant. *Water Res.*, 38(12), 2918, 2004.
31. Lishman. L., Smyth, S.A., Sarafin, K., Kleywegt, S., Toito, J., Peart, T., Lee, B., Servos, M., Beland, M., Seto, P. Occurrence and reductions of pharmaceuticals and personal care products and estrogen by municipal wastewater treatment plants in Ontario. *Canada. Sci. Total Environ.*, 367(2–3), 544, 2006.
32. Moldovan, Z. Occurrences of pharmaceuticals and personal care products as micropollutants in rivers from Romania. *Chemosphere.*, 64(11), 1808, 2006.
33. Rodil, R., Quintana, J.B., Concha-Graña, E., López-Mahía, P., Muniategui-Lorenzo, S., Prada-Rodrı´guez, D. Emerging pollutants in sewage, surface and drinking water in Galicia (NW Spain). *Chemosphere.*, 86(10), 1040, 2012.
34. Daughton, C.G., Ternes, T.A. Pharmaceuticals and personal care products in the environment: agents of subtle change? *Environ. Health Perspect.*, 107(6), 907, 1999.
35. Ziylan, A., Ince, N.H., The occurrence and fate of anti-inflammatory and analgesic pharmaceuticals in sewage and fresh water: treatability by conventional and non-conventional processes. *J. Hazard. Mater.*, 187(1–3), 24, 2011.
36. Ternes, T.A., Meisenheimer, M., McDowell, D., Sacher, F., Brauch, H.J., Gulde, B.H., Preuss, G., Wilme, U., Seibert, N.Z. Removal of pharmaceuticals during drinking water treatment. *Environ. Sci. Technol.*, 36(17), 3855, 2002.

37. Rodil, R., Quintana, J.B., Concha-Graña, E., López-Mahía, P., Muniategui-Lorenzo, S., Prada-Rodrı′guez, D. Emerging pollutants in sewage, surface and drinking water in Galicia (NW Spain). *Chemosphere.*, 86(10), 1040, 2012.
38. Malato, S., Fernandez-Ibanez, P., Maldonado, M.I., Blanco, J., Gernjak, W. Decontamination and disinfection of water by solar photocatalysis: recent overview and trends. *Catal. Today.*, 147(1), 1, 2009.
39. Calza, P., Pazzi, M., Medana, C., Baiocchi, C., Pelizzetti, E. The photocatalytic process as a tool to identify metabolitic products formed from dopant substances: the case of buspirone. *J. Pharm. Biomed. Anal.*, 35(1), 9, 2004.
40. Li, G., Nie, X., Gao, Y., An, T. Can environmental pharmaceuticals be photocatalytically degraded and completely mineralized in water using *g*-C_3N_4/TiO_2 under visible light irradiation? Implications of persistent toxic intermediates. *Appl. Catal. B: Environ.*, 180, 726, 2016.
41. Aydin, H., Alireza, K., Semra, K., Mehrangiz, F. Degradation of mixture of three pharmaceuticals by photocatalytic ozonation in the presence of TiO_2/montmorillonite nanocomposite: Simultaneous determination and intermediates identification. *J. Environ. Chem. Eng.*, 5, 1964, 2017.
42. Justin Chun-Te, L., Mark Daniel G, L., Graziel L, A., Ming-Chun, L. Degradations of acetaminophen via a $K_2S_2O_8$-doped TiO_2 photocatalyst under visible light irradiation. *Chemosphere,* 155, 388, 2016.
43. Subhan, S., Daria Juretic, P., Martina, B., Hrvoje, K., Sandra, B., Urska Lavrencic, S., Dionysios D, D., Ana Loncaric, B. Diclofenac removal by simulated solar assisted photocatalysis using TiO_2-based zeolite catalyst; mechanisms, pathways and environmental aspects. *Chem. Eng. J.*, 304, 289, 2016.
44. Mehdi, A., Hojjatallah Ramezani, M., Nematollah, J., Azar Mostoufi, R.S., Gelavizh Barzegar, S.J. Enhanced photocatalytic degradation of tetracycline and real pharmaceutical wastewater using MWCNT/TiO_2 nano-composite. *J. Environ. Manage.*, 186, 55, 2017.
45. Wang, X., Liu, Y., Hu, Z., Chen, Y., Liu, W., Zhao, G. Degradation of methyl orange by composite photocatalysts nano-TiO_2 immobilized on activated carbons of different porosities. *J. Hazard. Mater.*, 169, 1061, 2009.
46. Mohamed, G.A., Ahmed, T., Shinichi, O. Enhancement of photocatalytic activity of TiO_2 by immobilization on activated carbon for degradation of pharmaceuticals. *J Environ. Chem. Eng.*, 4, 1929, 2016.
47. Aydin, H., Alireza, K., Semra, K. Photocatalytic degradation of ciprofloxacin by synthesized TiO2 nanoparticles on montmorillonite: Effect of operation parameters and artificial neural network modelling. *J. Mol. Catal. A Chem.*, 409, 149, 2015.
48. Aboel-Magd A.W., Al-Sayed, A.S., Omima, M., Osama, N. Photocatalytic degradation of paracetamol over magnetic flower-like TiO_2/Fe_2O_3 core-shell nanostructures. *J. Photochem. Photobiol. A Chem.*, 347, 186, 2017.
49. Zhou, K., Xie, X.D., Chang, C.T. Photocatalytic degradation of tetracycline by Ti-MCM-41 prepared at room temperature and biotoxicity of degradation products. *Appl. Surf. Sci.*, 416, 248, 2017.

50. Vaiano, V., Sacco, O., Sannino, D., Ciambelli, P. Photocatalytic removal of spiramycin from wastewater under visible light with N-doped TiO_2 photocatalysts. *Chem. Eng. J.*, 261, 3, 2015.
51. Rodrigo, P.C., Renato, F.D., Heberton, W., Bernardí, B., Oscar, G., Jaime, G., Santiago, E., Amilcar, M. Jr. Photocatalytic treatment of metoprolol with B-doped TiO_2: Effect of water matrix, toxicological evaluation and identification of intermediates. *Appl. Catal. B: Environ.*, 176–177, 173, 2015.
52. Bożena, C., Waldemar, B. Photocatalytic treatment of pharmaceutical wastewater using new multiwall carbon nanotubes/TiO_2/SiO_2 nanocomposites. *Environ. Res.*, 137, 176, 2015.
53. Majeda, K., Jongkyu, K., Luiza, C., Ala'a H., A.M., Alaa, A.H., Mohammad, A.G., Gavin, M.W. Removal of pharmaceutical and personal care products (PPCPs) pollutants from water by novel TiO_2–Coconut shell powder (TCNSP) composite. *J. Ind. Eng. Chem.*, 20, 979, 2014.

6

Nanosilica Particles in Food: A Case of Synthetic Amorphous Silica

Rookmoney Thakur and Shalini Singh*

Department of Operations and Quality, Durban University of Technology, Durban, South Africa

Abstract

Additives have been introduced to food to preserve flavor or improve its taste and appearance. With the advent of processed foods, many more additives have been sought from both natural and artificial origins. The sizes of the additives are in the nano-range, 1–100 nm, and are found in salt, spices, sweets, coffee, coffee creamer, soup and sauce powders, and seasoning mixes, typically as an anti-caking agent and in beers and wines as a stabilizing agent. This chapter focuses on a food additive, E551 (silicon dioxide) or nanosilica, which is synthetic amorphous in nature and consists of micrometer-sized aggregates and agglomerates in the micrometer-size range. Nanosilica boasts wide applications despite suggestions from the literature that ingested nanoparticles can travel to the liver, the kidneys, and the brain, disrupting DNA and potentially leading to the development of cancer and lesions. The different forms of silica, its properties, and methods of manufacturing and potential hazards to human health are discussed.

Keywords: Nanosilica, food additives, E551, SAS, toxicology

6.1 Introduction

Additives have been introduced to food for centuries to enhance flavors or improve taste and appearance. However, with the advent of processed foods, many more additives have been sought from both natural and artificial origins. Additives such as silicon dioxide, calcium silicate, magnesium silicate,

**Corresponding author*: shalinis@dut.ac.za

Suvardhan Kanchi, Shakeel Ahmed, Myalowenkosi I. Sabela and Chaudhery Mustansar Hussain (eds.) Nanomaterials: Biomedical, Environmental, and Engineering Applications, (153–164)

potassium aluminum silicate, and aluminum calcium silicate are used and are open to debate on whether they should be allowed at all. Their sizes are in the nano-range, 1–100 nm, and are found in common household products such as salt, spices, sweets, coffee, soups, and seasoning mixes.

- Food contains many nanostructured materials [1]. Three main classes of nanomaterials identified in the literature are:
- Normal food structures containing naturally occurring biopolymers (carbohydrates, proteins, or lipids) that possess at minimum one dimension in the nanometer range [2, 3]
- Engineered NMs whose components are wholly metabolized inside the body or expelled, such as nanoemulsions or nanoencapsulations of nutrients (vitamins) [4]
- Persistent or gradually soluble engineered particulate ÉNMs such as synthetic amorphous silica (E551), nanosilver (antimicrobial agent), and titanium dioxide (food additive) [4].

As such, the introduction of nanotechnology has not only found numerous applications in various aspects of human life from engineering, electronics, and medicine but more recently in food. Studies show that nanoparticles are progressively being used in a number of consumer products [2,3,5,6]. The many benefits associated with this technology are in the areas of food packaging and improving food safety, taste, and texture.

Chaudhry and Groves [27] listed the currently known applications of nanoparticles in food as follows:

- Where food ingredients have been processed or formulated to form nanostructures, for example, to reduce the amount of salt, fat, color, or other additives to promote healthy option foods
- Where nano-sized, nano-encapsulated, or engineered nanoparticles have been used in food, for example, to improve the properties of food by altering flavor, color, texture, and consistency
- Where nanomaterials have been incorporated to develop improved, "active," or "intelligent" materials for food packaging, for example, to sense when a food product has passed its use-by-date.
- Where nanotechnology-based devices and materials have been used for nanofiltration, water treatment, and nanosensors for food safety and traceability.

As a result, governments and businesses have begun to invest heavily in nanotechnology. However, Aschberger and Christensen [7] observed that the safety of food products containing engineered nanomaterials (ENMS) has attracted widespread concern. Although Potter and Hotchkiss [8] concurred that "molecular engineering" could potentially revolutionize the food market, they expressed concern regarding its potential to cause harmful health effects on humans. Other studies [7, 9] reported that the surface area of a nanoparticle appears to be the chief activator for its toxic effects. Nogi, Naito, and Yokoyama [10] described an ENM as a microscopic particle or powder with at least one dimension of less than 100 nm. Trybula and Newberry [11] reported that there was a lack of scientific information on ENM exposure.

One such ENM is food-grade silica, synthetic amorphous silica (SAS). Scientific articles and reviews [12–16] established that SAS, also known as food additive E551, exhibits novel and improved physical, chemical, and biological properties compared to their bulk counterparts. This is due to its nanoscale size of between 1 nm and 100 nm. This chapter discusses the different forms of silica, its properties, and methods of manufacturing and potential hazards to human health.

6.1.1 The Different Forms of Silica

Silica is the name given to a group of materials composed of silicon dioxide (SiO_2). Fruitjtier-Polloth [13] refers to three main types of silica that are all found under the Chemical Abstracts Service (CAS No.) 7631-86-9. They are crystalline silica (a natural material found in sand, stone, and quartz), amorphous silica (naturally occurring or as a by-product in the form of fused silica or silica fume), and synthetic amorphous silica (SAS), which includes silica gel, precipitated silica, pyrogenic (fumed) silica, and colloidal silica.

Crystalline silica occurs in various forms including the well-known material, quartz, and more specifically α-quartz [17]. Quartz exists in natural and synthetic forms. McWham [18] observed two forms of amorphous silica, either as a natural form such as diatomaceous earth, opal, and silica glass or man-made products such as synthetic amorphous silica. Silica nanoparticles are extensively applied in a variety of industries and are manufactured on an industrial scale as additives to cosmetics, drugs, and food. Recently, Mamaeva, Sahlgren, and Linden [19] reported on the application of nanosilica in the medical sector as an aid in drug delivery and cancer therapy.

According to Napierska *et al.*, [34], quartz is a widespread and well-known material which upon heating is transformed into b-quartz, trydimite, and cristobalite. Porosil is the family name for porous crystalline silica.

However, with the emerging marketability of nano-enabled products, there is also growing concern on the human exposure to nanoparticles. These trepidations on consumer safety are related to the nanoscale of these particles [20]. While past studies explored the crystalline forms of silica particles in the nanoscale range, now, however, it has been observed that nanosilica may have different toxicological properties when compared to larger particles. Despite the unique physico-chemical properties of nano-sized silica that make them more appealing for the industry, there is budding potential that it may present hazards to human health, including a greater aptitude to infiltrate cellular barriers in major organs in the human body.

Street [21] noted that amorphous silica was less studied than the crystalline form. Warheit [22] described some toxicity information associated with the inhalation of amorphous silica particulates and established that some forms of amorphous silica are more powerful in generating pulmonary threats as compared to others. In light of this, he accentuated the urgency for greater toxicological testing of many of these amorphous silicates considering their significance in commercial development. Significantly, Vitusm *et al.*, [23] reported evidence of pulmonary fibrosis in workers exposed to amorphous silica dust manufactured as a byproduct of silicon metal production. In contrast to larger particles, nanoparticles may be able to pass cellular barriers such as the gastrointestinal epithelium, which can make them become systemically accessible and enter cells. This may be a result of it being potentially more reactive than the corresponding non-nanosized chemical substances, probably due to their large surface area. The above findings are significant because in the case of daily exposure, nanoparticles may accumulate over time in the human body. It is therefore important that such possible accumulation be considered in risk assessments.

6.1.2 Synthetic Amorphous Silica

Fruijtier-Polloth [13] described synthetic amorphous silica (SAS) as a distinct, manufactured form of silicon dioxide, consisting of nano-sized primary particles of nano-sized aggregates and agglomerates. Studies considered the application of SAS in consumer products as safe if occupational standards and recommended usage levels were adhered to [12, 28, 29].

Further studies described E551 as a nanostructured material, consisting of aggregates and agglomerates of primary particles in the nano-range [15,30–32]. Dekkers *et al.*, [33] first used the term "nanosilica" to describe silica particles and agglomerates/aggregates with an exterior size in the nanometer range (in principle between 1 and 100 nm, but due to analytical issues a range between 1 and 200 nm is considered). They further pointed out that this morphology and dimension of the silica particles are not usually stated on food labels. As such, consumers may not be informed of the presence of ENMs in their food.

However, several recent studies raised concerns about the hazards and health risks of nanosilica particles such as E551 in food products [33,35–37]. These studies found that products containing E551 may have high toxicity that could be injurious to human health. Consequently, it was observed that this was mainly size-related due to a much larger surface-to-mass-ratio when compared to the larger-sized bulk counterpart materials [38]. Furthermore, Martirosyn and Schneider [39] suggested that the possible accumulation of nanosilica particles in humans may be responsible for compromised gastrointestinal (GI) functioning.

6.1.3 Physical and Chemical Properties of SAS

SAS is described as a white fluffy powder or granule, hygroscopic and slightly soluble in water. It is distinguished from other forms of silica by its high chemical purity and its finely particulate nature [13]. Typical physicochemical properties for SAS are illustrated in Table 6.1.

6.1.4 Silica Applications in the Food Industry

In the food industry, SAS has been used for decades as a stabilizing agent to clear beers and wines, and as an anti-caking agent to maintain flow properties of powder products, and to thicken pastes. It is generally recognized

Table 6.1 Physical and chemical properties of E551 [13].

Property	Result
Physical State	Solid
Form	Powder, granules
Color	White
Melting point	>1700 °C
Flammability	Non-flammable
Vapor pressure	Not applicable
Water solubility	Slightly soluble

as safe (GRAS) by Codex Alimentarius and has been approved for use as a food or animal feed ingredient [12, 13].

Despite the wide applications of SAS, literature [12–14] suggests that ingested nanoparticles can travel to the liver, the kidneys, and the brain, disrupting DNA and potentially leading to the development of cancer and lesions.

Calzolai, Gilliland, and Rossi [24] reported that although there was limited evidence of the deliberate use and presence of nanoparticles (NPs) in commercially available food and food packaging, titanium dioxide (E171) and (E551) are most widely used as food additives containing nanosized particles.

According to the Codex Alimentarius, food additive means: "*any substance not normally consumed as a food by itself and not normally used as a typical ingredient of the food, whether or not it has nutritive value, the intentional addition of which to food for a technological (including organoleptic) purpose in the manufacture, processing, preparation, treatment, packing, packaging, transport or holding of such food results, or may be reasonably expected to result, (directly or indirectly) in it or its by-products becoming a component of or otherwise affecting the characteristics of such foods*" [25].

According to Passagne *et al.*, [26], SAS which is food grade silica has been incorporated into selected foods since the 1960s as well as in some pharmaceutical products.

6.1.5 Toxicity

Despite the wide applications of SAS in food products, there are still growing concerns about its effects on the human body. Pillai *et al.*, [40] found that the toxicity of nanoparticles such as SAS are dependent on their properties, including size and size distribution, surface area, shape, aggregation/agglomeration state, and chemical composition. It has been reported that although E551 has been a permitted ingredient for application in food for decades, it now seems that more information is available on the behavior and potential risks of nanoparticles in general, suggesting that the health risk of exposure to SAS may have to be reassessed in view of the current information [33].

According to Silva *et al.*, [41], the potential routes of SAS exposure may occur by means of: (1) inhalation via the respiratory tract that can occur during exposure in the workplace; (2) dermal exposure via the skin; or (3) ingestion/oral exposure via the gastrointestinal tract (GIT). This is aligned to an earlier study [42] which reported the same three potentially harmful possible routes for NPs to enter into the body.

It has been suggested that in whatever form engineered nanomaterials are in food, whether a nanostructured food ingredient, nanocarrier, or NPs incorporated in food packaging, some form of human exposure is likely to occur [39]. Furthermore, due to the huge surface area of the gastrointestinal tract (GIT), ingestion was possibly the most common route of intentional exposure to various nanoparticles.

Although there is currently a scarcity of the literature regarding metabolism or biotransformation of ENMs upon oral administration in the human model, Martirosyan and Schneider [39] reported on a possible association between high levels of dietary SAS and Crohn's disease, which is an inflammatory bowel disease (IBD) that causes inflammation in the intestinal tract.

They further inferred that the possible accumulation of SAS in humans may be responsible for compromised GIT functioning. An earlier study by Buzea *et al.*, [43] implied that contact exposure to some nanoparticles can be linked with the occurrence of autoimmune diseases such as systemic lupus erythematous, scleroderma, and rheumatoid arthritis. This was supported by other studies [36,44–46] that stated that nanosilica particles have high toxicity that could be injurious to human health.

In vivo studies [47, 48] showed that high doses of SAS fed to mice caused a higher value of alanine aminotransferase activity and that the ingestion of 70-nm SAS particles induced fetal reabsorption and restricted the growth of fetuses in pregnant mice. Related studies [49, 50] showed that high doses of SAS induced oxidative stress-dependent cytotoxicity in multiple cultured mammalian cell lines.

Exposure to certain NPs (carbon black, silicates, titanium dioxide, and iron oxide) may lead to oxidative damage and inflammatory reactions of the gastrointestinal tract in humans [51]. Silvestre *et al.*, [52] found that long-term exposure to some NPs such as SAS has been associated with acute toxic response including lesions of the kidney and liver, as well as numerous forms of cancer.

Considering the increasing use of SAS in food products, Bouwmeester *et al.*, [38] noted that some foodstuffs that contain nanoparticles may not have their safety claims tested before they are available in the global market and accessed through the internet. As a result, this created challenges in developing a standardized safety-testing method for nano-food products [53].

6.1.6 Conclusion

Interest in using silica nanoparticles is growing worldwide, especially in the medical and commercial sector. Although the application of nanoparticles in food products offers many benefits, the health risks of using nano-sized particles are relatively unknown. Studies have highlighted that high doses of SAS may result in acute pulmonary inflammatory responses. This may be attributed to the novel properties of nanoparticles ascribed to their small size, physico-chemical properties, chemical composition, and surface-to-mass ratio. It is these characteristics that makes it different from their conventional counterparts, and as a result, may lead to unexpected toxicological effects that need to be addressed by risk assessors. However, one of the challenges facing risk assessment is the lack of data. As a result, this leads to uncertainties in the characterization of nanomaterials and its effects on humans and the environment. In food safety, information is needed on correct dose metrics to use, the state of SAS during and after food processing, and its potential exposure to workers and consumer. Presently, current food safety standards do not specifically address the data requirements and measurement approaches to assess potential risks at nanoscale level.

References

1. Cockburn, A., Bradford, R., Buck, N., Constable, A., Edwards, G., Haber, B., Hepburn, P., Howlett, J., Kampers, F., Klein, C. Approaches to the safety assessment of engineered nanomaterials (ENM) in food. *Food Chem. Toxicol.*, 50(6), 2224, 2012.
2. Chaudhry, Q. and Groves, K. Nanotechnology applications for food ingredients, additives and supplements. In: Chaudhry, Q., Castle, L and Watkins, R. (eds). *Nanotechnologies in Food.* London: Royal Society of Chemistry. 69, 2010.
3. Chaudhry, Q. and Castle, L. Food applications of nanotechnologies: An overview of opportunities and challenges for developing countries. *Trends Food Sci. Technol.*, 22(11), 1, 2011.
4. Morris, V.J. Emerging roles of engineered nanomaterials in the food industry. *Trends Biotechnol.*, 29(10), 509, 2011.
5. Alfadul, S.M., Elneshwy, A.A. Use of nanotechnology in food processing, packaging and safety–review. *Afr. J. Food Agric. Nutr. Dev.*, 10(6), 2720, 2010.
6. Basford, K. and Harch, B. Statistics critical in securing our food supply. *ATSE Focus*, 1(182), 10, 2014.
7. Aschberger, K., Johnston, H.J., Stone, V., Aitken, R.J., Hankin, S.M., Peters, S.A., Tran, C.L., Christensen, F.M. Review of carbon nanotubes toxicity and exposure - Appraisal of human health risk assessment based on open literature. *Crit. Rev. Toxicol.*, 40(9), 759, 2010.
8. Potter, N.N., Hotchkiss, J. H. *Food Science.* 2nd edn. New York: Springer Science & Business Media, 2012.
9. Abbott, L.C., Maynard, A.D. Exposure assessment approaches for engineered nanomaterials. *Risk Anal.*, 30(11), 1634, 2010.

10. Nogi, K., Naito, M., Yokoyama, T. *Nanoparticle Technology Handbook*. 2nd ed. Spain: Elsevier, 2012.
11. Trybula, W., Newberry, D. Nanotechnology risk assessment. In: Asmatulu, R. (ed.) *Nanotechnology Safety*. Amsterdam: Elsevier, 195, 2013.
12. Lewinson, J., Mayr, W., Wagner, H. Characterization and toxicological behavior of synthetic amorphous hydrophobic silica. *Regul. Toxicol. Pharmacol.*, 20, 37, 1994.
13. Fruijtier-Pölloth, C. The toxicological mode of action and the safety of synthetic amorphous silica - A nanostructured material. *Toxicology.*, 294(2), 61, 2012.
14. Dekkers, S., Bouwmeester, H., Bos, P.M., Peters, R.J., Rietveld, A.G., Oomen, A.G. Knowledge gaps in risk assessment of nanosilica in food: evaluation of the dissolution and toxicity of different forms of silica. *Nanotechnology.*, 7(4), 367, 2013.
15. Athinarayanan, J., Periasamy, V.S., Alsaif, M.A., Al-Warthan, A.A. and Alshatwi, A. Presence of nanosilica (E551) in commercial food products: TNF-mediated oxidative stress and altered cell cycle progression in human lung fibroblast cells. *Cell Biol. Toxicol.*, 30(2), 89, 2014.
16. Higashisaka, K., Yoshioka, Y., Tsutsumi, Y. Applications and safety of nanomaterials used in the food industry. *J. Food Saf.*, 3(2), 39, 2015.
17. Tang, C., Zhu, J., Li, Z., Zhu, R., Zhou, Q., Wei, J., Tao, Q. Surface chemistry and reactivity of SiO_2 polymorphs: A comparative study on α-quartz and α-cristobalite. *Appl. Surf. Sci.*, 355, 1161, 2015.
18. McWhan, D. *Sand and Silicon: Science that Changed the World*. Oxford: OUP, 2012.
19. Mamaeva, V., Sahlgren, C., Linden, M. Mesoporous silica nanoparticles in medicine—Recent advances. *Adv. Drug Deliv. Rev.*, 65(5), 689, 2013.
20. Maynard, A.D., Aitken, R.J., Butz, T., Colvin, V., Donaldson, K., Oberdorster, G., Philbert, M.A., Ryan, J., Seaton, A., Stone, V., Tinkle, S.S., Tran, L., Walker, N.J., Warheit, D.B. Safe handling of nanotechnology. *Nature.*, 444, 267, 2006.
21. Street, R. *Technology and Applications of Amorphous Silicon*. Springer Science & Business Media, Springer, NY, 37, 2013.
22. Warheit, D.B. Inhaled amorphous silica particulates: what do we know about their toxicological profiles? *J. Environ. Pathol. Toxicol. Oncol.*, 1, 133, 2001.
23. Vitums, V.C., Edwards, M.J., Niles, N.R., Borman, J.O., Lowry, R.D. Pulmonary fibrosis from amorphous silica dust, a product of silica vapor. *Arch Environ Health.*, 32, 62, 1997.
24. Calzolai, L., Gilliland, D., Rossi, F. Measuring nanoparticles size distribution in food and consumer products: a review. *Food Addit. Contam. Part A.*, 29(8), 1183, 2012.
25. Furia, T. *CRC Handbook of Food Additives*. Boca Raton: Florida Press, 1980.
26. Passagne, I., Morille, M., Rousset, M., Pujalté, I., L'azou, B. Implication of oxidative stress in size-dependent toxicity of silica nanoparticles in kidney cells. *Toxicology.*, 299(2), 112, 2012.

27. Chaudhry, Q., Groves, K. Nanotechnology applications for food ingredients, additives and supplements. In: Chaudhry, Q., Castle, L and Watkins, R. (eds.) *Nanotechnologies in Food*. London: Royal Society of Chemistry, 69, 2010.
28. Organization for Economic Cooperation and development (OECD). SIDS dossier on synthetic amorphous silica and silicates (online). Available at: http://www.inchem.org/documents/sids/sids/SolubleSilicates.pdf., 2004.
29. Becker, M., Fernandes, L., Rothhardt, M., Bruckner, S., Schuster, K., Kobelke, J., Marques, P.V. Inscription of fiber Bragg grating arrays in pure silica suspended core fibers. *Photonic Tech. L J.*, 21(19), 1453–1455, 2009.
30. Aureli, M., Basaran, M.E., Porfiri, M. Nonlinear finite amplitude vibrations of sharp-edged beams in viscous fluids. *J. Sound Vibration.*, 331(7), 1624–1654, 2012.
31. Bosch, A., Maier, M., Morfeld, P. Nanosilica? Clarifications are necessary! *Nanotoxicology.*, 6(6), 611, 2012.
32. De Temmerman, P.J., Van Doren, E., Verleysen, E., Van der Stede, Y., Francisco, M.A.D., Mast, J. Quantitative characterization of agglomerates and aggregates of pyrogenic and precipitated amorphous silica nanomaterials by transmission electron microscopy. *J. Nanobiotechnol.*, 10(1), 1, 2012.
33. De Temmerman, P.J., Van Doren, E., Verleysen, E., Van der Stede, Y., Francisco, M.A.D., Mast, J. Quantitative characterization of agglomerates and aggregates of pyrogenic and precipitated amorphous silica nanomaterials by transmission electron microscopy. *J. Nanobiotechnol.*, 10(1), 1, 2012.
34. Napierska, D., Thomassen, L.C.J., Lison, D., Martens, J.A., Hoet., P.H. The nanosilica hazard: another variable entity. *Part Fibre Toxicol.*, 7(1), 1, 2010.
35. Asmatulu, R., Zhang, B. and Asmatulu, E. Nanotechnology safety. In: Asmatulu, R. (ed.) *Nanotechnology Safety*. San Diego, CA: Elsevier, 31, 2013.
36. Dekkers, S., Bouwmeester, H., Bos, P.M., Peters, R.J., Rietveld, A.G. and Oomen, A.G. Knowledge gaps in risk assessment of nanosilica in food: evaluation of the dissolution and toxicity of different forms of silica. *Nanotechnology.*, 7(4), 367, 2013.
37. Yang, Y.X., Song, Z.M., Cheng, B., Xiang, K., Chen, X.X., Liu, J.H., Wang, H. Evaluation of the toxicity of food additive silica nanoparticles on gastrointestinal cells. *J. Appl. Toxicol.*, 34(4), 424, 2014.
38. Bouwmeester, H., Brandhoff, P., Marvin, H.J., Weigel, S., Peters, R.J. State of the safety assessment and current use of nanomaterials in food and food production. *Trends Food Sci. Technol.*, 40(2), 200, 2014.
39. Martirosyan, A., Schneider, Y.J. Engineered nanomaterial in food: implications for food safety and consumer health. *Int. J. Environ. Res. Publ. Health.*, 11(6) 5720, 2014.
40. Pillai, K.V., Hunt, P.R., Duncan, T.V. Nanoparticles in polymer nanocomposite food contact materials: Uses, potential release, and emerging toxicological concerns. In: *Toxicants in Food Packaging and Household Plastics*. Springer, London, 95, 2014.

41. Silva, P., Reis, C.M., Ferreira, J., Oliveira, C. Nanoparticles characterization and potential hazard assessments. In: Arezes, P.M., Baptista, J.S., Barroso, M.P., Carneiro, P., Cordeiro, P., Costa, N., Melo, R.B., Miguel, A.S., Perestrelo, G. (eds.) *Occupational Safety and Hygiene*. London: Taylor and Francis, 453, 2015.
42. Chau, C.-F., Wu, S.-H., Yen, G.-C. The development of regulations for food nanotechnology. *Trends Food Sci. Technol.*, 18(5), 269, 2007.
43. Buzea, C., Pacheco, I.I., Robbie, K. Nanomaterials and nanoparticles: sources and toxicity. *Biointerphases.*, 2(4), 17, 2007.
44. Bouwmeester, H., Dekkers, S., Noordam, M.Y., Hagens, W.I., Bulder, A.S., De Heer, C., Ten Voorde, S.E., Wijnhoven, S.W., Marvin, H.J., Sips, A.J. Review of health safety aspects of nanotechnologies in food production. *Regul. Toxicol. Pharmacol.*, 53, 52, 2009.
45. Busk, S.A. Nanostructured titanium dioxide: Fate in the aquatic environment and effects on the blue mussel Mytilus edulis (online). *Master's Thesis*, University of Stavanger. https://brage.bibsys.no/xmlui/bitstream/handle/11250/182444/Busk,%20Siw%20Anette.pdf?sequence=1, 2011.
46. Asmatulu, R., Zhang, B., Asmatulu, E. Nanotechnology safety. In: Asmatulu, R. (ed.) *Nanotechnology Safety.* San Diego, CA: Elsevier, 31, 2013.
47. So, M., Xu, C., Loening, A.M., Gambhir, S.S., Rao, J. Self-illuminating quantum dot conjugates for *in vivo* imaging. *Nat. Biotechnol.*, 24(3), 339, 2006.
48. Yamashita, K., Yoshioka, Y., Higashisaka, K., Mimura, K., Morishita, Y., Nozaki, M., Yoshida, T., Ogura, T., Nabeshi, H., Nagano, K. Silica and titanium dioxide nanoparticles cause pregnancy complications in mice. *Nat. Nanotechnol.*, 6(5), 321, 2011.
49. Chang, J.-S., Chang, K. L. B., Hwang, D.-F., Kong, Z.-L. *In vitro* cytotoxicity of silica nanoparticles at high concentrations strongly depends on the metabolic activity type of the cell line. *Environ. Sci. Technol.*, 41(6), 2064, 2007.
50. Wu, J., Wang, C., Sun, J., Xue, Y. Neurotoxicity of silica nanoparticles: brain localization and dopaminergic neurons damage pathways. *ACS Nano.*, 5(6), 4476, 2011.
51. Momin, J.K., Jayakumar, C., Prajapati, J.B. Potential of nanotechnology in functional foods. *Emir. J. Food Agric.*, 25, 10, 2013.
52. Silvestre, C., Duraccio, D., Cimmino, S. Food packaging based on polymer nanomaterials. *Prog. Polym. Sci.*, 36(12), 1766, 2011.
53. Cushen, M., Kerry, J., Morris, M., Cruz-Romero, M., Cummins, E. Nanotechnologies in the food industry–Recent developments, risks and regulation. *Trends Food Sci. Technol.*, 24(3), 30, 2012.

7

Bio-Sensing Performance of Magnetite Nanocomposite for Biomedical Applications

Rajasekhar Chokkareddy, Natesh Kumar Bhajanthri, Bakusele Kabane and Gan G. Redhi*

Electroanalytical Laboratories, Department of Chemistry, Durban University of Technology, Durban South Africa

Abstract

Previously, the focus of interest in magnetic nanoparticles had a very significant part in biomedical applications and has been the topic of much interest in research groups. Physico-chemical properties of magnetic nanoparticles, i.e., nanoparticle size, surface chemistry, and, composition, vary widely with the impact of their biological and pharmacological properties, and finally, their medical usages. Furthermore, in cellular imaging and molecular application of various magnetic nanoparticles which include super paramagnetic iron oxide nanoparticles were initiated to nontoxic nature and used as contrast agents in magnetic resonance imaging. In addition, drug conveyance through hyperthermia, magnetic targeting, as well as labeling of stem cells have also remained as the source of travel and a prospective therapeutic choice. Recent advancement in the evolution and categorizing of active biomagnetic nano-materials, and their interactions with biological molecules, and their usage in bioanalytical sensors have been discussed in this chapter. Lastly, the surface coating of magnetic nanoparticle procedures is shortly described and various magnetic nanomaterials that are utilized as surface coatings are displayed in features with illustrations from the literature.

Keywords: Magnetic nanoparticles, synthetic routes, surface modifications, magnetic hyperthermia, targeted drug delivery, gene delivery

**Corresponding author*: redhigg@dut.ac.za

Suvardhan Kanchi, Shakeel Ahmed, Myalowenkosi I. Sabela and Chaudhery Mustansar Hussain (eds.) Nanomaterials: Biomedical, Environmental, and Engineering Applications, (165–196)

7.1 Introduction

Various types of nanoparticle composites containing magnetic components that include cobalt, nickel, iron, gadolinium, manganese, as well their alloys, oxide compounds, cationic compounds together with polymers, etc., which are known to exhibit paramagnetism or even superparamagnetism or ferromagnetism, are known as magnetite nanoparticles. For many years, interest in magnetic nanomaterials have enlarged attentiveness as an appropriate contender for usage in different applications because of their wide-ranging properties such as easy separation under external magnetic area, superparamagnetism, and huge surface-to-volume ratio, and high surface area Fe_3O_4 nanoparticles have enormous possibility in the discipline including immobilization of biomaterials [1]. Prior to their use in any determination procedure, most magnetic nanoparticles are essentially functionalized with enzymes, metal oxides, or metals in order to improve their stability and physiochemical properties. Furthermore, in recent decades, magnetic nanomaterials have enlarged nanotechnology by simple initiation of special character for the development of modern motives such as biomedical sciences generated by their distinctive characteristics [2, 3]. Applications of magnetic nanomaterials containing cations, e.g., Fe, Ni, Co, Cr, and their oxides, are frequently used, and can be formed naturally, e.g., hematite (α-Fe_2O_3), maghemite (γ-Fe_2O_3), magnetite (Fe_3O_4), cobalt ferrite (Fe_2CoO_4), and chromium di-oxide (CrO_2) [4]. Whereas more of these types show some positive properties that include biocompatibility and a comparatively low level of toxicity in human body, less sensitivity to oxidation, possibility of transfer to superparamagnetic formed by particle sizes that are decreasing, high stability in magnetic response, and ease of synthesis method and treatment of surface, the magnetite nanoparticles have more suitable performances [5–7]. A minimum value of coercive field (Hc) shows an appropriate effectiveness in numerous biomedical uses that include the targeting of drug delivery and contrast agent substance in magnetic resonance imaging (MRI). In this regard, nanoparticles would be unmasked to high value of saturation magnetization (Ms) and remnant magnetization (Mr); therefore, owing to higher Ms, the magnetite nanomaterials can be superior applicants [8, 9]. Some of the significant magnetic parameters of transition metal oxides (ferrites) utilized in biomedical applications are shown in Table 7.1.

7.1.1 Hematite

Below ambient conditions, hematite is the most stable iron oxide with a hexagonal closely packed structure (Figure 7.1) and an n-type semiconductor.

Table 7.1 Some of the important magnetic parameters which includes (room temperature saturation magnetization, first degree anisotropy constants, Curie temperatures, and superparamagnetic transition sizes of ferrites.

Ferrites	RT saturation magnetization M_s (emu/g)	Anisotropy constant K_1 ($\times 10^4$ J/m^3)	Curie temperature T_c (°C)	Superparamagnetic size D_{SP} (nm)
Fe_3O_4	90–100	−1.2	585	25
$NiFe_2O_4$	56	−0.68	585	28
$CoFe_2O_4$	80–94	18–39	520	14
$MnFe_2O_4$	80	−0.25	300	25

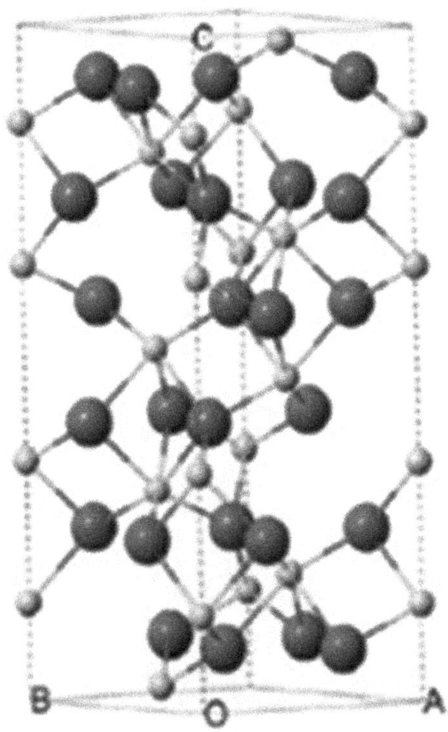

Figure 7.1 Crystal structure of hematite rhombohedral, R3c.

Due to low costs as well as high resistance to corrosion, hematite (α-Fe_2O_3) is commonly utilized in pigments, catalysts, as well as gas sensors. The band gap of hematite is known to be 2.3eV, with the conduction band composed of vacant Fe^{3+} d-orbitals and a valence band containing occupied $3d$ crystal field orbitals of Fe^{3+}, as well as an approximate mixture from the non-bonding 2p oxygen orbitals. Hematite shows antiferromagnetism at Neel temperature (T_N) of 948 K; hematite is also paramagnetic at this temperature. M_S for hematite approximately equals 2.5 kA/m or 0.4 Am^2/kg, and this low magnetization is because of the canted basal plane and defect. As a result of this, hematite shows an analytical transition temperature at 250 K, called the Morin transition temperature (T_M). At this temperature, an exchange of magnetic moments from the basal plane occurs, aligning along the *c*-axis [10]. At low T_M, hematite is perfectly antiferromagnetic, with the exact T_M being a function of particle size and induced internal pressure [11, 12].

7.1.2 Maghemite

Maghemite has a structural formula of Fe^{3+} $[Fe^{3+}Fe^{3+}_{2/3—1/3}]$ O_4. It is the end member of a solid solution sequence with magnetite (Figure 7.2). Maghemite is an *n*-type semiconductor with a band-gap of 2.0 eV and can also be considered as entirely oxidized magnetite. Oxygen anions give rise to a cubic close-packed array while ferric ions are distributed over tetrahedral sites (eight Fe ions per unit cell) and octahedral sites (the remaining Fe ions and vacancies). Hence, the maghemite can be considered as fully oxidized magnetite and it act as a n-type semiconductor. The removal occurs

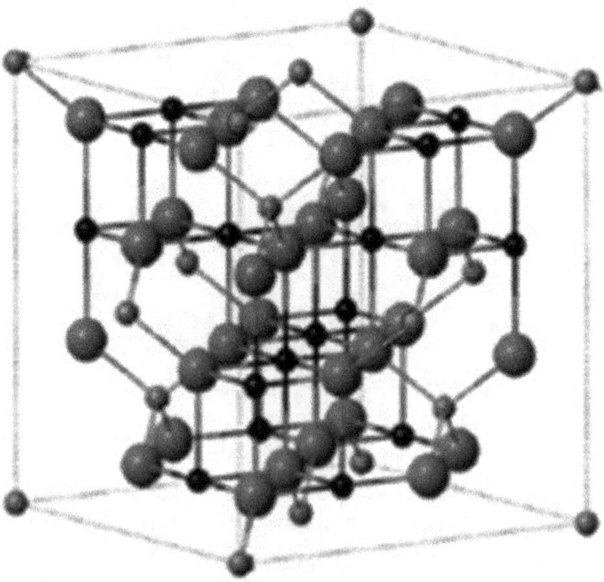

Figure 7.2 Crystal structure of magnetite cubic, Fd3m.

by diffusion where it produces vacancies (—) in the spinel structure where Fe^{2+} cation had been resided [13]. Moreover, the magnetization saturation of maghemite is 380 kA/m or ≈80 Am^2/kg. At elevated temperatures, it is not stable enough to make detection of its Curie temperature.

7.1.3 Magnetite

The structure is shown in (Figure 7.3) which has a reverse spinel with oxygen creating a face-centered cubic crystal system. $Fe^{3+}[Fe^{3+}Fe^{2+}]O_4$ is the structural formula for magnetite, where, on the octahedral sublattice, the initiates are Fe^{2+} and Fe^{3+} while the tetrahedral lattice is occupied with only Fe^{3+}. On the octahedral sublattice, it is shown that Fe^{2+} is due to the net magnetic moment of magnetite. At Curie temperature (T_C) of 853 K, magnetite is ferromagnetic, and at higher temperatures, it displays paramagnetism. The pure stoichiometric magnetite has a saturation magnetization (M_S) of 480 kA/m or 92 Am^2/kg, and the divalent irons could be partially or completely substituted by other divalent ions (Co, Mn, Zn, etc.). In Mohs scale, sedimentary rocks with hardness of about 5.5 to 6.5, a natural magnetite with a density of 5.2 g/cm^3 can be established as fine grains. Therefore, Fe_3O_4 can be either an *n*- or *p*-type semiconductor. However, between iron oxides, Fe_3O_4 has the lowest resistance because of its negligible bandgap of (0.1 eV). Pure multidomain (MD) magnetite through the magnetocrystalline anisotropy shows a great transition (T_V) around 120 K [14].

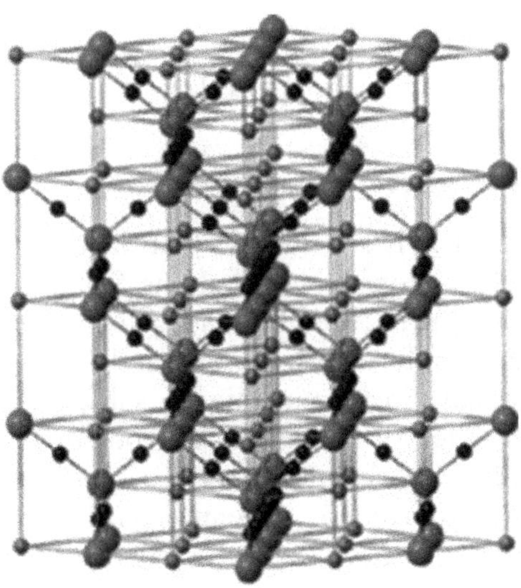

Figure 7.3 Crystal structure of maghemite cubic, $P4_332$/Tetragonal, $P4_12_12$.

7.1.4 Magnetism and Magnetic Materials

Magnetism is generally well known to most of us as an occurrence by which some substances attract or repel other substances from a certain distance; these substances include lodestone, iron, and various steels. The movement of charged particles results in magnetic forces, foremost to the magnetic fields. As a result, iron oxide magnetic properties can be defined by the dependence of the magnetic induction (B) on the magnetic field (H). Dipoles contain magnetic dipole moments which then respond to an external magnetic field. Certain field paths are required in order to recognize this response [15]. The magnetic field H (units A/m) represents the external magnetic field strength, where B (unit tesla) denotes the magnetic induction in the substance and the magnetization by M (units A/m):

$$B = \mu \times H. \tag{1}$$

In the equation above, μ represents the magnetic permeability of free space of the particles (with magnitude value of 1.257×10^{-6} H/m). When $\mu > 1$, iron oxide particles show paramagnetism, but when $\mu < 1$, it shows diamagnetism. In characterization of these NPs, at $\chi = \mu - 1$, the magnetic susceptibility is also considered: in this regard, at $\chi > 0$, NPs are paramagnetic, and diamagnetic substances at $\chi < 0$ [16]. Magnetization is mainly based on the type of substance and the temperature, which can be connected to the field H via the volumetric magnetic susceptibility χ by the relation:

$$M = \chi H \tag{2}$$

7.1.5 Types of Magnetic Substances

Based on the magnetism basis, it shows that the magnetism lies between the spin motion of electrons and orbitals, as well as how interactions of electrons occur with one another. No aggregate magnetic interactions are shown for substances in the first two groups and are also not in a magnetic arrangement. Below distinct temperatures, substances in the last three groups display a magnetic arrangement in a long range. Some of the substances that we recognize to be magnetic (i.e., possess iron behavior) are ferrimagnetic and ferromagnetic substances [17]. The three outstanding magnetic substances are weakly in such a way that they are considered as "nonmagnetic". Based on the magnetic performance of substances, they are categorized into the following five significant groups:

a) Paramagnetic materials
b) Diamagnetic materials
c) Ferri magnetic materials
d) Ferro magnetic materials
e) Anti-ferro magnetic materials

7.1.5.1 *Paramagnetic Substances*

In this group of substances, some of the atoms or ions have unpaired electrons and incompletely filled orbitals. The Langevin classification, which is applicable to substances with non-interacting localized electrons, stipulates that each atom has a randomly orientated magnetic moment resulting from thermal agitation (Figure 7.4). Moreover, the atomic magnets experience no interaction among each other. An incomplete orientation of these atomic magnetic moments in the direction of applied magnetic field results in a net positive magnetization and positive susceptibility in the presence of a magnetic field [18]. Moreover, when the temperature of paramagnetic materials increases, the orientation of the atomic magnets is disturbed. This simply means that the susceptibility of the magnet is inversely proportional to the absolute temperature.

7.1.5.2 *Diamagnetic Substances*

An essential property of all material is diamagnetism, which is categorized as a weak magnetism and is in the direction opposite to that of the applied field. There is no permanent dipole moment in each atom. It is because of the non-cooperative behavior of orbiting electrons when visible to an applied magnetic field. Moreover, in diamagnetic materials, all of the atoms have paired electrons and contain no unpaired electrons in the shells. Hence, the net magnetic moment of the atom for a diamagnetic

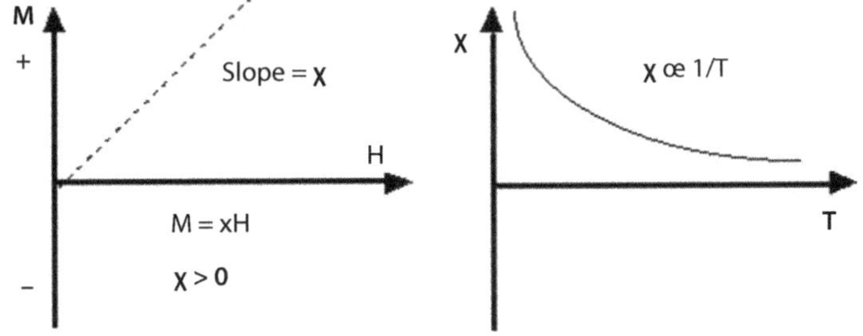

Figure 7.4 Plot of M vs. H for paramagnetism.

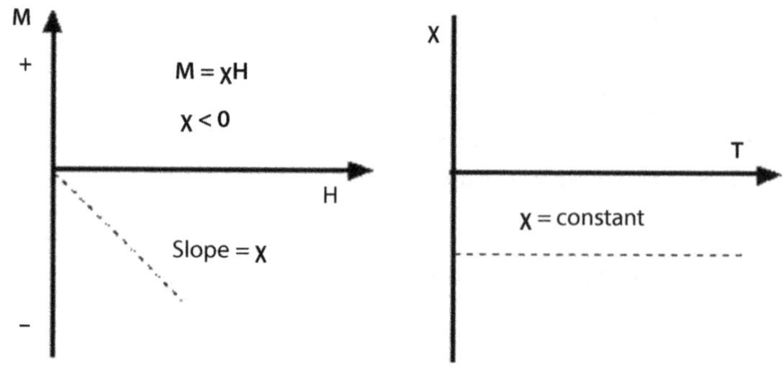

Figure 7.5 Plot of M vs. H for diamagnetism.

substance is zero; therefore, for all diamagnetic materials, susceptibility is negative. The additional characteristic behavior of diamagnetic substances is that their susceptibility is independent of temperature. If we plot M vs. H, we see Figure 7.5.

7.1.5.3 Ferri Magnetic Substances

In ionic complexes, such as oxides (certain oxides of Fe), other complex forms of magnetic ordering can occur as a result of the crystal structure. One type of magnetic ordering is called ferrimagnetism. A simple alignment of magnetic spins in a ferrimagnetic oxide is shown in Figure 7.6. In addition, the material breaks down into magnetic domains, such as a ferromagnetic material, and the magnetic behavior is also very similar, while ferrimagnetic materials generally have lesser saturation magnetizations. The magnetic structure in a ferrimagnetic oxide consists of two magnetic sub-lattices separated by oxygen. For example, in barium ferrite ($BaO.6Fe_2O_3$), the unit cell contains 64 ions of which the barium and oxygen ions have no magnetic moment, 16 Fe^{3+} ions have moments aligned parallel while 8 Fe^{3+} and aligned anti-parallel giving a net magnetization parallel to the applied field. The amplitude of the net magnetization is relatively low as only 1/8 of the ions contribute to the magnetization of the material.. Ferrimagnetic substances also show spontaneous magnetization, Curie temperature, hysteresis, and retentivity.

7.1.5.4 Ferro Magnetic Substances

When atoms are in a sequence in atomic magnetic and lattice moments, ferromagnetism individual potential interacts in alignment similar to one

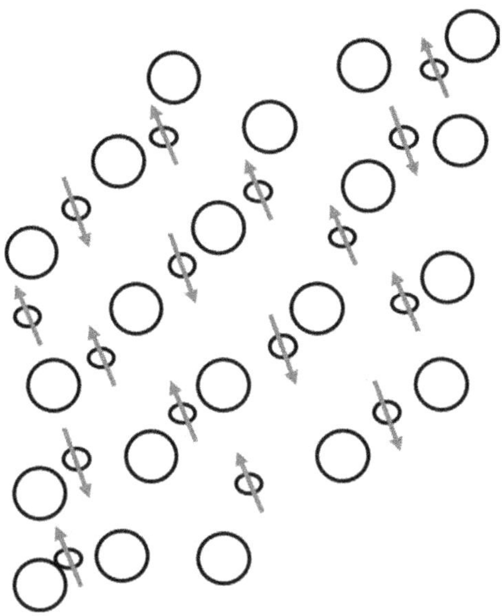

Figure 7.6 Magnetic arrangement ferromagnetic material.

another (Figure 7.7). The classical theory describes these results by the existence of a molecular field in ferromagnetic substances, which was proposed in 1907 by Weiss. This arena is enough to magnetize the substance to saturation. Furthermore, the interaction exchange between the neighboring of the magnetic moments in parallel alignment is explained by the Heisenbergs model of ferromagnetism in quantum mechanics. Between the forces, the type of exchanges are very huge and contain a magnitude of 1000 Tesla, and this type of magnetic strength is nearly 10^8 times the earth's magnetic field strength. The abnormal properties of ferromagnetic substances are spontaneously magnetization in critical temperatures.

7.1.5.5 Anti-Ferro Magnetic Substances

Antiferromagnetic and ferromagnetic substances are both parallel to one another, but surprisingly, the interchange interaction between atoms close to each other lead to an anti-parallel orientation of atomic magnetic moments (Figure 7.8). When magnetic field stops, the substances act in a similar way as the paramagnetic material. Similar to ferromagnetic materials, these substances are converted into paramagnetic material beyond transition temperatures, which are also known as the Neel temperature, T_N. (Cr: T_N = 37 °C). Furthermore, the paramagnetic susceptibility of

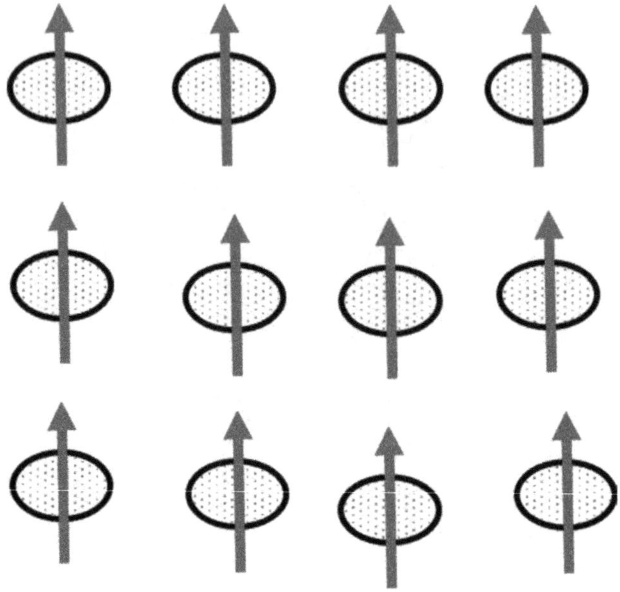

Figure 7.7 Parallel alignment in ferromagnetism.

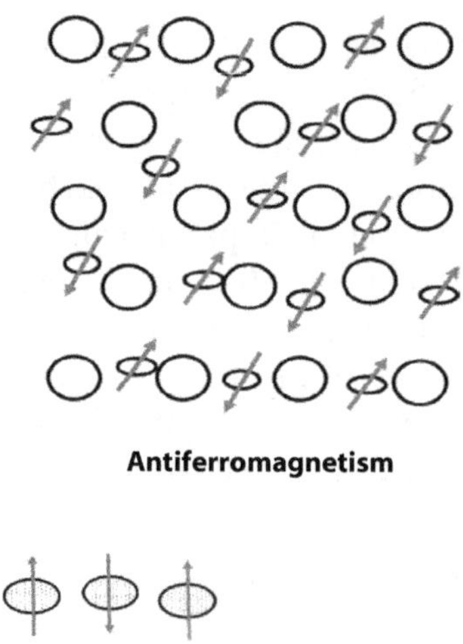

Figure 7.8 Magnetic ordering in the antiferromagnetic material.

materials follows the Curie–Weiss law, through a negative intercept denoting the existence of negative exchange interactions.

The importance of magnetic susceptibility falls through a particular range for each type of substance and this is displayed in Table 7.2 with examples.

Table 7.2 Summary of different types of magnetic behavior.

Types of magnetism	Susceptibility	Atomic/magnetic behavior		Example/ susceptibility	(m. mol^{-1})
Diamagnetism	Negative and small	No magnetic moment for atoms	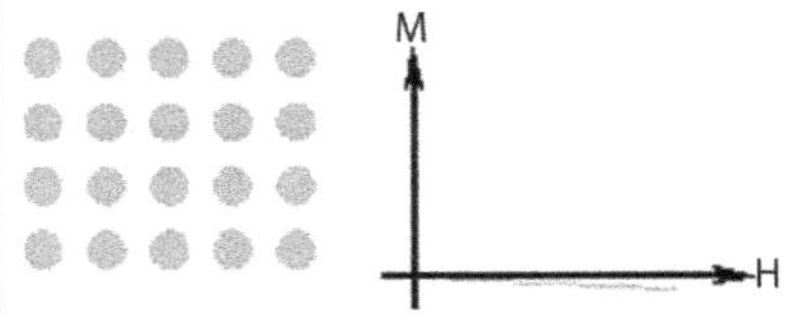	Au Cu	-2.74×10^{-6} -0.77×10^{-6}
Paramagnetism	Positive and small	Random oriented magnetic moments shown by atoms	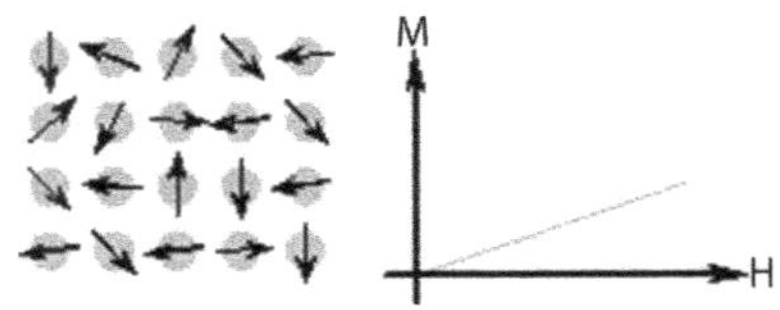	β-Sn Pt Mn	0.19×10^{-6} 21.04×10^{-6} 66.10×10^{-6}
Ferromagnetism	Positive and large function of micro-structure dependent, applied field	Parallel aligned magnetic moments shown by atoms	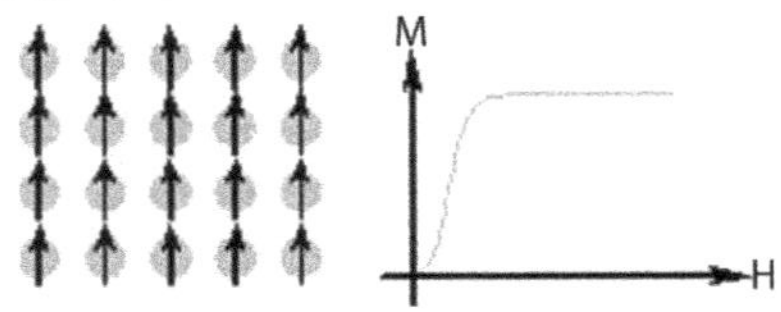	Fe	~100,000

(*Continued*)

Table 7.2 Cont.

Types of magnetism	Susceptibility	Atomic/magnetic behavior		Example/ susceptibility	(m. mol^{-1})
Antiferro magnetism	Positive and small	Parallel and anti-parallel aligned magnetic moments shown by atoms	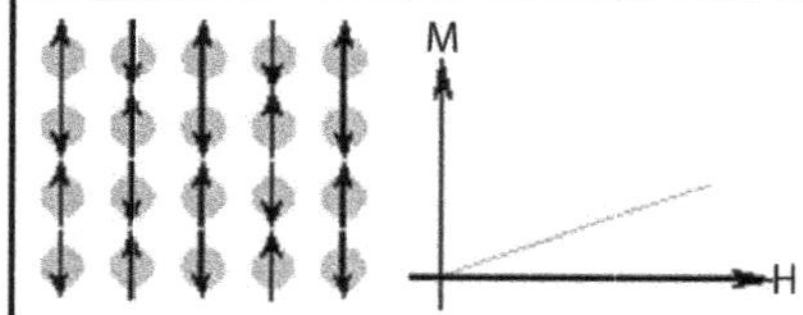	Cr	3.6×10^{-6}
Ferrimagnetism	Positive and large function of applied field, microstructure dependent	Atoms display an anti-parallel aligned magnetic moments	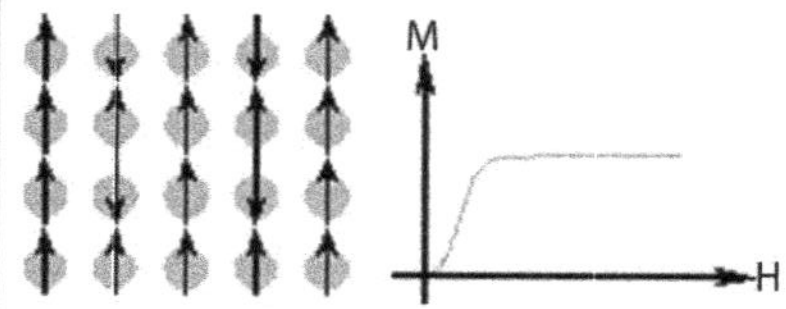	Ba ferrite	~3

7.1.6 Shape, Size, and Magnetic Properties

The prerequisite for extensive utilization of magnetism in data storage as well in bio-separation areas is the correlation between magnetic properties as well as the size and shape of iron oxide nanoparticles [19]. At ambient temperature, a weak ferromagnetism is shown by α-Fe_2O_3; in this, the saturation magnetization is frequently reduced by 1 emu g^{-1}. At room temperature γ-Fe_2O_3 and Fe_3O_4 show ferrimagnetism, with saturation magnetization reaching up to 92 emu g^{-1} [19]. It is notable that various properties of magnetic nanoparticles are determined based on their shape and size. When the size of nanoparticles is less than 15 nm at room temperature, a wide range of magnetic nanoparticles are transformed to superparamagnetic, this means that the thermal energy can prevail the anisotropy energy wall of a single nanoparticle. But, aggregation between superparamagnetic nanoparticles is a usual occurrence. Magnetic nanoparticle size plays an important role in different magnetic biomaterial uses, and we will now consider the outcomes of particle size on magnetic properties shown in Figure 7.9.

Additionally, in order to protect basic magnetic nanoparticles against aggregation, coating substances, such as Ag, CuO, Au, and Co_3O_4, are used to tailor the magnetic properties. The outside magnetic field actively supports the reorientation of the times of the particular particle throughout the useful field at lower temperatures. Therefore, when increasing the temperature, a maximum is reached when all zero filed magnetic moments are increased; here, the temperature is referred to as the blocking temperature.

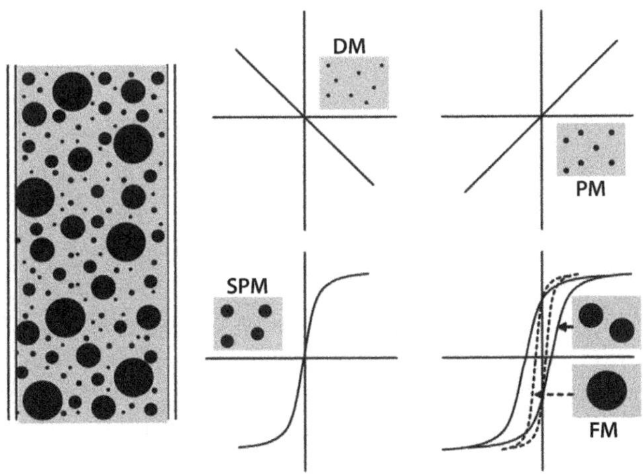

Figure 7.9 Particle size hugely affects the magnetic properties (DM = diamagnetic, PM = paramagnetic, SPM = superparamagnetic, FM = ferromagnetic) [20].

7.1.7 Synthesis Methods of Magnetic Nanoparticles

Many synthetic methods are used to prepare the metal oxide nanoparticles, which can be widely categorized into three: chemical, biological, and physical methods. Electron ray lithography [21], gas-phase deposition [22], and mechanical techniques are all part of physical methods. While physical methods are not difficult to complete, it is easy for them to control the size particle. Wet chemical preparation technique includes oxidation methods [23], sol–gel synthesis [24], chemical co-precipitation [25], reduction method [26], thermal decomposition method [27], hydrothermal reactions [28], flow injection synthesis [29], solvothermal method [30], aerosol/vapor phase technique [31], electrochemical technique method [32], sonochemical decomposition reactions [33], and supercritical fluid technique. Hence, in the case of wet chemical preparation technique, comparatively less energy is consumed and this is associated with that of physical methods. Many magnetic nanomaterials with various morphologies have been manufactured with rods, wires, and particles. The magnetic nanoparticle morphology and size can be measured by particularly indicating the reaction media, the reaction physical parameters, which include reactant concentration, precursors, base (NaOH, ammonium hydroxide, and CH_3NH_2), ionic strength (CH_3NH^{3+}, $N(CH_3)^{4+}$, Na^+, NH^{4+}, Li^+ and K^+), reaction temperature, pH of the media, and also some additional factors. The microbial process denotes a functional process technology regarding to high yield, great scalability, and good reproducibility, as well as low energy input, which result to a low cost, but the fermentation method is rather time-consuming. The summary for several techniques for preparing iron oxide nanoparticles is shown in Table 7.3.

7.1.8 Advantages of Magnetic Nanomaterials

Magnetic nanoparticles have various advantages and applications in the fields of biology and medicine. Initially, their sizes are easily controlled from few to tens of nanometers. These sizes are mostly equal to those of a virus (20–450 nm), a cell (between 10–100 μm), a protein, (5–50 nm), and a gene (2 nm wide). Magnetic nanoparticles contain enough ability and size to highly interact with biological entities. Additionally, because they contain a magnetic nature, they easily comply with Coulomb's inverse square law. Hence, these particles are able to respond to an external magnetic field. In immobilization and transporting of magnetic nanoparticles, this idea can be utilized. This method can be successful in drug delivery to infected regions of the body such as tumors, cancer tissues, etc. Magnetic

Table 7.3 Comparison between methods for the synthesis of magnetic nanoparticles.

	Methods	**Advantages**	**Disadvantages**
	Sol–gel synthesis	Correctly controlled in aspect ratio, size, and internal structure	Weak bonding, low wear-resistance, high permeability
	Oxidation method	Constant size and narrow size distribution	Small-sized ferrite colloids
	Reduction method	Simple	High reaction temperature
	Chemical coprecipitation	Well organized and simple	Not suitable for the preparation of high pure, accurate stoichiometric phase
	Hydrothermal reactions	Easy to control particle size and shapes	High pressure, high reaction temperature
	Solvothermal method	Easy to control particle size and shape	High reaction temperature
Wet chemical preparation methods	Thermal decomposition method Flow injection synthesis	Easy to control particle size and shape Good reproducibility and high mixing homogeneity together with a precise control of the process	Includes multiple steps Need continuous or segmented mixing of reagents under a laminar flow regime in a capillary reactor
	Electrochemical method	Easy to control particle size	Poor reproducibility
	Aerosol/vapor phase method	High yields	Very high temperatures

(*Continued*)

Table 7.3 Cont.

	Methods	**Advantages**	**Disadvantages**
	Sonochemical decomposition reactions	Narrow particle size distribution	Mechanism not still understood
	Supercritical fluid method	Effectively controlled of the particle size, no organic solvents involved	Critical pressure and temperature
	Synthesis using nanoreactors	Correctly controlled of the particle size	Complex condition
Physical methods	Electron beam lithography	Well-controlled inter-particle spacing	Costly and highly complex machines needed
	Gas-phase deposition	Easy to perform	Not easy to control the particle size
	Mechanical techniques	No chemicals involved	Highly complex machines needed and too much time
Microbial methods	Microbial incubation	Environmental friendly, increased yield, great reproducibility, and great scalability, inexpensive	Too much time

nanoparticles have an increased surface area. By transforming their surface area, biological and chemical agents can be involved. In order for nano-magnetic particles to bind easily to a biological entity, they can be coated with biochemical and chemical molecules. Under significant conditions, when time change is applied on magnetic fields in a nanoparticle, there is an exchange of energy from field to the nano-particle. This results in an increased heat on the nanoparticle. These properties allow them to be used as hyperthermia agents. The thermal energy is delivered to targeted bodies such as tumors. Due to the novel physical properties of magnetic nanoparticles mentioned above, they show possible applications in biomedicine.

7.1.9 Surface Modifications of Magnetic Nanoparticles

For practical applications, magnetic nanoparticles are not suitable because of their tendency to form aggregates and similarly aggregation, which might result in the modification of magnetic properties. These setbacks can be overcome by the use of an exact coating stabilizer. To avoid aggregation of the magnetic nanoparticles, stabilizers such as surfactants, or polymers, organic molecules and enzymes are frequently added throughout or after the synthesis. Some of the essential issues to be addressed is the stability of magnetic nanoparticles in a physical and biological aqueous environment; in this regard, external kinetics performs an outmost role. Moreover, magnetic nanoparticles are prepared by the use of two methods: in the first method, bare paramagnetic nanoparticles are synthesized by adding a concentrated base to di- and trivalent Fe salt solutions. Here, bare paramagnetic naoparticles are coated in a monomer and polymers through nonspecific adsorption, and then it is followed by purification in order to make them extra biocompatible. Otherwise, to stop aggregation of the nanoscale particulate, co-precipitation steps are introduced to stabilizers. Finally, it is highly proposed to reduce these hydrophilic nanoparticles for biomedical applications as the body can easily identify hydrophobic units as foreign and are quickly occupied by a mononuclear phagocytic system [34, 35].

7.2 Potential Applications of Magnetic Nanoparticles

In previous decades, a wide number of applications have been recognized for magnetic nanoparticles especially for magnetite ones. This enhances them to be tailored for precise utilization as shown in Figure 7.10. Moreover, for successful potential application, separate properties are required from magnetic nanoparticles, i.e. data packing, which is one of the inexpensive and has many

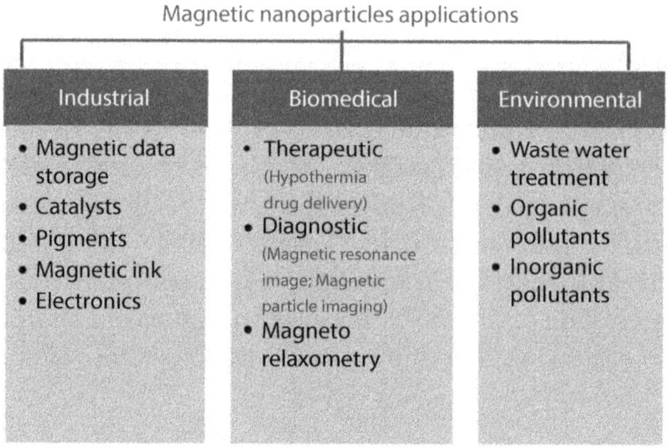

Figure 7.10 Illustrations of high performance abilities of magnetic nanoparticles in several fields of application.

significant applications, which require magnetic nanoparticles with switchable magnetic and constant states. Economically, biomedical applications have vital attraction, i.e. magnetic nanomaterials found use in hyperthermia action; it is also active for cancer therapy, mainly tumors. The principle used to construct this technique is in such a way that when applying AC fields to the magnetic nanoparticles, it can produce a heat in the following order range (42–46) °C, and the cancer cells are terminated [36]. In addition, magnetic nanoparticles are used similarly in several environmental applications. For example, in contaminated sites, pollutants can be easily removed by the magnetic extraction technique only, when functionalized to attract them [37].

The exceptional magnetic properties as well as suitable dispersibility, biocompatibility, and linking ability of magnetic nanomaterials are produced to existing novel bio applications that can be classified into two groups such as "*in vitro*" and "*in vivo*" applications. *In vitro* applications involved the actions that are completed in the laboratory environment and external of living organisms. The main ones of these applications are the magnetic recognition and separation of cells, DNA, proteins, and so forth by the use of magnetic nanoparticles [38]. On the other hand, the significant part of bio-applications is associated with *in vivo* (refer to living samples) ones, that is, the disease analysis methods like MRI, and the treatment methods such as magnetic hyperthermia and gene/drug delivery systems.

7.2.1 Magnetic Separation

Existence of species from environments can be isolated by the use of magnetic nanomaterials; therefore, the surroundings can be purified or

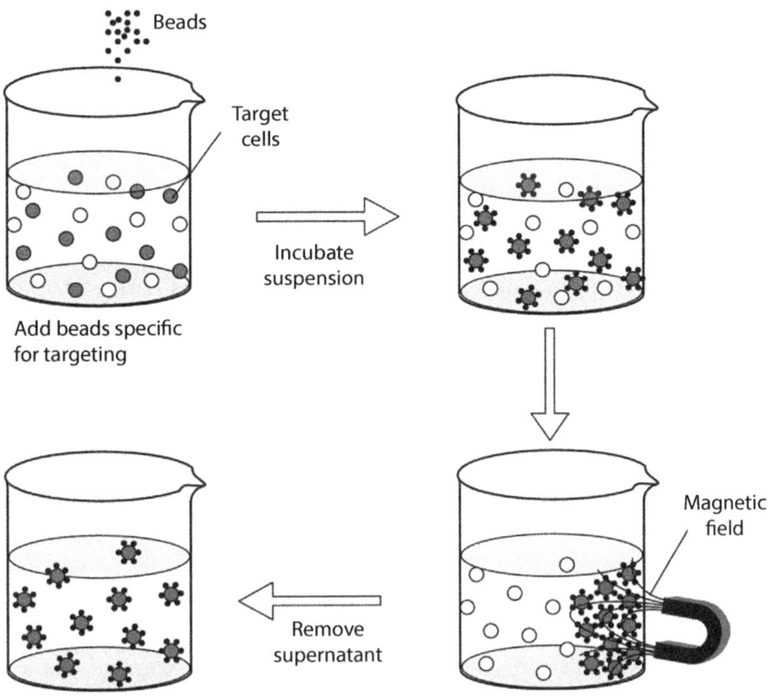

Figure 7.11 Magnetic separation [39, 40].

concentrate on the entities for further study. This usage is found on the transformation of susceptibility between a magnetically characterized material and the surrounding medium.

In addition, this principle is based on the magnetic cell arrangement for cellular treatment and immunoassay, which is a process that measures and identifies a specific biological ingredient such as an antigen. Species can consist of bacteria, cells, and some groups of vesicles. As shown in Figure 7.11, it is advised to first label the entities consisting of particles that are then followed by magnetic separation of the labeled entities. Most of the magnetically treated particles will be utilized in this process; the layer will help with the assistance to tie the atoms to entities such as cells. From the cell surfaces, particular spots can be targeted for extra antibodies; this is used as the labeling method because antibodies tie easily to their identical antigen. Hence, a magnetic field gradient is used to separate these labeled entities, because it can strongly attract and hold the species in particular regions, and then it is followed by elimination of these species. For the selection of tumor cells from blood, this process has been functional, as well as in separation of enzymes, RNA and DNA from several sources as well as body fluids.

7.2.2 Magnetic Resonance Image

Magnetic resonance image (MRI) was first introduced by Bloch and Purcell in 1930s (Nobel Prize in Physics 1952); it based is mainly on a physics principle named as nuclear magnetic resonance, where atomic nuclei magnetic properties are studied. In the year 1971, Damadian exposed the starting point on how to use magnetic resonance imaging as a tool for medical analysis. He initiates that various kinds of animal tissue produce response signals with a variable distance, and a response signals from carcinogenic tissue last longer as compared to the non-cancerous tissue [41]. In 1974, Damadian was granted the world's first patent in the field of MRI [42]. Discoveries concerning MRI were made by Lauterbur and Mansfield in the year 2003, and they were awarded a Nobel Prize in Medicine. MRI is a non-invasive technique significantly depending on the relaxation properties of proton nuclei in water and lipids showing images of the inside of a material. MRI found use in displaying image in pathological or other physiological deviations of living tissues in the body. Hence, magnetic nanomaterials are used as contrast enhancement agents [43, 44]. The enhanced contrast in MRI permits well defined and particularly in locating the unwanted tissues (such as tumors) by capturing and monitoring the results of the applied therapy. In comparison with other medical imaging techniques which include positron emission tomography (PET), computed tomography (CT), radiological imaging, and optical imaging, MRI has more advantages: (i) ability to detect many characteristics in tissues through different scanning parameters, (ii) use nonionizing radio frequency (RF) signals to attain its images which correspond to non-calcified tissues in the body, (iii) greater ability to detect and recognize tumors, (iv) ability to process cross-sectional images in any images as well as oblique planes, (v) time effective, (vi) able to do multiple contrast mechanisms, i.e., T1weighted, T2weighted, and T2* weighted MRI [45]. Young *et al.*, introduced T1 contrast agents *t* in MRI that mainly depended on gadolinium constituents. Work done by Levy and coworkers established that there is an improvement in the magnetic resonance field. Gadolinium (Gd)-based MRI contrast agents (CAs) of many sizes and chemical properties equipped through comparatively simple chemistry and are capable of contributing enough contrast improvement for many applications. In addition, Gd-based contrast agents have a high magnetic momentum of 7.94 μB and is one of the higher magnetic momentum used in MRI. Furthermore, Gd components show several purposes that include contrast agents with a hydrophobic core of polypropylenimine diaminobutane (DAB) dendrimer, which are used easily to gather in the liver and utilize as liver contrast agents; and

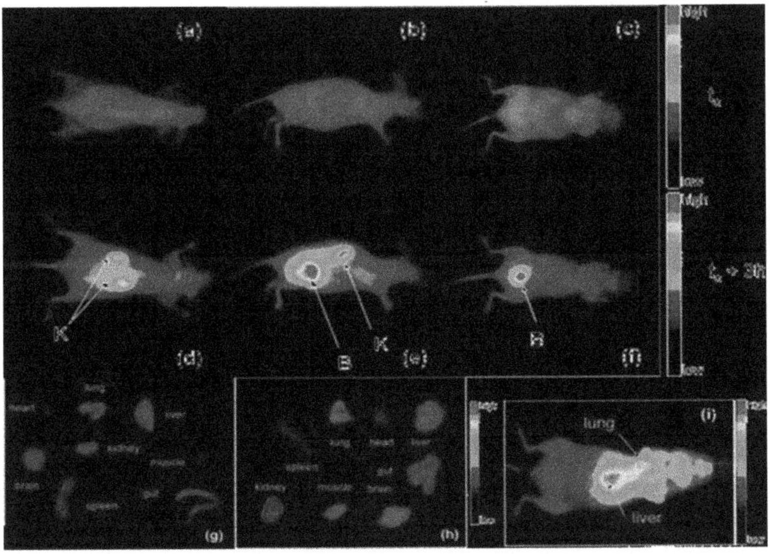

Figure 7.12 (a, b, c) The fluorescence reflectance imaging of a nude mouse before and (d, e, f) 3h after the injection of GadoSiPEG2C (K: kidneys; B: bladder) [48].

in lymphatic imaging, a hydrophilic contrast agent can be used. Finally, antibodies are also targeted by contrast agents [46], DNA receptors [47], or functionalized peptides can act as tumor-particularly agents with double diagnostic and therapeutic applications which are depended on gadolinium component. The investigational data exhibited that these atoms induced an improvement of the positive contrast of MRI as in comparison to the frequently utilized positive contrast agents such as Gd-DOTA in clinical MRI practices shown in Figure 7.12.

Also, when water-soluble Gd_2O_3 surface is doped with MnO nanoparticles, it provides greater performance as confirmed by the *in vivo* T1 MRI of a mouse shown in Figure 7.12. In 1978, Ohgushi *et al.* produced a T2/T2* contrast agent and superparamagnetic particles were used by the Lauterbur group and other groups for MRI. In 1990, Weissleder and coworkers introduced an ultra-small superparamagnetic iron-oxide nanoparticles for T2/T2* contrast agents, which are still currently used. Furthermore, the ultra-small superparamagnetic iron-oxide nanoparticles through non-targeted or targeted ways were extensively used in divergently clinical or biological applications, which include targeted-receptors [49], target of small molecules by imaging, cell migration, magnetically labeled cells, atherosclerotic plaque, cell inflammation, tissue inflammation, reticuloendothelial

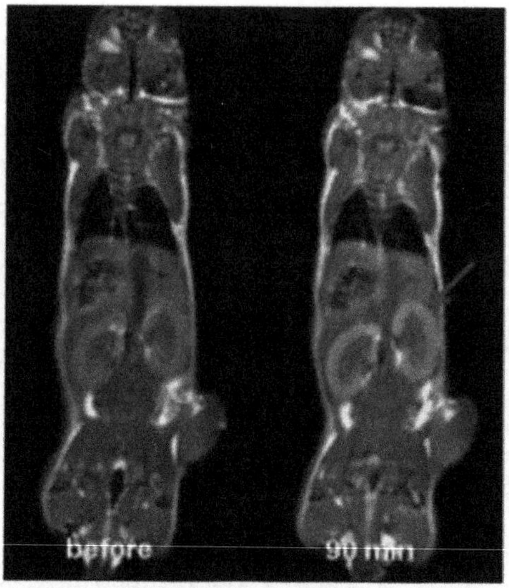

Figure 7.13 (Left) T *in-vivo* T1 MRimages of a mouse before and injection after 90 min (right) of the sample solution into the tail vein of the mouse; it also shows a clear contrast improvement in the kidneys (illustrated by an arrow) [55].

systems (RES) including liver, spleen, pancreatic islets, lung and lymph nodes, perfusion imaging of brain [50], myocardium [51], cartilage and kidney [52], MR angiography [53], and tumor vascular imaging [54].

In addition to that, a double emulsion solvent evaporation interfacial deposition (water-in oil-in-water emulsion) technique was used to produce the micro-bubble, which has nitrogen in its core (Figure 7.13). Exhibited *in vivo* in rat liver and improved images fulfills the optimization of magnetic nanomaterials in the shell and it had appropriate echogenicity for the determination of existence used as an ultrasonography (US) contrast agent. Figure 7.14 shows the magnetic nanoparticle-used MRI images. Table 7.4 shows the several parameters affecting the contrast among various tissues.

7.2.3 Targeted Drug Delivery Systems

The impression of using magnetic nanoparticles as a transporter tool for drug delivery was considered in the late 1970s by Widder, Senyei, and their coworkers. As mentioned previously, in order to enhance innovative applications, the magnetic nanoparticles are attached with various multifunctional materials and agents like DNA and RNA segments or drugs. Hence, the use of solution techniques can be submitted to improve drug delivery systems and decrease side effects of the therapy process [58]. It is well

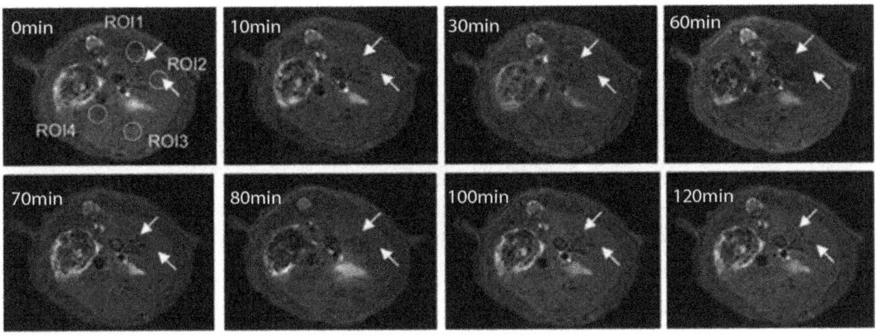

Figure 7.14 Equivalent anatomical image structures from the same rat at two adjacent slice locations, during magnetic nanoparticles present in microbubble injection. After injection, when the time lapse, the images display that the T_2 signal in liver decreases at rest and then increases [57].

Table 7.4 MRI parameters: components which have impact on the signal from an individual location [56].

Parameter	Description
T_1	Longitudinal spin-lattice/composure time. The T_1 composure time constant is a substance property reporting the properties of how this energy is given back to the surroundings.
T_2	Transverse relaxation time. T_2 relaxation time constant stating the energy shift among adjacent protons.
T_2^*	Same as T_2, but also consist of heterogeneities in the environment
ρ	Spin density: the concentration of H nuclei in the tissue

identified that most methods of chemotherapy are relatively non-specific. As a result, drugs are "wasted" by distributing to areas where they are not essential and important, and this can lead to undesirable side effects. However, new virus-influenced physiological diseases and nonpathogenic disorders are now converted and statistically important to be the interest in medical science. Now, 'AIDS' and 'cancer' induce the equal dreaded feeling as 'leprosy' and 'plague' would produce in the 13th century in Europe. But, though viruses have altered their form and manner, medicines and drugs have still continued the easiest and conventionally the utmost secure therapy or relief to all diseases. As per a substitute, the magnetic nanoparticle-targeted drug delivery organizations can expand these situations. In this

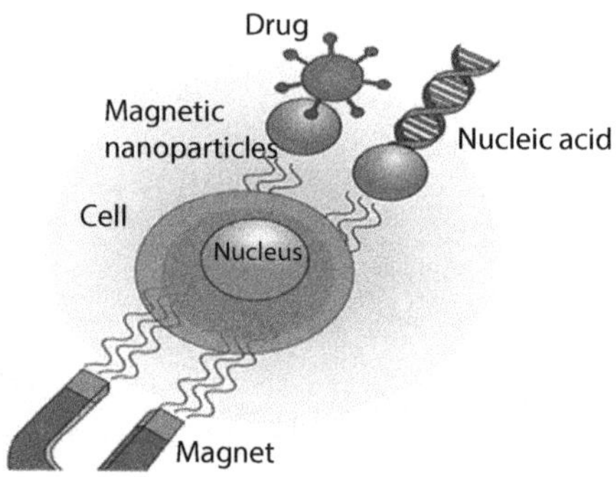

Figure 7.15 The graphical illustration of magnetic nanoparticle-targeted drug delivery mechanism [60].

process, the collections of drug/magnetic transporters (magnetic nanoparticles) are vaccinated to blood circulation, and then by applying the outside magnetic field that generates a magnetic slope in special spots of the body, i.e., tumors, the drug/carrier groups are removed and demonstrated in tumors [59]. The schematic magnetic nanoparticles targeted by the drug delivery mechanism are shown in Figure 7.15. Furthermore, in other systems, their lease methods contain osmolality changing, enzymatic activity, temperature varying, and specially pH changing.

Moreover, the primary advantages of magnetic nanomaterials are the target of drug delivery systems that contain (i) reducing of therapy side effects that arise from the targeting process, (ii) increasing of therapy effectiveness due to reduction of drug losses, (iii) ability to work in combination with other systems for further associated applications like MRI and hyperthermia, and (4) presenting novel modification abilities such as magnetic thermal releasing mechanisms. Based on these advantages, Figure 7.16 displays the target delivery mechanism of drug by magnetic nanoparticles to the tumor (cancer) cell by receptor-mediated endocytosis. From this method, the blood stream accepts the magnetic nano-particles carried by the drug to the specific tumor cells where they arrive by the development of the endosome. Therefore, the osmotic pressure increase results in endosome swells and finally, separation occurs in tumor cells to release the drug. The benefits of this strategy are that it can provide a demand on drug release profiles, affording the needs of each patient.

7.2.4 Magnetic Hyperthermia

In the year 1957, Gilchrist *et al.*, proposed an idea of using small atoms in magnetic nanoparticle hyperthermia [62], but utmost studies showed

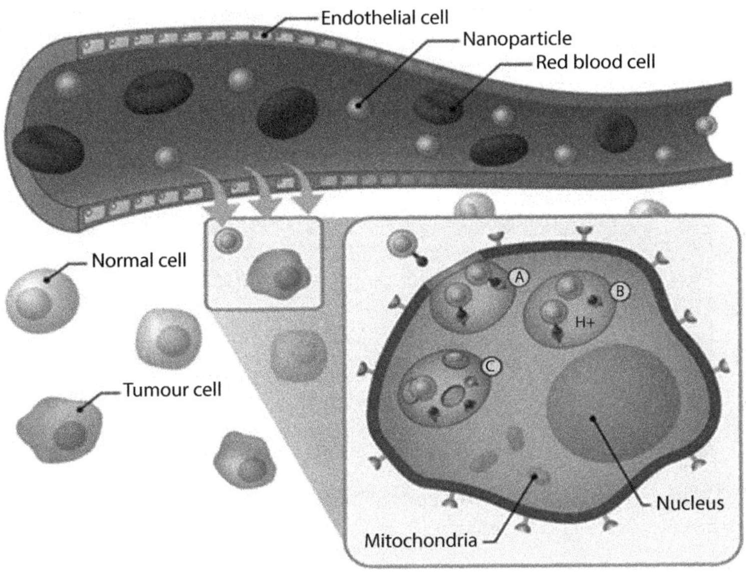

Figure 7.16 Specific tissue delivery of magnetic nanoparticles via active targeting, which is facilitated by "leaky" vasculature. Nanoparticle internalization by (A) formation of an endosome and receptor-mediated endocytosis. (B) Endosomal acidification by proton pumps that results in elevated swelling, osmotic pressure, and (C) rupture of the endosome allowing the release of the nanoparticle and conjugated therapeutic agents reprinted from [61].

incorrect thermometry and bad/undefined AC magnetic field parameters in animal models. Later, iron oxide nanoparticles were initiated in 1993 by Jordan and his coworkers, which showed a remarkable particular absorption rate (PAR), which clinically acceptable H_0f mixtures in comparison to hysteresis heating of increased multidomain magnetic nanoparticles. Hence, thermal energy is then released to the neighboring of the targeted implant, mixed with the size of the magnetic nanomaterial used and the strength of the functional magnetic field. Hyperthermia is one of the favorable biomedical applications of magnetic nanoparticles for cancer treatment. Magnetic initiation hyperthermia means the description of cancer cells to a repeated magnetic field of exact frequency and amplitude; when magnetic nanoparticles are placed around or inside the tumor area, this increases the temperature of the tumor. Temperatures above 45 °C are to highly destroy the tumor cells by necrosis. Hence, if temperature reaches 42 °C, it is able to enlarge the effectiveness of chemotherapy, in which temperature (typically about 43 °C) is formed due to magnetic hysteresis loss.

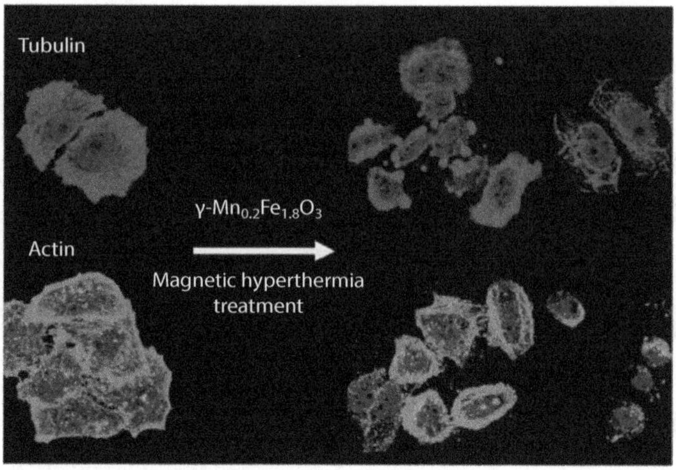

Figure 7.17 Mechanism of cell death induced by magnetic hyperthermia with nanoparticles of γ-Mn_xFe_2–xO_3 [63].

Furthermore, the revolution of the particles or the rotation of the atomic magnetic moments can increase the heat of superparamagnetic particles. Some of the non-magnetic techniques of hyperthermia similarly exist. An AC magnetic field application that is done in the presence of the Acrypol 934 stabilized γ-$Mn_xFe_{2-x}O_3$ suspension produced by the death of HeLa cells is able to induce hyperthermia. Figure 7.17 shows the exhibited cells by changing the degrees of membrane blabbing with substantial disturbance of the actin and tubulin cytoskeletons, followed by magnetic nanomaterial hyperthermia treatment which finally leads to death of cells. The cell death was observed to be corresponding to the duration of the applied AC magnetic field and the quantity of the particles. Similarly, cancer tissues or cells of animals and humans can be treated by the use of magnetic hyperthermia. Not long ago, Thomas *et al.*, observed that the iron oxide nanoparticles produced with tiopronin as the ligand in hyperthermia treatment exhibited notable heating properties to commercially presented samples [62]. At concentrations between 6.25 and 50 mg/mL of tiopronin, stabilized nanoparticles can significantly kill the bacteria. This was the first reported usage of magnetic hyperthermia to get rid of bacteria. These techniques can find use in the treatment of a wide range of transferable diseases in future.

7.2.5 Gene Delivery

A huge number of syndromes can be described or understood with one or more detailed genetic information, which can then be used either for early

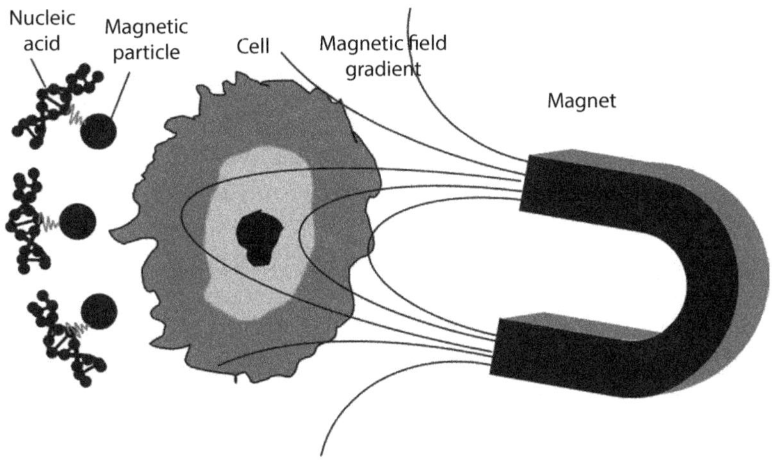

Figure 7.18 The gene delivery principle by the usage of magnetic particles. The cells are to be transfected and positioned between the nucleic acids and hemagnetic field gradient which are then attached to the particles. The applied field is the reason for the particles to progress towards the target cells; here, the cell entry is achieved, e.g., by endocytosis [64].

determination of such diseases or even for their treatment. Hence, a system is essential for gene delivery applications which can easily control some setbacks, such as quick DNA degradation by endonuclease or exonuclease and bad intracellular uptake of the targeted DNA [100,101]. This method is also known as magnetofection, because it includes the usage of magnetic nanoparticles to enlarge the effectiveness of gene transfection (introducing foreign DNA into host cell) and expression (the process by which a gene's coded information is changed into the structures' existence and operating in the cell) [7]. A virus related to a vector that is carrying the gene is treated on the surface of the magnetic nanoparticle; by applying a magnetic field, this particle can then be held at the target area. For an increased duration, the tissue is in interaction with the virus and also increases the transfection efficiency (Figure 7.18).

7.3 Conclusion

In developing an efficient drug delivery system, the use of nanotechnology is necessary to involve in some of the biomedical fields. To deliver medicine, the subsequent development of nanotechnology for *in vivo* uses such as implanting multifunctional particles in biological tissue will be used; this damages tumors and increases immune responses. Magnetic nanoparticles have converted a gradually significant tool in therapy and disease diagnosis. Most of the clinical usage of magnetic nanoparticles has changed focus to superparamagnetic iron oxide because they possess a good biocompatibility, chemical stability, and relative ease of production. The occurrence of magnetism has attracted and excited many scientists for centuries. For a number of biomedical uses, magnetic biomaterials can be successfully applied. Many of the applications that are presently being examined include immunoassay, hyperthermia, magnetic cell separation, radionuclide, gene delivery, and MRI contrast drug and agents. One of the greatest advantages of these substances is their capability to respond and be operated by the external magnetic fields. In this field, continuous improvement on nano magnetism will enhance more interest and development in nanomedicine and biomedical research.

References

1. Laurent, S., Forge, D., Port, M., Roch, A., Robic, C., Vander Elst, L., Muller, R.N. Magnetic iron oxide nanoparticles: synthesis, stabilization, vectorization, physicochemical characterizations, and biological applications. *Chem. Rev.* 108, 2064–2110, 2008.
2. Sharifi, I., Shokrollahi, H. Structural, magnetic and Mössbauer evaluation of Mn substituted Co–Zn ferrite nanoparticles synthesized by co-precipitation. *J. Magn. Magn. Mater.* 334, 36–40, 2013.
3. Sharifi, I., Shokrollahi, H., Doroodmand, M.M., Safi, R. Magnetic and structural studies on $CoFe_2O_4$ nanoparticles synthesized by co-precipitation, normal micelles and reverse micelles methods. *J. Magn. Magn. Mater.* 324, 1854–1861, 2012.
4. Teja, A.S., Koh, P.-Y. Synthesis, properties, and applications of magnetic iron oxide nanoparticles. *Prog. Cryst Growth Charact. Mater.* 55, 22–45, 2009.
5. Neuberger, T., Schöpf, B., Hofmann, H., Hofmann, M., Von Rechenberg, B. Superparamagnetic nanoparticles for biomedical applications: possibilities and limitations of a new drug delivery system. *J. Magn. Magn. Mater.* 293, 483–496, 2005.
6. Lübbe, A.S., Bergemann, C., Riess, H., Schriever, F., Reichardt, P., Possinger, K., Matthias, M., Dörken, B., Herrmann, F., Gürtler, R. Clinical experiences with magnetic drug targeting: a phase I study with 4′-epidoxorubicin in 14 patients with advanced solid tumors. *Can. Res.* 56, 4686–4693, 1996.
7. Tartaj, P., Morales, M., Gonzalez-Carreno, T., Veintemillas-Verdaguer, S., Serna, C. Advances in magnetic nanoparticles for biotechnology applications. *J. Magn. Magn. Mater.* 290, 28–34, 2005.
8. Murad, E. Properties and behavior of iron oxides as determined by Mössbauer spectroscopy. *Iron in Soils and Clay Minerals*. Springer, Netherlands, 309–350, 1988.

9. Meisen, U., Kathrein, H. The influence of particle size, shape and particle size distribution on properties of magnetites for the production of toners, NIP & Digital Fabrication Conference. *Soc. Imag. Sc. Techn.* 556–560, 1999.
10. Morin, F. Magnetic susceptibility of α-Fe_2O_3 and α-Fe_2O_3 with added titanium. *Phys. Rev.* 78, 819, 1950.
11. Kündig, W., Bömmel, H., Constabaris, G., Lindquist, R. Some properties of supported small α-Fe_2O_3 particles determined with the Mössbauer effect. *Phys. Rev.* 142, 327, 1966.
12. Muench, G., Arajs, S., Matijević, E. The morin transition in small α-Fe_2O_3 particles. *Phys. Status Solidi* (a) 92, 187–192, 1985.
13. Peng, H.-P., Liang, R.-P., Qiu, J.-D. Facile synthesis of Fe_3O_4–Al_2O_3 core–shell nanoparticles and their application to the highly specific capture of heme proteins for direct electrochemistry. *Biosens. Bioelectron.* 26, 3005–3011, 2011.
14. Verwey, E., Haayman, P. Electronic conductivity and transition point of magnetite ("Fe_3O_4"), *Phys.* 8, 979–987, 1941.
15. Zhang, Z., Kong, J. Novel magnetic Fe_3O_4-C nanoparticles as adsorbents for removal of organic dyes from aqueous solution. *J. Hazard. Mater.* 193, 325–329, 2011.
16. Sadat, M., Patel, R., Sookoor, J., Bud'ko, S.L., Ewing, R.C., Zhang, J., Xu, H., Wang, Y., Pauletti, G.M., Mast, D.B. Effect of spatial confinement on magnetic hyperthermia via dipolar interactions in Fe_3O_4 nanoparticles for biomedical applications. *Mater. Sci. Eng.* C 42, 52–63, 2014.
17. Shen, T., Weissleder, R., Papisov, M., Bogdanov, A., Brady, T.J. Monocrystalline iron oxide nanocompounds (MION): physicochemical properties. *Magn. Res. Med.* 29, 599–604, 1993.
18. Majewski, P., Thierry, B. Superparamagnetic magnetite (Fe_3O_4) nanoparticles for bio-applications. *Recent Patents Mater. Sci.* 1, 116–127, 2008.
19. Cobley, C.M., Skrabalak, S.E., Campbell, D.J., Xia, Y. Shape-controlled synthesis of silver nanoparticles for plasmonic and sensing applications. *Plasmonics* 4, 171–179, 2009.
20. Pankhurst, Q.A., Connolly, J., Jones, S., Dobson, J. Applications of magnetic nanoparticles in biomedicine. *J. Phys. D: App. Phys.* 36, 167, 2003.
21. Rishton, S., Lu, Y., Altman, R., Marley, A., Bian, X., Jahnes, C., Viswanathan, R., Xiao, G., Gallagher, W., Parkin, S. Magnetic tunnel junctions fabricated at tenth-micron dimensions by electron beam lithography. *Microelectron. Eng.* 35, 249–252, 1997.
22. Reddy, L.H., Arias, J.L., Nicolas, J., Couvreur, P. Magnetic nanoparticles: design and characterization, toxicity and biocompatibility, pharmaceutical and biomedical applications. *Chem. Rev.* 112, 5818–5878, 2012.
23. Amemiya, Y., Arakaki, A., Staniland, S.S., Tanaka, T., Matsunaga, T. Controlled formation of magnetite crystal by partial oxidation of ferrous hydroxide in the presence of recombinant magnetotactic bacterial protein Mms6. *Biomaterials.* 28, 5381–5389, 2007.

24. Da Costa, G., De Grave, E., De Bakker, P., Vandenberghe, R.E. Synthesis and characterization of some iron oxides by sol-gel method. *J. Solid State Chem.* 113, 405–412, 1994.
25. Massart, R. Preparation of aqueous magnetic liquids in alkaline and acidic media. *IEEE Trans. Magn.* 17, 1247–1248, 1981.
26. Chueh, Y.L., Lai, M.W., Liang, J.Q., Chou, L.J., Wang, Z.L. Systematic study of the growth of aligned arrays of α-Fe_2O_3 and Fe_3O_4 nanowires by a vapor–solid process. *Adv. Fun. Mater.* 16, 2243–2251, 2006.
27. Liu, X., Guo, Y., Wang, Y., Ren, J., Wang, Y., Guo, Y., Guo, Y., Lu, G., Wang, Y., Zhang, Z. Direct synthesis of mesoporous Fe_3O_4 through citric acid-assisted solid thermal decomposition. *J. Mater. Sci.* 45, 906, 2010.
28. Chen, F., Gao, Q., Hong, G., Ni, J. Synthesis and characterization of magnetite dodecahedron nanostructure by hydrothermal method. *J. Magn. Magn. Mater.* 320, 1775–1780, 2008.
29. Salazar-Alvarez, G., Muhammed, M., Zagorodni, A.A. Novel flow injection synthesis of iron oxide nanoparticles with narrow size distribution. *Chem. Eng. Sci.* 61, 4625–4633, 2006.
30. Li, Y., Jiang, R., Liu, T., Lv, H., Zhou, L., Zhang, X. One-pot synthesis of grass-like Fe_3O_4 nanostructures by a novel microemulsion-assisted solvothermal method. *Ceram. Int.* 40, 1059–1063, 2014.
31. Strobel, R., Pratsinis, S.E. Direct synthesis of maghemite, magnetite and wustite nanoparticles by flame spray pyrolysis. *Adv. Powder Technol.* 20, 190–194, 2009.
32. Cabrera, L., Gutierrez, S., Menendez, N., Morales, M., Herrasti, P. Magnetite nanoparticles: electrochemical synthesis and characterization. *Electrochim. Acta.* 53, 3436–3441, 2008.
33. Dang, F., Enomoto, N., Hojo, J., Enpuku, K. Sonochemical synthesis of monodispersed magnetite nanoparticles by using an ethanol–water mixed solvent. *Ultrason. Sonochem.* 16, 649–654, 2009.
34. Lawaczeck, R., Menzel, M., Pietsch, H. Superparamagnetic iron oxide particles: contrast media for magnetic resonance imaging. *Appl. Organomet. Chem.* 18, 506–513, 2004.
35. Bulte, J.W., Kraitchman, D.L. Iron oxide MR contrast agents for molecular and cellular imaging. NMR in *Biomed.* 17, 484–499, 2004.
36. Berry, C.C., Curtis, A.S. Functionalisation of magnetic nanoparticles for applications in biomedicine. *J. Phys. D: Appl. Phys.* 36, 198, 2003.
37. Elliott, D.W., Zhang, W.-X. Field assessment of nanoscale bimetallic particles for groundwater treatment. *Environ. Sci. Technol.* 35, 4922–4926, 2001.
38. Mahmoudi, M., Stroeve, P., Milani, A.S., Arbab, A.S. Superparamagnetic iron oxide nanoparticles: *Synthesis, Surface Engineering, Cytotoxicity and Biomedical Applications*. Nova Science Publishers, Inc. 2011.
39. Tartaj, P., Veintemillas-Verdaguer, S., Serna, C.J. The preparation of magnetic nanoparticles for applications in biomedicine. *J. Phys. D: Appl. Phys.* 36, 182, 2003.

40. Shinkai, M. Functional magnetic particles for medical application. *J. Biosci. Bioeng.* 94, 606–613, 2002.
41. Damadian, R. Tumor detection by nuclear magnetic resonance. *Science*, 171(3976), 1151–1153, 1971.
42. Damadian, R. Apparatus and method for detecting cancer in tissue. *Google Patents*, 1974.
43. Casula, M.F., Floris, P., Innocenti, C., Lascialfari, A., Marinone, M., Corti, M., Sperling, R.A., Parak, W.J., Sangregorio, C. Magnetic resonance imaging contrast agents based on iron oxide superparamagnetic ferrofluids. *Chem. Mater.* 22, 1739–1748, 2010.
44. Umut, E., Pineider, F., Arosio, P., Sangregorio, C., Corti, M., Tabak, F., Lascialfari, A., Ghigna, P. Magnetic, optical and relaxometric properties of organically coated gold–magnetite (Au–Fe_2O_3) hybrid nanoparticles for potential use in biomedical applications. *J. Magn. Magn. Mater.* 324, 2373–2379, 2012.
45. Pollacco, D.A., Magnetic resonance imaging, BSc Maths and Physics University of Malta. 1–11, 2016.
46. Mulder, W.J., Strijkers, G.J., Briley-Saboe, K.C., Frias, J.C., Aguinaldo, J.G.S., Vucic, E., Amirbekian, V., Tang, C., Chin, P.T., Nicolay, K. Molecular imaging of macrophages in atherosclerotic plaques using bimodal PEG-micelles. *Magn. Reson. Med.* 58, 1164–1170, 2007.
47. Endres, P.J., Paunesku, T., Vogt, S., Meade, T.J., Woloschak, G.E. DNA–TiO_2 nanoconjugates labeled with magnetic resonance contrast agents. *J. Am. Chem. Soc.* 129, 15760–15761, 2007.
48. Bridot, J.-L., Faure, A.-C., Laurent, S., Rivière, C., Billotey, C., Hiba, B., Janier, M., Josserand, V., Coll, J.-L., Elst, V.L. Hybrid gadolinium oxide nanoparticles: multimodal contrast agents for *in vivo* imaging. *J. Am. Chem. Soc.* 129, 5076–5084, 2007.
49. Chen, X., Pan, H., Liu, H., Du, M. Nonenzymatic glucose sensor based on flower-shaped Au@ Pd core–shell nanoparticles–ionic liquids composite film modified glassy carbon electrodes. *Electrochim. Acta.* 56, 636–643, 2010.
50. Torchilin, V.P. PEG-based micelles as carriers of contrast agents for different imaging modalities. *Adv. Drug Delivery Rev.*54, 235–252, 2002.
51. Li, Z., Zhang, Y., Jiang, S. Multicolor core/shell-structured upconversion fluorescent nanoparticles. *Adv. Mater.* 20, 4765–4769, 2008.
52. Rodrigues, J., Santos-Magalhaes, N., Coelho, L., Couvreur, P., Ponchel, G., Gref, R. Novel core (polyester)-shell (polysaccharide) nanoparticles: protein loading and surface modification with lectins. *J. Controlled Release.* 92, 103–112, 2003.
53. Kim, J.H., Randall Lee, T. Discrete thermally responsive hydrogel-coated gold nanoparticles for use as drug-delivery vehicles. *Drug Dev. Res.* 67, 61–69, 2006.
54. Sahiner, N., Ilgin, P. Synthesis and characterization of soft polymeric nanoparticles and composites with tunable properties. *J. Polym. Sci. A: Polym. Chem.* 48, 5239–5246, 2010.

55. Vuong, Q.L., Van Doorslaer, S., Bridot, J.-L., Argante, C., Alejandro, G., Hermann, R., Disch, S., Mattea, C., Stapf, S., Gossuin, Y. Paramagnetic nanoparticles as potential MRI contrast agents: characterization, NMR relaxation, simulations and theory. *Magn. Reson. Mater. Phys. Biol. Med.* 25, 467–478, 2012.
56. Sharma, P., Brown, S., Walter, G., Santra, S., Moudgil, B. Nanoparticles for bioimaging. *Adv. Colloid Interface Sci.* 123, 471–485, 2006.
57. Yang, F., Li, Y., Chen, Z., Zhang, Y., Wu, J., Gu, N. Superparamagnetic iron oxide nanoparticle-embedded encapsulated microbubbles as dual contrast agents of magnetic resonance and ultrasound imaging. *Biomaterials.* 30, 3882–3890, 2009.
58. Wu, B., Yin, J., Texier, C., Roussel, M., Tan, K.S.-W. Blastocystis legumain is localized on the cell surface, and specific inhibition of its activity implicates a pro-survival role for the enzyme. *J. Biol. Chem.* 285, 1790–1798, 2010.
59. Briley-Saebo, K., Bjørnerud, A., Grant, D., Ahlstrom, H., Berg, T., Kindberg, G.M. Hepatic cellular distribution and degradation of iron oxide nanoparticles following single intravenous injection in rats: implications for magnetic resonance imaging. *Cell Tissue Res.* 316, 315–323, 2004.
60. Plank, C. Nanomedicine: silence the target. *Nat. Nanotechnol.* 4(9), 544–545, 2009.
61. Sun, C., Lee, J.S., Zhang, M. Magnetic nanoparticles in MR imaging and drug delivery. *Adv. Drug Delivery Rev.* 60, 1252–1265, 2008.
62. Thomas, L.A., Dekker, L., Kallumadil, M., Southern, P., Wilson, M., Nair, S.P., Pankhurst, Q.A., Parkin, I.P. Carboxylic acid-stabilised iron oxide nanoparticles for use in magnetic hyperthermia. *J. Mater. Chem.* 19, 6529–6535, 2009.
63. Prasad, N., Rathinasamy, K., Panda, D., Bahadur, D. Mechanism of cell death induced by magnetic hyperthermia with nanoparticles of γ-$Mn_xFe_{2-x}O_3$ synthesized by a single step process. *J. Mater. Chem.* 17, 5042–5051, 2007.
64. Plank, C., Anton, M., Rudolph, C., Rosenecker, J., Krötz, F. Enhancing and targeting nucleic acid delivery by magnetic force. *Exp. Opin. Biol. Ther.* 3, 745–758, 2003.

8

The Importance of Screening Information Data Set in Nanotechnology

Khan Ameera Bibi, Suruj Gitesh and Shalini Singh*

Department of Operations and Quality, Durban University of Technology, Durban, South Africa

Abstract

Screening Information Data Set (SIDS) conducted by the Organization for Economic Co-operation and Development (OECD) is an initial screening or risk assessment of a chemical or substance manufactured in high volumes. Engineered nanoparticles (ENPs) have not been put on the SIDS list for evaluation as it is not considered a high production volume substance. Yet, ENPs are man-made substances, just like lead, gasoline, asbestos, and polychlorinated biphenyls (PCBs). Experience shows that chemicals that have not undergone extensive risk assessment and are used by consumers are harmful to fauna and flora. Products such as sunscreen and beauty cosmetics, among others, contain nano-enhanced particles that are already being sold to, and are being used by consumers globally. This chapter aimed to show the need for ENPs to be placed on the SIDS list. The objectives of this chapter are to define the potential risks of using ENPs, to review risk assessment already conducted on other man-made harmful substances, and conduct comparative analysis between them to show the need for this technology to be on the SIDS list. ENP's (nanosilver and multi-walled carbon nanotubes) behavior and interaction are not completely understood and are shown to be harmful; however, they are still manufactured and used in products. There are alarming similarities between asbestos and mutli-walled carbon nanotubes. Thus, ENPs should be included onto the SIDS list despite that it may not be manufactured or imported in excess of 1000 tons per annum. This minimum requirement for SIDS qualification should therefore be re-evaluated in the case of ENPs, due to its exceptionally small size.

**Corresponding author*: shalinis@dut.ac.za

Suvardhan Kanchi, Shakeel Ahmed, Myalowenkosi I. Sabela and Chaudhery Mustansar Hussain (eds.) Nanomaterials: Biomedical, Environmental, and Engineering Applications, (197–216)

Keywords: Engineered nanoparticles, screening information data set, risk assessment, nano-enhanced silver preservatives

8.1 Introduction

Balbus *et al.*, [1] define nanotechnology as the design and manipulation of materials on a molecular and atomic scale with nanoparticles (NPs) at 100 nanometers or less in size. Stern and McNeil [2] categorize NPs as either being incidental or engineered depending on its origin. Stern and McNeil [2] cite Barregard *et al.*, (2006), Chang *et al.*, (2004), and Fang *et al.*, (2005), who concluded that incidental NPs can be present in wood smoke (particles generated in forest fires) and automobile furnace exhausts (diesel exhaust particles). This points to the notion that humans have been exposed to NPs in their everyday environment for centuries without knowing or understanding their presence or impact, if any engineered nanoparticles (ENPs) on the other hand are manmade substances, manufactured for its unique attributes which allow for a variety of potential uses. These substances are presently applied in the manufacturing process of many common household items. Schmidt [3] stated that roughly over 2000 nano-materials were in use or development in the year 2009.

ENPs are manmade materials and are commonly seen as nanotubes, dendrimers, and quantum dots. Lam *et al.*, [4] suggests that ENPs can be generated to exploit their size-related properties. For example, carbon nanotubes (CNTs) are ENPs that have thermal and electrical properties, and are lightweight with a high tensile strength expected to be 100 times stronger than steel.

Drawing on Schmidt [3], NPs have unique physical properties that can influence their uptake, distribution, and behavior in the body. Another school of thought from Balbus *et al.*, [1] is that ENPs have the potential to deliver numerous benefits to the society and science, and may also have the potential to inflict harm, due to their inherent ability to damage skin, brain, lung tissue, and to be mobile and persistent in the environment. This brings to the fore Kane and Hurt [5], Ribak and Ribak [6], and Langer [7] studies, which show that certain manmade chemicals such as asbestos, that did not undergo extensive risk assessment (RA) before being used by consumers, were later discovered to inflict irreversible harm. Studies that were comparatively analyzed by Kane and Hurt [5] of multi-walled (MW) CNTs directly injected into the abdominal cavities of mice showed that both studies produced inflammation and granulomas (nodular lesions) and early fibrosis. Acknowledging that these results are similar to those produced by long fibers of brown asbestos (amosite), of concern is the extent of the current use ENPs in products to enhance their performance and effectiveness. According to Schmidt [3], products such as sunscreen and beauty cosmetics contain nano-enhanced silver preservatives that are already being sold to, and are used by consumers globally. He is of the view that conducting risk assessment of ENPs is becoming more important and relevant, especially since an estimated 2000 nano-materials are in commercial use today.

It is against this backdrop that this chapter will outline a type of risk assessment that can be conducted on chemicals or substances called Screening Information Data Set (SIDS). Gelbke *et al.,* [8] affirms that Organization for Economic Co-operation and Development [9] defines SIDS as a type of risk assessment designed to collect information on high production volume (HPV) substances.

Initiated in 1993 as a cooperative effort by OECD countries and industry, SIDS was designed to include information on the identity of each chemical, uses, sources, and extent of exposure; physical and chemical properties; environmental fate; and certain limited toxicity data for humans and the environment. Drawing on Gelbke *et al.,* [8], SIDS is regarded as the minimum information needed to assess whether a HPV chemical should be further evaluated. SIDS is an initial screening process that is conducted by the OECD on chemicals or substances that are manufactured or imported in quantities of more than 1000 tons per year. This would qualify as a HPV substance, and it would immediately be picked up as a substance [8, 9] have been corrected...other references have been checked they are fine as is as they directly reference the author that requires risk assessment by the OECD. A SIDS list is a register of chemicals or substances that have undergone extensive risk assessment. This list is available on the Environmental Protection Agency (EPA) website.

Stern and McNeil [2] describe ENPs as having at least one dimension at 100 nanometers or less. Due to the significantly small size of ENPs, a few grams of engineered nanoparticles are extremely concentrated or dense. Therefore, used ENPs are added in comparatively small ratios to its bulk material.

Referring to the work by Gelbke *et al.,* [8], SIDS was designed to include information on the identity of each chemical, its uses, sources, and extent of exposure; physical and chemical properties; environmental fate; and certain limited toxicity data for humans and the environment. It is regarded as the minimum information needed to assess whether or not HPV chemicals should be further evaluated. It can be inferred that including ENPs on SIDS will provide the necessary understanding for its handling, use, and disposal.

The minimum data necessary for evaluation within the SIDS guidelines as explained by Gelbke *et al.,* [8] can be summarized as follows: environmental fate (photo-degradation, stability in water, transport, and distribution between environmental compartments including distribution pathways, and aerobic biodegradability), environmental toxicology (fish, daphnia, algae, and in some cases terrestrial organisms), mammalian toxicology (acute and repeat dose toxicity by the most relevant route of exposure, point mutation and chromosomal aberration genetic toxicity, developmental toxicity, and reproductive toxicity), and any available data on human exposure, skin irritation, eye irritation, and sensitization or other relevant information should also be included.

Drawing on the information above, SIDS can be used by any organization as a guideline within a production or manufacturing environment. Understanding the uses and handling requirements for any substance, ENP can ensure the safety of the employees when using the substance, acknowledging that this will also influence the manner in which it is treated or disposed of after being used, thereby possibly preventing possible negative impacts on the environment and humans.

Some ENPs such as carbon nanotubes (CNTs) and nanosilver have displayed significant pulmonary toxicity to humans [2]. Stern and McNeil [2] cite the work by Thomas *et al.,* (2006) who believed that exposure to NPs could occur during their development, manufacture, use, or following disposal. Thus, the health and safety of those who manufacture, handle, store, and use ENPs can be open to potential harm. The challenge lies in that ENPs have not undergone extensive risk assessment but are currently being used to manufacture products. In spite of this, ENPs have not been put onto the SIDS list as it is not considered to be a high production volume substance because it is not produced or exported in excess of 1000 tons per annum.

The aim of the chapter is to ascertain the importance of including ENMs onto the SIDS register. This will be accomplished by presenting the intention of the register and highlighting the reasons for suggesting the inclusion ENPs on it. The risks associated with the manufacture, handling, storage, and use of nano-engineered materials established through the literature review will be presented. Furthermore, a comparative analysis highlighting the similarities between a previously known harmful substance and ENPs will be undertaken.

The rationale for qualification of ENMs, onto the SIDS register for risk assessment, should not only be quantity as is with other materials. Recognizing the unknown properties of ENMS, the criteria on inclusion should be based on other important factors such as unknown behavior, novelty with regard to its extremely unique characteristics, and significant potential uses and its significantly small size. Failure to do so is of great concern as these ENPs are not included onto the SIDs register and are already widely used in manufacturing of "improved" and novel products.

The motivation of this chapter is that there is currently minimal information available to understand the effects of using ENPs. It is hoped that this chapter fills the dearth in the literature by bringing to the fore the importance of SIDS in nanotechnology.

8.2 Review of the Literature

It is highly probable that the production of ENPs is a fast-growing industry and likewise it can be assumed that its production volume has increased exponentially since 2009. However, studies show that ENPs have the potential to be harmful to humans when it comes into direct contact with skin and when inhaled. It may therefore be imperative to conduct risk assessment analysis as an indication of the potential risk so that steps can be taken to mitigate the identified risk. This chapter will look at CNTs and nanosilver's potential environmental and biological impact, and conduct a comparative analysis of asbestos to carbon nanotubes and show the significance of exhaustive risk assessment that still needs to be conducted on ENPs.

8.2.1 Carbon Nanotubes

The differentiation between naturally occurring NPs and ENPs, according to Schmidt [3], is that ENPs are manmade materials that have uniformly identical shapes including spheres, tubes, wires, rings, and planes, whereas NPs do not. One such example of ENPs is CNTs. It has a cylindrical structure, such as that of a tube. These crystalline carbon structures are extremely unique. Lam *et al.*, [4] stated that CNTs are light weight and have the strongest tensile strength of any synthetic fiber and that some forms of CNTs can conduct electricity better than copper. These observations are consistent with Ema *et al.*, [10] who reported that there was growing development for CNT use in electronics, magnetics, biomedicine, pharmaceuticals, cosmetics, energy, and catalytic and environmental detection and monitoring. However, Lam *et al.*, [4] stated that CNT production was still used at a small scale in 2003.

Murashov *et al.*, [11] stated that ENPs can be further differentiated into second-generation nano-materials or active nano-materials. ENPs that react to a stimulus external to themselves are active nano-materials. The distinguishing feature of active nano-materials from other nano-materials is that their properties change or evolve during their functional operation in response to a stimulus or signal external to themselves. Of concern, it is believed that its intended and unintended reactions to the external environment can result in variable and potentially unstable behavior.

Muller *et al.*, [12] stated that Maynard *et al.*, (2004) observed that when handlers were gentle during the synthesis of the CNTs, it reduced the risk of particles becoming airborne and losses of this expensive material were minimized. These facilities had implemented exceptional industrial hygiene measures. As expected, the airborne concentrations of CNTs in these work environments were found to be low at 53 $\mu g/m^2$. Lam *et al.*, [4] cited the work by Bearden (2003) who predicted that huge amounts of CNTs would be produced in the years to follow. Correspondingly, he suggested that such a large production volume would involve a very large work force, and that many workers would likely be exposed during CNT synthesis, post-synthetic material collection, handling, purification, and packaging. Furthermore, the occupational risk of exposure of a worker will be directly associated with the different phases at which the product is handled.

Stern and McNeil [2] cite the work by Thomas *et al.*, (2006) who also caution that exposure to ENPs could occur during their development, manufacture, use, or following disposal. Thus, they further emphasized that the lack of exposure data available versus the considerable consumer products that are present in the market suggests that significant research is needed. Also cited, Bailey (1994) proposed the possibility that inhalation is a likely route of NP exposure as they can travel significant distances in air by Brownian diffusion, are respirable, and can deposit within the alveolar region of the lung.

It can be gleaned from the above literature that ENPs' behavior has not been explored to its full depth. The fact that it is easily dispersed implies that it has a potential to be hazardous during manufacturing and handling. Without the proper risk assessment and guidelines, there is very little assurance for the health and safety of those exposed to ENPs during manufacturing, handling, storage, and use. It is even more alarming to note that CNTs behavior can be likened to asbestos. They are both easily diffused in air, exceptionally small in size, and are persistent in the environment as they do not breakdown easily. There is a notion that CNTs' harmful effects may not be easily reversible due to its small particle size that can penetrate the respiratory system.

8.2.2 Nanosilver

A further example of ENPs is silver NPs, which are often referred to as nanosilver. Nanosilver can be manufactured in various sizes and shapes such as nanosilver spheres, rods, wires, and plates depending on the method used to produce it. Nanosilver may be in colloidal form, dissolved in water, or as a suspension. Table 8.1 shows the different forms of silver as well as their approximate size and charge. Stebounova *et al.*, [13] note that nanosilver is used in a variety of applications and is known to have antimicrobial properties. They also recognize that nanosilver is used in the treatment of burns, wounds, air disinfection, and as the coating on textiles. By contrast, Bar-Ilan *et al.*, [14] found that nanosilver is toxic and can be harmful to health and furthermore have biological effects. Concomitantly, there is a need to ensure that the effect of exposure to nanosilver on the environment and humans is understood [15].

8.2.3 Carbon Nanotubes vs. Asbestos

Asbestos was known to be an innovative substance in the 19th century. It was widely used in the manufacture of various heat-resistant materials and fabrics as a constituent of asbestos cement and insulation and

Table 8.1 Forms of silver and approximate size and charge (adapted from [16]).

Type of silver	Approximate size	Attributes
Elemental/metallic (single atom)	0.288 nm	Not found normally as in single atom; normally found as an aggregate; has no oxidation number
Silver ion	0.258 nm	Toxic may dissolve in water
Nanosilver	1–100 nm	May release ions/may be toxic on its own
Colloidal	1–1000 nm	Mixture of different size particles, suspended in fluid, may have nano-particulate silver, or silver ions or both
Inorganic silver compounds	–	Not easily dissolved, can be nanosized
Organic compounds	–	Covalent, most impossible to dissolve

friction products. Asbestos can be characterized as fine flexible fibers that occur naturally in nature and has a high thermal stability and high tensile strength. An asbestos fiber was defined as a particle that is greater than 5 micrometers, and less than 100 micrometers, with an aspect ratio (length to width of 3:1 or greater). The standard for exposure to asbestos in air was set at 5 fibers per mm [7].

According to Ribak and Ribak [6], asbestos, which was widely used in industries and in commercial products, became a health hazard as it was found to cause chronic lung illnesses and cancer in humans [5]. Studies on the effects of historical exposure of asbestos to humans from three different factories have shown on average a 17.2% mortality rate. Furthermore, grunerite asbestos (amosite) has been shown to cause lung cancer in epidemiological and experimental animal studies.

According to Kane and Hurt [5], the nanotube and asbestos analogy have several points of material similarity, such as long length and chemical stability in physiological environments (bio persistence), and a small fiber diameter. There are also properties that differentiate these materials, such as their chemical composition and surface properties.

Kane and Hurt [5], Langer [7], and Ribak and Ribak [6] advocate that risk assessment for asbestos was not conducted adequately, if at all, by any independent governing bodies, organizations, or companies. For decades it was mined, stored, handled, and used within its many end products. In-depth analysis was not conducted on asbestos particles before the fatal consequences of its use were discovered. The biological and toxicological effects of asbestos's microscopic airborne particles on humans and animals, exposure during mining, storage, handling, and use were not taken into account. Ribak and Ribak [6] reported that its consequences led to hundreds of thousands of workers developing chronic respiratory diseases by the 1970s. The first National Asbestos Standard (NAS) was circulated in the United States through the Occupational Health and Safety Administration (OSHA) in 1972. The protocols and techniques in the NAS were found to be inadequate by the Food and Drug Administration (FDA). This was mainly attributed to the nature of the substance, with its morphological characteristics. The testing and verification were imperative in order to use these protocols within mines to determine asbestos pollution levels. In 1976, the EPA found that the OSHA's protocol was limited for its purpose after studies for asbestos pollution were conducted. This prompted the asbestos standard to be modified [10]. It is highly unfortunate that all this work was prompted by the realization that asbestos is extremely harmful and fatal to humans. This was only realized in the 20th century after being used for over a decade [6].

By comparative analyses, Kane and Hurt [5] found that multi-walled CNTs directly injected into the abdominal cavities of mice produced inflammation and granulomas (nodular lesions) and early fibrosis. These results were similar to those produced by long fibers of brown asbestos (amosite).

There is an incomplete understanding of ENPs in the literature and thus highlights the need for in-depth toxicology and investigation on CNTs and nanosilver, to provide for a better understanding of the ENPs toxicity with regard to its potential environmental and biological impact. It is evident from the literature that the similarities between these ENPs and asbestos leave room for potential health and safety risks. It provides adequate basis for concern and the need for in-depth risk assessment, such as SIDS.

8.2.4 Density

According to Sang [17], density is a macroscopic property of matter portraying how concentrated the matter is. Density is calculated as the mass of a material divided by its volume. Due to the significantly small size of ENPs, a few grams of ENPs are extremely concentrated or dense. Therefore, when used in bulk materials, ENPs are added in comparatively small ratios to the bulk material. It is therefore important that ENPs not be assessed for acceptance to SIDS as other bulk materials t based on volume but rather on surface area.

8.2.5 Risk Assessment

Sang [17] is of the view that conducting risk assessment of ENPs is becoming more important and relevant, especially since an estimated 2000 nanomaterials are in commercial use. Stern and McNeil [2] define risk assessment as being the estimation of the potential for exposure and characterization of hazard.

The Department of Engineering Health and Safety Risk Assessment [18] instructs that the following procedure should be carried out for any risk assessment conducted:

- Identify the hazards associated with a procedure and consider who may be exposed and what the maximum possible exposure to that hazard is. Include storage waste, disposal, and cleaning, if appropriate.
- List existing control measures
- Consider emergency procedures (including first aid)
- If further control measures are required, list and set actions.

8.2.6 Using SIDS as a Risk Assessment Tool for ENPs

A lack of understanding surrounding exposure of CNTs and nanosilver to humans and the environment can cause manufacturers to neglect the use of safe procedures. This was highlighted by Schmidt [3] who stated that there is a greater chance of producing something uniformly dangerous when particles with precise characteristics are engineered. Resonating from this, although ENPs may have many novel attributes, it can also create more novel problems than it can solve if used without a complete understanding.

Previously known harmful substances that have caused devastating long-term effects after being used worldwide within vast arrays of applications have been critiqued against ENPs. Global guidelines for risk assessment (SIDS) were evaluated.

Data discussed was collected from articles obtained from peer-reviewed journals.

8.3 Behavioral Patterns of Engineered Nanoparticles

ENP behavior and interaction between humans, animals, and the environment is not completely understood. The extensive biological and toxicological testing and research, together with the necessary health and safety protocols and guidelines for those exposed to ENPs during manufacturing, handling, storage, and use, has been partially or not been conducted. Yet, existing test results from several independent studies provide conflicting opinions and schools of thought. Sterna and McNeil [2] believe that humans have been exposed to NPs in their everyday environment for centuries without knowing or understanding their presence or impact, if any. Balbus *et al.*, [1], by contrast, believe that ENPs have the potential to deliver numerous benefits to the society and science. They may also have the potential to inflict harm due to their inherent ability to damage skin, brain, lung tissue, and to be mobile and persistent in the environment. Kane and Hurt [5] are of the same opinion due to the analysis of independent studies conducted on laboratory mice (Table 8.2). They showed strikingly similar characteristics and behavior found between asbestos and ENPs, in particular MWCNTs.

The ENPs (MWCNTs) proved to be harmful in laboratory tests conducted on mice when injected into the abdominal cavity, which produced inflammation, granulomas, and early fibrosis. These results are similar to that of asbestos causing severe lung damage leading to chronic illness or cancer.

Table 8.2 Comparative analysis of engineered nanoparticles and asbestos.

	Nano-engineered particles	**Asbestos**
Size	Microscopic, 100 micrometers or less	Microscopic between 5 and 100 micrometers
Benefits	High tensile strength, thermal, and electrical properties	Heat-resistant properties
Likely forms of exposure	Skin penetration Inhalation	Inhalation
Possible effects of exposure	Unknown	Penetrates respiratory system
Occurrence	Synthetic and naturally occurring	Naturally occurring
Concerns	ENPs (MWCNTs) proven to be harmful in laboratory tests conducted on mice when injected into the abdominal cavity, which produced inflammation, granulomas, and early fibrosis. These results are similar to that of asbestos.	Severe lung damage leading to chronic illness or cancer.

With current research and technology available, the oversights that were made during the 19th century with asbestos should not repeat itself. In fact, more caution should be taken with ENPs, considering the long-term consequences of not understanding the effects of asbestos before exposure to the substance, and the frightening similarities found between asbestos behavior and MWCNTs behavior in mice. The rush to commercialize ENPs within everyday products and exploit their inherent size-related properties may lead to the same downfall as experienced with asbestos.

8.3.1 Products Containing Nanosilver

The project on emerging nanotechnologies is an online inventory site that contains a list of manufactured goods that contain nano-materials. The use of nano-materials is growing and this is evident from the Woodrow Wilson database, which has increased from 54 in 2005 to 1628 in 2013 [19]. One of the most widely used nano-materials is nanosilver due to its antibacterial properties. It has been used in textiles, shoes, and electronics, among others. Table 8.3 illustrates the categories, examples of consumer products containing nanosilver, and the types of exposure routes.

Table 8.3 Products containing nanosilver with subcategories and routes of exposure (adapted from [16] and [20]).

Categories	Subcategories	Examples	Exposure route
Personal care and cosmetics	Skin care Oral hygiene Hair care Cleaning Coating Baby care	Cream, hand sanitizer Tooth brush, toothpaste Hair brush, hair musk Elimination wipes and spray Watch chain Pacifier, teeth developer	Dermal and oral
Textile and shoes	Clothing Other textiles	Socks, shirts, caps, fabrics Sheets, towels, shoe care	Dermal
Electronics	Personal care Household appliance Computer hardware Mobile devices	Wavers, irons, shavers Washing machine Keyboard, mouse Mobile phone	Dermal
Household products/ home improvement	Cleaning Coating Furnishing	Detergents, fabric softner Paint supplements Pillows	Inhalation, dermal
Filtration, purification, neutralization, sanitation	Filtration Cleaning	Air filters, ionic sticks Disinfectants and aerosol sprays	Inhalation,
Food and beverages	Cleaning Cooking utensils Coatings supplements	Sterilizing spray Cutting boards, baby bottle brush Storage bags and containers Silver particles in water	Inhalation, dermal and oral
Medical products	Breathing masks Wound dressing pharmaceuticals	Masks Band aids Coating on medical instruments	Inhalation, dermal and oral

8.3.2 Toxicity Effects of Nanosilver on Humans

The National Institute for Occupational Safety and Health (NIOSH) notes that products containing nano-materials such as nanocomposites, materials comprising nanostructures, and surface-coated materials are not likely to cause exposure risks during handling as these materials are non-inhalable in size [21]. During the production process, however, exposure might occur as cutting or grinding of the products may lead to the release of respirable-size nanoparticles. Additionally, engineered nanoparticles are difficult to characterize in terms of size, shape, and surface area as there is a lack of baseline information and the particles produced tend to be non-uniform leading to novel properties when compared to the bulk form of the material. Reportedly, the skin, the respiratory tract, and oral digestion have been identified as routes of exposure to nanosilver. A study conducted on a boy who had 30% of his body burnt and was treated with nanosilver-coated wound dressings presented argyia-like symptoms and liver toxicity. This was caused by the adsorption of nanosilver into the blood stream via skin pores leading to a build-up of silver, which led to toxic effects [22]. Burd *et al.*, [36] concur with Trop *et al.*, [22] that silver-based dressings show toxic effects where silver is passed into the blood stream from the silver dressing. A further example of adsorption through skin would be the application of face and hand creams at 0.8 g three times a day. Von Goetz [23] calculated that 4.5 μg silver/day is absorbed through the skin; yet the concentration at which it is said to have toxic effects on human is still to be determined. Based on the fact that nanoparticles have an element of non-uniformity in its particle size, the rate of adsorption that might occur via skin varies. It is shown by Larese *et al.*, [24] that skin proves to be an effective barrier against nanoparticles and showed penetration rates less than 0.01% for nanoparticle size of greater than 10 nm.

As stated previously, the respiratory tract is also mooted as a route of exposure to nanosilver. Ji *et al.*, [25] showed that inhaled 15 nm nanosilver particles resulted in the adsorption of nanosilver into the lungs and then into the systemic circulation of rats. Panyala *et al.*, [26] cited the work by Limbach *et al.*, (2007) and Sharma *et al.*, (2007) who showed that exposure to nanoparticles can induce oxidative stress in lung epithelial cells. It was further supported by Limbach *et al.*, (2007) that intensive catalytic activity caused toxic effects due to the greater surface area of the nanoparticle. Price *et al.*, [27] used mathematical models and deduced that nanoparticles smaller than 100 nm when inhaled will have 30% to 80% deposited into the respiratory tract. This is of concern because the nanosilver will get in the blood stream and have toxic effects on the lungs and may cause other disease-like symptoms such as argyia.

According to Wijnhoven *et al.*, [20], nanosilver is well renowned for its antimicrobial properties in curative and preventive medicine. They also mention that silver salts, silver complexes, and metallic silver are most widely used in pharmaceutical and homeopathic products. Nanosilver is used for controlling infections and is deposited or coated on medical

Table 8.4 Reported cases of over-the-counter colloidal medicine (adopted from [16]).

Preparation used	Disease treated	Observed effect
Silver-coated protein-containing vasoconstrictor	Allergic rhinitis	Sever argyria
Silver-containing nose drops over 2–3 years	Unknown	Death
Chronic administration of silver-containing nose drops	Unknown but possibly rhinitis	Sever argyria, silver deposits in liver, kidney, arteries, pituitary, and choroids plexus
Colloidal silver (homemade), used for 4 months	Prostate cancer	First irreversible neurological toxicity then coma and finally death
Silver nitrate	Tongue ulcers	Argyria, manic depression, died 6 years later from aortic aneurism
Unknown silver preparation for 18 years	Unknown	Arygria, died of cardiac failure, probably due to long-term silver consumption

devices or fabrics. However, according to Drake and Hazelwood [28], the human exposure of nanosilver is generally higher through the oral administration of medication as compared to exposure such as occupational inhalation of nanosilver. This is a concern as nanosilver is used predominately in the medical sector and is readily available to consumers even though there are various case studies highlighting the negative effects of nanosilver. Literature were reported on a few cases of people found suffering from argyia, using medication containing silver compounds (bulk) (Table 8.4).

The above literature shows that humans exposed to nanosilver may result in various health effects. It must be appreciated that the concentration and period of exposure need to be further investigated in order to determine more conclusive results on human exposure to nanosilver.

8.3.3 Toxicity Effects on the Environment

Silver particles in the nanoscale are not readily available in the environment. This is in accordance with Dos Santos [29] who explained that the

Table 8.5 Predicted silver in the environment in Europe (adopted from [16]).

Location of silver	Total amount of silver	Amount of biocidal silver
Natural waters	20–130 tons	20 tons
Terrestrial ecosystems	80–190 tons	29 tons

increased use of nanoparticles in consumer products is a concern for environmental regulators and consumer advocates as these nano-materials are expected to return to the environment via effluents, waste streams, and sewer lines. This is due to these materials being incorporated into filters, socks, pesticides, toothpaste, creams, and washing machines (refer to Table 8.2). These silver nanoparticles are said to be released from these products and returned to the terrestrial ecosystem, yet the transformation that the particles will undergo in the real world is still largely unknown due to the uncertainty of its chemical reactivity. This leads to the concern around the amount of silver expected to be released via the products (refer to Table 8.5).

A study by Hund-Rinke [30] revealed that a Samsung washing machine contained 10 g of silver-released silver ions into water via electrolysis. According to the manufacturer, 2.75 mg of silver ions are released but about half to a third remains in the textiles, leaving approximately 2 mg being drained into the sewage system. They also argued that it is difficult to calculate the contribution to the environment, though they calculate an estimated 12.2 kg silver being washed into the environment alone, which might not seem a lot but is from one manufacturer with one product only. Benn and Westerhoff [31] found that great amounts of nanosilver were lost from socks that contained the nanoparticle and estimated that more than half were dissolved into ionic silver. They further reported that these ions may eventually react with sulfur in the environment causing a harmful formation of silver sulfide. Raising concerns with the effect of an accumulation of silver sulfide in our water treatment systems, Limbach *et al.*, (2007) in Panyala [26] notes that the toxicity of silver in water is determined by the concentrations of silver ions, which is currently low in waste water treatment systems and the environment and could be due to silver forming strong bonds with chlorides and dissolved organic carbon. This is further supported by Zheng *et al.*, [32]. According to Benn and Westerhoff [31], 15% of the total silver released came from receiving outlets of textiles and plastics containing the NP with an estimated amount between 4 and 40 μg silver per liter. This raises further concerns of an accumulation of silver that may affect the bacteria that is present in waste water treatment plants. Senjen and Ian [16] quote Choi and Hu [2008] "The results of nanosilver toxicity to environmentally sensitive nitrifying micro-organisms suggest that stringent regulations of silver nanoparticles entering waste water treatment plants are necessary. Nitrifying micro-organisms involved in nitrification are critical to biological nutrient removal in modern waste water treatment." However, very little is known about the mobility or formations of agglomerates that may occur with nanosilver, thus leading to a need for further experimentation and investigation on the effects that nanosilver has on waste water. It is evident though that with the use of nanosilver being so prevalent in consumer products, a reservoir of silver ions could be released into the environment.

The literature further documents that nanosilver is harmful to aquatic life such as zebra fish, algae, and daphnia. Several studies showed the toxic effects that nanosilver has on aquatic life for instance Kennedy *et al.*, [33] showed that toxicity of $AgNO^3$ nanoparticles with different particle sizes from the range of 10–80 nm on daphnia for a 48 h period with concentrations 0.002–0.126 μg/ml had been detected in the embryos yielding abnormality. Furthermore, Wijnhoven *et al.*, [20] stated that the chemical form and availability of free silver ions from silver determines acute toxicity. They found that concentrations of 1–5 $\mu g\ l^{-1}$ are harmful to aquatic organisms and insects, while trout and flounder may be killed. Asharani *et al.*, [34] reported that nanosilver negatively impacted on daphnia and zebra fish mortality, caused delayed hatching, caused abnormal body axes, slowed blood flow, decreased heart rate, and led to growth retardation when being exposed to 5–20 nm diameter of silver nanoparticles with a capping agent. They also elaborated that different types of malformation such as edema, heart malformations, and defects were also seen. This is further supported by Powers *et al.*, [35]. Wijnhoven *et al.*, [20] suggested that further studies need to be conducted to better understand and characterize nanosilver by using higher doses, longer exposure periods, as well as various particle sizes.

It is evident that large amount of nanosilver is expected to be released into the environment, yet the true effects it might have is still not fully understood. It is also seen that nanosilver has detrimental effects on humans and aquatic life, which should be of concern to environmentalists, governments, regulators, as well as consumers.

Time should be taken to consider the possibility that ENPs may cause potential harm to those exposed to it directly and indirectly now that there is a better understanding of the consequences of breathing microscopic particles that can invade lung tissue and trigger immune responses within the body. In doing so, the necessary cautionary steps should be taken as is with any potentially hazardous material.

Substantial evidence has been presented that ENPs should undergo extensive risk assessment, most preferably through the SIDS program, even though it is not being produced and imported/exported over 1000 tons per annum. The inherently small size of ENPs and its correlating almost insubstantial weight will not allow it to qualify for the SIDS program, unless it is produced in extreme quantities. It should be understood that millions of ENPs can be found in a small dense area. The weight of ENPs should not determine if it is a high production volume substance; instead, the number of particles should be considered. It would be prudent to wait for ENPs to be produced in extreme quantities in order to conduct proper risk assessment.

8.4 Conclusions and Recommendations

It is evident from the literature available that ENPs' behavior and interaction is not completely understood; however, they are still being manufactured and used in products despite this fundamental lack of knowledge. Even with the reasonable doubts created from the alarming similarities between asbestos and MWCNTs, and various cases studies and experiments conducted using nanosilver, protocols and guidelines for its use and manufacture have not been implemented by the OECD, FDA, EPA, or other bodies. This is mainly due to the lack of consolidated and definite risk information on the biological and toxicological behavior of ENPs.

SIDS should therefore be implemented to fully explore and consolidate testing methods, results, and recommendations to create uniform protocols and guidelines for manufacturing and use of ENPs. The fundamental characteristic of ENPs that make them such novel innovative materials is its size; however, this is now its main drawback. ENPs should be included onto the SIDS list despite the fact that it may not be manufactured or imported in excess of 1000 tons per annum. This minimum requirement for SIDS qualification should therefore be overlooked in the case of ENPs, due to its exceptionally small size.

References

1. Balbus, J., Florini, K., Denison, R., Walsh, S. Getting nanotechnology right the first time. *Issues Sci. Technol.*, 21(4), 10, 2013.

2. Stern, S.T., McNeil, S.E. Nanotechnology safety concerns revisited. *Toxicol. Studies.*, 101(1), 4, 2008.
3. Schmidt, C.W. Nanotechnology-related environment, health, and safety research: Examining the national strategy. *Environ. Health Perspect.*, 117(4), 158, 2009.
4. Lam, C., James, J.T., McCluskey, R., Arepalli, S., Hunter, R.L. A review of carbon nanotube toxicity and assessment of potential occupational and environmental health risks. *Crit. Rev. Toxicol.*, 36, 189, 2006.
5. Kane, A.B., Hurt, R.H. Nanotoxicology: The asbestos analogy revisited. *Nat. Nanotechnol.*, 3, 378, 2008.
6. Ribak, J., Ribak, G. Human health effects associated with the commercial use of Grunerite asbestos (amosite). *Regul. Toxicol. Pharmacol.*, 52, 82, 2007.
7. Langer, M. Identification and enumeration of asbestos fibers in the mining environment: Mission and modification to the Federal Asbestos Standard. *Regul. Toxicol. Pharmacol.*, 52, 207, 2008.
8. Gelbke, H., Fleig, H., Meder, M. SIDS reprotoxicity screening test update: testing strategies and use. *Regul. Toxicol. Pharmacol.*, 39, 81, 2004.
9. OECD Secretariat: Manual for Investigation of High Production Volume Chemicals (online), 2007. Available at http://www.oecd.org/document/7/0,3343,en_2649_34379_1947463_1_1_1_1,00.html. (January 2015), 2007.
10. Ema, M., Matsuda, A., Kobayashi, N., Naya, M., Nakanishi, J. Evaluation of dermal eye irritation and skin sensitization due to carbon nanotubes. *Regul. Toxicol. Pharmacol.*, 61, 276, 2011.
11. Murashov, V., Schulte, P., Howard, J. Progression of occupational risk management with advances in nanomaterials. *J. Occup. Environ. Hyg.*, 9, 12, 2011.
12. Muller, J., Huaux, F., Moreau, N., Misson, P., Heilier, J., Delos, M., Arras, M., Fonseca, A., Nagy, J.B., Lison, D. Respiratory toxicity of multi-wall carbon nanotubes. *Toxicol. Appl. Pharmacol.*, 207, 221, 2005.
13. Stebounova, L.V., Dodd, A.A., Kim, J.S., Park, H., O'Shaughnessy, P.T., Grassian, V.H., Thorne, P.S. Nanosilver induces minimal lung toxicity or inflammation in a subacute murine inhalation model. *Part Fibre Toxicol.*, 8, 5, 2011.
14. Bar-Ilan, O., Albrecht, R.M., Fako, V.E., Fuegeson, D.Y. Toxicity assessments of multisized gold and silver nanoparticles in zebrafish embryos. *Small.*, 5(16), 189, 2009.
15. Warheit, D.B. How meaningful are the results of nanotoxicity studies in the absence of adequate material characterization. *Toxicol. Sci.*, 101(2), 183, 2008.
16. Senjen, R, *Nano and Biocidal Silver*: extreme germ killers present a growing threat to public health, This is a report by FoE Australia and FoE United States, 2009.
17. Sang, D. *Basic Physics: 1 and 2.* 1st edn. Cambridge: Press Syndicate, 1995.
18. Department of Engineering Health and Safety Risk Assessment Procedure (online). 2015. Available: http://safety.eng.cam.ac.uk/procedures/riskassessment/riskassessmentprocedure (21 August 2015).

19. Johari, S.A., Kalbassi, M.R., Soltani, M., Yu, I.J. Toxicity comparison of colloidal silver nanoparticles in various life stages of rainbow trout (Oncorhynchus mykiss). *Iran J. Fish Sci.,* 12(1), 2013.
20. Wijnhoven, S.W.P., Peijnenburg, W.J.G.M., Herberts, C.A., Hagens, W.I., Oomen, A.G., Heugens, E.H.W., Roszek, B., Bisschops, J., Gosens, L.M., van de, D., Dekkers, S., Jong, W., De Zijverden, M., Sips, Adrienne, J.A.M., Geertsma, R.E. Nanosilver: a review of available data and knowledge gaps in human and environmental risk assessment. *Nanotoxicology.,* (3), 109, 2009.
21. National Institute for Occupational Safety and Health. Approaches to safe nanotechnology managing the health and safety concerns associated with engineered nano materials (online). Available: http://www.cdc.gov/niosh/docs/2009-125/pdfs/2009-125.pdf. (June 2015), 2009.
22. Trop, M. Novak, M. Rodl, S. Helibom, B. Kroell, W., Goessler, W. Silver-coated dressing acticoat caused raised liver enzymes and argyia-like symptoms in burn patient. *J. Trauma.,* 60, 648, 2006.
23. Von Goetz, N., Fabricius, L., Glaus, R., Weitbrecht, V., Gunther, D., Hungerbuhler, K. Migration of silver from commercial plastic food containers and implications for consumer exposure assessment. *Food Addit. Contam. Part A.,* 23: 30(3), 612, 2013.
24. Larese, F.F., D'Agostin, F., Crosera, M., Renzi, N., Bovenzi, M., Adami, G. Human skin penetration of silver nanoparticles through intact and damaged skin. *Toxicology.,* 255, 233, 2009.
25. Ji, J.H., Jung, J.H., Kim, S.S., Yoon, J.U., Park, J.D., Choi, B.S., Chung, Y.H., Kwon, I.H., Joeng, J., Han, B.S., Shin, J.H., Song, K.S., Yu, I.J. Twenty-eight day inhalation toxicity study of silver nanoparticles in Spague–Dawley rats. *Inhal. Toxicol.,* 19, 857, 2007.
26. Panyala, N.R., Pene-Mendez, E.M., Havel, J. Silver or silver nanoparticles: hazardous threat to the environment and human health. *Appl. Biomed.,* 117, 2008.
27. Price, O.T., Asgharian, B., Miller, F.J., Cassee, F.R., de Winter-Sorkina, R. Multiple path particle dosimetry model (MPPD v1.0): A model for human and rat airway particle dosimetry. RIVM Report 650010030, 2002.
28. Drake, P.L., Hazelwood, K.L. Exposure related health effects of silver and silver compounds: A review. *Ann. Occup. Hyg.,* 49, 575, 2005.
29. Dos Santos, C.A., Seckler, M.M., Ingle, A., Gupta, I., Galdiero, S., Gladiero, M., Gade, A., Rai, M. Silver nanoparticles: Therapeutical uses, toxicity and safety issues. *Pharm. Sci.,* 103(7), 1931.
30. Hund-Rinke, K., Werdemann, F.M., Kemper, M. Beurteilung der Gesamturnweltexposition von Silberion aus Biozid-Produkten. *Forschungsbericht des Umweltbundesamtes,* text 43/08, 103(7), 2008.
31. Benn, T.M., Westerhoff, P. Nanoparticle silver released into water from commercially available sock fabrics. *Environ. Sci. Technol.,* 42, 4133, 2008.
32. Zheng, J., Wu, X., Wang, M., Ran, D., Xu, W., Yang, J. Study on the interaction between silver nanoparticles and nucleic acids in the presence of cetyl

trimethyl ammonium bromide and its analytical application. *Talanta.*, 74, 526, 2008.

33. Kennedy, A.J., Hull, N.S., Bednar, A.J., Goss, J.D., Gunter, J.C., Bouldin, J.L., Vikesland, P.J., Steveens, J.A. Fractionating nanosilver: Importance for determining toxicity to aquatic test organisms. *Environ. Sci. Technol.,* 44, 9571, 2010.
34. Asharani, P.V., Wu, Y.L., Gong, Z., Valiyaveettil, S. Toxicity of silver nanoparticles in zebrafish models. *Nanotechnology.,* 19(25), 255102, 2008.
35. Powers, K.W., Brown, S.C., Krishna, V.B., Wasdo, S.C., Moudgil, B.M., Roberts, S.M. Research strategies for safety evaluation of nanomaterials: Part VI. Characterization of nanoscale particles for toxicological evaluation. *Toxicol. Sci.,* 90(2), 296, 2006.
36. Burd, A., Kwok, C.H., Hung, S.C., Chan, H.S., Gu, H., Lam, W.K., Huang, L. A comparative study of the cytotoxicity of silver-based dressings in monolayer cell, tissue explant and animal models. *Wound Repair Regen.*, 15(1), 94, 2007.

9

Nanomaterials for Biohydrogen Production

Periyasamy Sivagurunathan[1,2,*], Abudukeremu Kadier[3], Ackmez Mudhoo[4], Gopalakrishnan Kumar[5], Kuppam Chandrasekhar[6], Takuro Kobayashi[7] and Kaiqin Xu[7]

[1]*Green Energy Technology Research Group, Ton Duc Thang University, Ho Chi Minh City, Vietnam*
[2]*Faculty of Environment and Labour Safety, Ton Duc Thang University, Ho Chi Minh City, Vietnam*
[3]*Department of Chemical and Process Engineering, Faculty of Engineering & Built Environment, National University of Malaysia (UKM), Selangor, Malaysia*
[4]*Department of Chemical and Environmental Engineering, Faculty of Engineering, University of Mauritius, Republic of Mauritius*
[5]*Department of Environmental Engineering, Daegu University, South Korea*
[6]*School of Applied Biosciences, Kyungpook National University, Dong-Daegu, South Korea*
[7]*Center for Materials Cycles and Waste Management Research, National Institute for Environmental Studies, Tsukuba, Japan*

Abstract

The rapid growth of the biofuels sector address the key issues related with fossil fuels utilization, such as reducing the greenhouse gas emissions, and sustainable and renewable fuels production. Among various biofuels option, biohydrogen production is a novel biotechnological tool that can be converting the organic matter into a valuable energy with simultaneous waste disposal. Hydrogen is an excellent energy carrier with a greatest energy potential of 122 kJ/g and about 2.75 times higher than the hydrocarbon fuels; besides, the byproducts formed during combustion is only water vapor without any adverse carbon footprint. The biological mediated hydrogen production is categorized into two major groups namely (i) photo biological route and (ii) dark fermentation route, and both can be performed under moderate temperature and low pressure conditions. The low hydrogen yield

**Corresponding author*: periyasamy.sivagurunathan@tdt.edu.vn

Suvardhan Kanchi, Shakeel Ahmed, Myalowenkosi I. Sabela and Chaudhery Mustansar Hussain (eds.)
Nanomaterials: Biomedical, Environmental, and Engineering Applications, (217–238)

is a major obstacle needed to be overcome for a commercial scale-up of this technology and this can be improved via various strategies. Nano-based technology has been practiced in recent times for the significant improvement of hydrogen production. In the present chapter, the application of nanobased materials for biohydrogen and their potential scale-up option has been outlined.

Keywords: Biohydrogen, immobilization, nano particles, energy, hydrogen yield

9.1 Introduction

Currently, the world economy and energy consumption depend heavily on fossil fuels (FFs). This has led to increase in a rapid depletion of FFs as well as the increasing prices of its remaining reserves [1, 2]. Besides, the massive use of FFs has caused serious environmental issues such as emissions of greenhouse gases (GHG) and other toxic pollutants to the atmosphere. Consequently, an enormous GHG emission is causing global warming and climate change [3, 4]. To mitigate global warming and ensure sustainability of global energy supply, substantial effort is being made on global scale to explore alternative energy sources that could replace FFs.

Biohydrogen is one of the cleanest energy sources with high energy content (142 MJ/kg), which is about 2.75 times higher than that of other petroleum or hydrocarbon fuels [5, 6]. Currently, approximately 96% of global H_2 production is mainly produced from FFs, 48% from natural gas, 30% from oil, 18% from coal, while 4% of total global H_2 production comes from electrolysis of water [3, 7]. There are varieties of technologies for biohydrogen production pathways, including biophotolysis, photo-fermentation (PF), dark-fermentation (DF), photo-dark coupled fermentation, and microbial electrolysis (MEC)-based on H_2 production processes [8]. Biohydrogen production is not yet practical because of limitations inherent to each method. Biophotolysis or photosynthetic H_2 production involves converting sunlight energy into H_2 by using photosynthetic bacteria. However, the practical applicability of H_2 production is affected by the requirement of high-cost bioreactor design, poor light transfer efficiency, and slow hydrogen production rates (HPR) [7]. In addition, the dark fermentative hydrogen production provides rapid HPR, simpler reactor operation, and the utilization of the diverse range of feedstock, making them an attractive method for the sustainable and clean hydrogen production [9].

The rapid development of nanomaterials has opened up a new research direction for the enhancement of biohydrogen process efficiency by stimulating the bioactivity of the microorganisms due to its exclusive physicochemical properties. The stimulation activity of the microbes is mediated by the electron to electron transport [10], direction of the favorable metabolic by products formation such as acetate and butyrate-mediated fermentation pathway [11], and the changes in the hydrogenase gene expression levels [12]. The trace amount of metal co-factors such as zinc, iron, nickel, and potassium ions is essential for microbial growth and metabolism [13]. Important parameters in different biohydrogen production processes, such as H_2 yield, energy or conversion efficiency, HPR, and capital cost, have all seen benefits from the application of nanoparticles or nanomaterials [14]. This chapter reviews latest advances in the application of nanoparticles for hydrogen generation via the above-mentioned methods. It mainly focuses on the role of nanomaterial or nanoparticle to the enhancement of biohydrogen performance of different biohydrogen production pathways.

9.2 Major Biohydrogen Production Pathways

The methods are classified as direct or indirect biophotolysis, photo-fermentation (PF), dark fermentation (DF), and microbial electrolysis cell (MEC) (Figure 9.1).

9.2.1 Biophotolysis

Clearly, biophotolysis provides a renewable and non-toxic way to produce bio-H_2 from renewable resources. Prokaryotic cyanobacteria or eukaryotic green microalgae split H_2O into H_2 and O_2 using sunlight with special conditions. They produce H_2 by direct photolysis of water under anaerobic conditions (Eq. 1) [15]:

$$2H_2O + \text{light energy} \rightarrow 2H_2 + 2O_2. \tag{1}$$

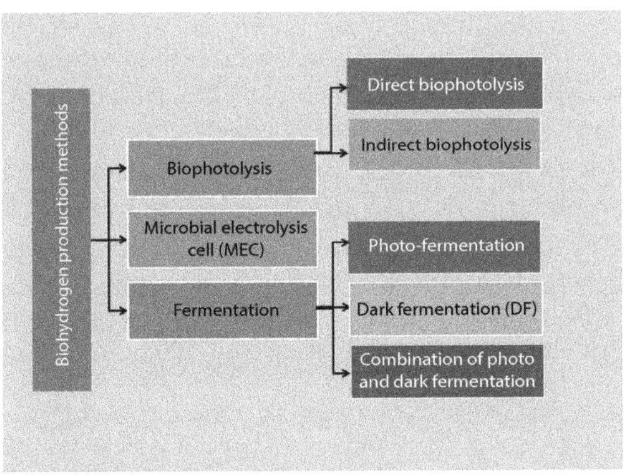

Figure 9.1 Major biohydrogen production methods.

The major advantages of biophotolysisis are that there is no requirement of adding substrate as nutrients. Water is the primary electron donor required for the production of H_2. Sunlight and CO_2 are the basic inputs needed to grow the cyanobacteria or microalga on the biophotolysis process through the hydrogenase enzyme. However, only with special conditions enzyme (hydrogenase or nitrogenase) Fe-hydrogenase plays its activity in H_2 which is exceedingly O_2 sensitive. In this case, inhibition of the enzyme activity due to O_2 release will inhibit the H_2 evolution process. Energy conversion efficiency of biophotolysis can be as high as 10% under low light intensities and very low partial pressures of O_2 correspond to conversion efficiency of 22% [16].

9.2.2 Photo-Fermentation

In photo-fermentation (PF), H_2 is formed by the bioconversion of organic substrates along with the generation of CO_2 with the help of the light energy source, although the H_2 production rate is relatively slower when compared to the dark fermentation reactions, the maximum substrate utilization rate, ability to transform the dark fermentation effluents rich in organic acids (butyric acid, acetic acid, lactic acid), and various waste organics. Fermentation of acetic acid is common in DFs and can produce four moles through the biophotolysis as in equation 2 as follows:

$$2CH_3COOH + 2H_2O \xrightarrow[\text{photosynthetic bacteria}]{\text{light}} 4H_2 + 2CO_2. \quad (2)$$

9.2.3 Dark Fermentation

Dark fermentation (DF) mainly differs from photo-fermentation in which it works without the presence of light. DF employs diverse groups of facultative and anaerobic bacteria such as *Escherichia coli*, *Eneterobacter cloacae*, and *Clostridium* Sp. for the efficient conversion of wide range of organic substrates. Most of the biologically mediated hydrogen productions have been examined with the DF technology due to the simpler reactor design and less energy requirement when compared to other hydrogen production technology. The most dominant hydrogen-producing route for the DF can be achieved with the acetate-mediated fermentative pathway with the generation of four moles of molecular hydrogen with one mole of hexose as shown in equation (3) below:

$$C_6H_{12}O_6 + 2H_2O \rightarrow 4H_2 + CO_2 + 2CH_3COOH \quad (3)$$

or

$$C_6H_{12}O_6 + 2H_2O \rightarrow 4H_2 + 2CH_3COO^- + 2HCO^{3-} + 4H^+.$$

9.2.4 Microbial Electrolysis Cell

Microbial electrolysis cell (MEC) is a novel bioelectrochemical tool for H_2 production that employs domestic and industrial wastes as a fuel source and uses electrochemically active bacteria (EAB) as a biocatalyst with the presence of electric current (Figure 9.2). Figure 9.2 shows the main components of MEC that consist of anode, cathode, membrane (optional), electrochemically active bacteria (EAB), and an electric power supply.

This technology was firstly discovered and named as "electrochemically assisted hydrogen generation" [17], then "biocatalyzed electrolysis" [18], "electrohydrogenesis" [19], and was finally accepted by experts as "microbial electrolysis cells (MECs)" [20]. MECs have several great advantages over other biohydrogen production methods. Firstly, the substrates can be from renewable and waste materials rather than fossil fuels: various organic matters such as cellulose, glucose, glycerol, acetic acid, sewage

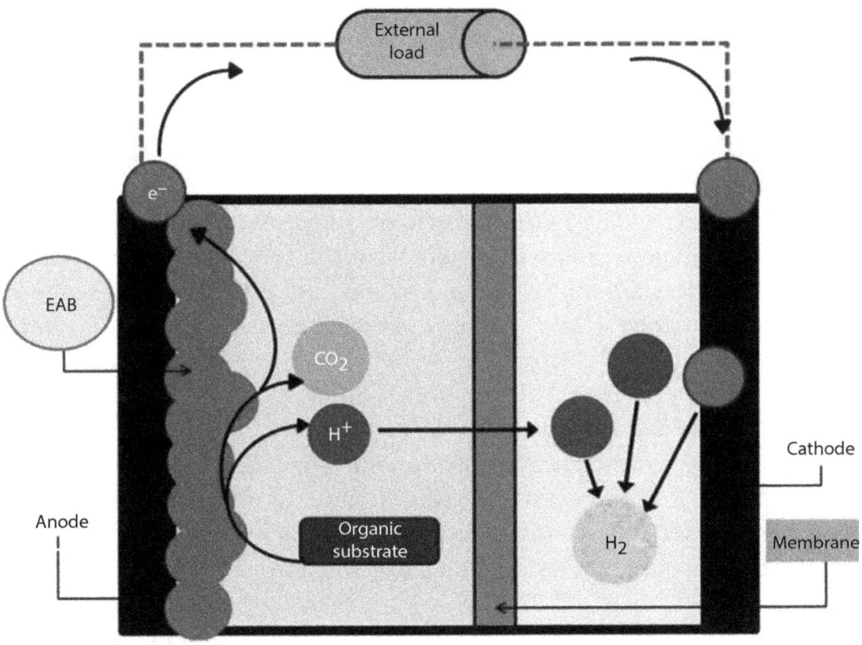

Figure 9.2 Schematic representation of a typical two-chamber MEC reactor and its operation.

sludge, varied wastewaters, and DF effluent can be converted into H_2 in MECs [17, 19–22]. Furthermore, the H_2 production efficiencies of MECs (80–100%) [23–25] are significantly higher than that of the DF process (33%) [26, 27] and water electrolysis (65%) [28]. Moreover, MECs need relatively low supplied or applied voltage (0.2–0.8 V) is much smaller than that needed for traditional water electrolysis (typically 1.8–2.0 V) [29, 30]. The phototrophic conversion of organic substrate to H_2 by algae and photosynthetic bacteria due to low solar efficiencies and large surface area requirements could not generate higher energy than MEC, which is 90% at the rate of 0.5 kW h/m^3-H_2 [20, 31].

9.3 Nanaparticle Effects on Biohydrogen Production

9.3.1 Dark Fermentative Hydrogen Production

Wimonsong *et al.* [32] have developed and tested various Au/Fe–Zn–Mg–Al–O hydrotalcites-supported gold catalysts in their potential to alter the production of biohydrogen. An improvement in the biohydrogen generation was noted by Wimonsong *et al.* [32] when the hydrotalcites-supported gold catalyst was employed namely in terms of the Au/Zn–Mg–Al hydrotalcite producing a peak H_2 yield (HY) of 2.74 mol H_2 per mol of sucrose. This performance being twice better than with the control experimental runs. Lin *et al.* [10] reported the addition of ferric oxide nanoparticles enhanced the hydrogen production from *Enterobacter aerogenes* over 17% than the tested control with no nanoparticle addition. Their results inferred that the addition of 200 mg/L of ferric oxide nanoparticles facilitated the improved hydrogen production with an acetate-mediated fermentative pathway with less amount of ethanol formation. Moreover, the scanning electron microscopy (SEM) images revealed the presence of bacterial nanowires for efficient electron transfers between adjacent microbial cells.

Gadhe *et al.* [33] reported that the co-addition of nickel and hematite nanoparticles enhanced the process efficiency of hydrogen production over 27% from dairy wastewater than the individual nanobioacatlysts. Moreover, Zhang *et al.* [34] demonstrated the addition of zero-valent iron-activated carbon microelectrolysis stimulated the enrichment of *Clostridium* sp. in a mixed consortium and showed an improvement in hydrogen yield over 50%. In another report, Han *et al.* [11] optimized the hematite nanoparticle dosage concentration (0–1600 mg/L) on the improvement of hydrogen production from sucrose with a wide range of initial pH (4–10.0) and the outcomes showed that under the optimal conditions (initial pH of 6.0 and hematite concentration of 200 mg/L), the HY of 3.57 mol H_2/mol sucrose was observed. Additionally, the gradual discharge of hematite nanoparticles monitored by transmission electron microscopy (TEM) revealed the variations in the shape of bacteria with an increase in length from 2.0–3.6 μm to ca. 2.6–5.6 μm. Furthermore, Zhang and Shen [35] reported the enhancement of hydrogen production from sucrose by mixed consortia strongly dependent on the size of the biocatalysts added. The addition of 5 nm gold particles improved the bioactivity of the hydrogen-producing microorganisms with a HY of 4.47 mol H_2/mol sucrose. Mullai *et al.* [36] reported that the addition of a low concentration of 5.67 mg/L nickel nanoparticles could stimulate the hydrogen production efficiency by 22.7% and resulted in a HY of 2.54 mol H_2/mol glucose. Recently, Hsieh *et al.* [12] monitored the activity of the hydrogenase enzyme by reverse-transcription polymerase chain reaction (RTPCR) on hydrogen production from glucose using *Clostridium pasteurianum* after the addition of the nanometal solutions into the nutrient medium and concluded that the addition of Fe-mediated nanoparticles stimulated the hydrogen production; however, the improvement was not observed at the gene level and the possible stimulatory response is attributed by the increased electron transport within the cells of *C. pasteurianum*. Hence, monitoring the activity of hydrogen producers after the addition of nanoparticles is essential for better understanding the stimulatory roles of nano-mediated biocatalysts on the process efficiency of the biohydrogen production system. The details of nanoparticles in dark fermentative hydrogen production are shown in Table 9.1.

9.3.2 Photo Fermentative Hydrogen Production

Tian *et al.* [37] have examined the efficiency of *Rhodopseudomonas palustris* CQK 01 immobilized in a PVA-boric acid gel granule in their effects on the production of hydrogen under light conditions. Tian *et al.* (2009) recorded peak hydrogen production rates in tune of 3.6 mmol/g cell dry weight/h and reflected that the use of *Rhodopseudomonas palustris* CQK 01 immobilized in the carrier tested here had significantly improved the photo-production of hydrogen.

Xie *et al.* [38] have modified the surface of activated carbon fibers using thermal and acid pretreatments in view to serve as a potential carrier for photo-fermentative generation of hydrogen, and observed that the new carrier presented excellent immobilization characteristics for the adsorption of the more effective photo producer involved in hydrogen synthesis. Xie *et al.* [39] have equally provided results that advocated the improvements in

Table 9.1 Applications of nanoparticles on dark fermentative hydrogen production.

Inoculum source	Substrate	Nanoparticles	Concentration mg/L	Hydrogen yield (HY) (mol/mol substrate)	References
Mixed consortia	Glucose	zero-valent iron activated carbon microelectrolysis	200	429 mL/ g glu	[34]
Mixed consortia	Sucrose	*Hematite*	200	3.57 mol/mol sucrose	[11]
Mixed consortia	Sucrose	*Gold*	10 nM	4.47 mol H2/mol sucrose	[35]
Mixed consortia	Glucose	*Nickel*	5.67	2.54 mol/mol glucose	[36]
Clostridium pasteurianum	Gluose	Hematite	800	2.2 mol/mol glucose	[12]
Mixed consortia	Distillery wastewater	*Hematite*	200	7.85 mmol/g COD	[66]
Mixed consortia	Distillery wastewater	*Co addition of hematite and nickel*	200, 5	8.83 mmol/g COD	[66]
Clostridium butyricum	Glucose	*Iron oxide nanoparticles encapsulated in porous silica*	(10^{-6} mol L^{-1})	1.08 mol/mol glucose	[67]
Mixed consortia	Starch	Fe^0 and Ni^0	37.5	147.3 mL/ g-starch	[68]

the production of hydrogen by *Rhodopseudomonas faecalis* RLD-53 immobilization on activated carbon fibers. The key enhancements reported by Xie *et al.* [39] refer to the improved external morphology of this new solid carrier of bacteria by virtue of having more adsorption/binding sites and a dense biofilm. Xie *et al.* [39] reported the hydrogen production performance under these conditions as follows: a peak yield reaching 3.08 mol H_2 per mol of acetate and a production rate of 32.85 ml l^{-1} h^{-1} of hydrogen for a specific surface area of 1500 m^2 g^{-1} at a dosage of 0.8 g l^{-1} of activated carbon fibers. Ren *et al.* [40] have tested an activated carbon fiber as a carrier for immobilizing *Rhodopseudomonas faecalis* RLD-53 during the photoproduction of hydrogen, and have deduced that their photo-bioreactor proved to be a reasonably effective configuration for the intended purpose.

Giannelli and Torzillo [41] have studied the impacts of using a suspension of silica nanoparticles for scattering light in a photobioreactor used for biohydrogen production by the *Chlamydomonas reinhardtii* microalga, and reported an average biohydrogen production of 3.1215 L. Nasr *et al.* [42] have examined the production of biohydrogen from starch-based effluents under anaerobic sequential dark-photo fermentative conditions with pretreated sludge immobilized on maghemite nanoparticles as the microbial inoculum, and have equally hinted the merits of having the nanoparticle carriers in improving the overall yield of biohydrogen generation.

Liao *et al.* [43] have studied the use of *Rhodopseudomonas palustris* CQK 01 immobilized in a photobioreactor for the production of biohydrogen by varying the intensities and wavelengths of illumination allowed in the system, and have observed that the type of illumination and its intensity significantly affected the morphological shape of the microbial biofilm and that the extent of microbial enrichment achieved in the biofilms directly determined the biohydrogen production biokinetics. Li *et al.* [44] had equally examined the effects of light intensity and the cell growth technique of *Rhodobacter sphaeroides* ZX-5 in an anaerobic photobioreactor, and concluded that their freshly developed approach that consisted in providing additional illumination with shaking had had positive effects in enhancing the net rate of photoproduction of biohydrogen, and if this approach be further optimized, it could become a viable and sustainable route toward high-efficiency phototrophic biohydrogen generation.

Rashid *et al.* [45] have assessed the influence of intensity of light, pH, and type of organic matter substrate on the biohydrogen production by algae, and reported that the best pH for an optimal biohydrogen production was 8.0 to reach a peak yield for a total volume of 1.315 L of biohydrogen evolved at a maximum rate of 24 ml/L h^{-1}) with fructose being the substrate.

Zagrodnik & Laniecki [46] also noted that a pH of 7.5 had improved the biohydrogen generation under light-assisted fermentation from 0.96 to 2.5 L biohydrogen for every liter of the medium in contrast with the uncontrolled system.

Guevara-López & Buitrón [47] have assessed the performance of high-density polyethylene cylinders, acrylic rods, and dispersed fibers and cubes for the immobilization of a *Rhodopseudomonas palustris* during the generation of biohydrogen by the anaerobic synthetic pathway in a continuously illuminated bioreactor. Guevara-López and Buitrón [47] observed that the dispersed fibers had produced the largest extent of immobilization of microbial biomass at an average of 19.6 mg VS/cm^3 seconded by dispersed cubes, and then the high-density polyethylene cylinders and acrylic bars (in decreasing order of immobilization capacity). While Guevara-López and Buitrón [47] stressed that the support materials more significantly affected and determined the extent of light distribution within the bioreactor, the kinetics of the biohydrogen production seemed to be have been independent of the type of support materials under consideration.

9.3.3 Photocatalytic Hydrogen (H2) Production

Hakamizadeh *et al.* [48] have designed mesoporous TiO_2/activated carbon, Pt/TiO_2, and Pt/TiO_2/activated nanocomposites and used them as potential photocatalysts in the production of hydrogen under ultraviolet light. Their results clearly spelt out the merits of the Pt with activated carbon in enhancing the hydrogen production kinetics assisted here by the water splitting route. Hakamizadeh *et al.* [48] also concluded that the mesoporous Pt/TiO_2/AC nanocomposite proved to be the most useful catalyst and had occasioned the highest production rate at 7490 μmol/h/g photocatalyst and which was a rate nearly 75 times more than those achieved with the conventional P25 photocatalyst [28, 49].

Taboada *et al.* [50] have developed cordierite honeycomb structures impregnated with variable quantities of Au/TiO_2 to study the production of hydrogen from ethanol/water–ethanol in light dependent systems. Taboada *et al.* [50] provided a favorable assessment of their work in that the production of hydrogen under light had been greatly increased by five times as compared to rates observed in a typical slurry photoreactor.

9.3.4 MEC-Based Hydrogen Production

As discussed in the last section, MEC provides a sustainable way for H_2 production from renewable resources. Anode is an indispensable component that affects the H_2 production capability of MECs. A study carried out by Qiao *et al.* [51] demonstrated that carbon nanotube/polyaniline nanostructure composite could enhance the electron transfer efficiency and electrode surface area when using as anode materials in MECs. Furthermore, Au and Pd nanoparticle-decorated graphite anode was synthesized and examined in a newly designed multi-anode MEC reactor [52]. Moreover, Xu *et al.* [53] investigated the effects of Fe nanoparticle-modified graphite disks on the H_2 production performance of *Shewanella oneidensis MR-1* in MECs as anode. The experimental results showed that MECs incorporated with Fe nanoparticle-decorated graphite anodes provided 5.89-fold higher current density than the plain graphite anode. On the other hand, cathode catalysts for proton (H^+) reduction play a key role in reducing energy input and increasing HPRs. MEC still suffers from the lack of a high efficient and inexpensive cathode catalyst. Huang *et al.* [54] used carbon paper coated with Pd nanoparticles as the cathodic catalyst in MEC to facilitate H_2 production. The novel nanoparticle cathode showed a lower overpotential than the carbon paper cathode coated with Pt. The coulombic efficiency, H_2 recoveries of the MEC with the Pd nanoparticles were slightly higher than that with Pt cathode, while the Pd loading was one order of magnitude less than Pt. Furthermore, Xiao *et al.* [55] investigated the performance of hydrogen production and catalyst stability of a novel nitrogen-containing core-shell-structured (N–Fe/Fe3C@C) nanocatalyst in a two-chamber MEC. The novel cathode catalyst significantly enhanced H_2 production performance MEC, and a great advantage of the N–Fe/Fe3C@C is extremely inexpensive (less than 5% of the Pt/C cathode catalyst), suggesting its promise for real-world MEC applications.

9.4 Biohydrogen Producing Associated with Immobilized Enzymes (Cellulases and Hydrogenases)

Cellulase and dehydrogenase are two very important enzymes that have been regularly encountered in a number of works related to the fermentation of biomass for the production of biofuels, not specifically addressing the metabolism of biohydrogen generation. These two enzymes have been proving helpful in the hydrolysis of cellulose, an active component which is broken down during anaerobic fermentative bioprocess of a number of biomass types, and a breakdown to produce more bioavailable sugars that in turn find their way toward more efficient biofuel production. Coupled with the need to enhance the bioavailability of cellulosic biomass and their derivatives of improved hydrolysis, research efforts have also been geared lastly toward using particularly chitosan-based immobilization for promoting the enzymatic action of the cellulase and dehydrogenase moieties in biofuel production, but much less being reported, and possibly being done, for biohydrogen production by fermentation. A number of findings have indeed advocated the merits of standalone and combined chitosan-based enzyme immobilization, and it is more than natural and imperative to initiate robust research toward using this interesting and useful technique for enhancing the biohydrogen generation metabolism. Zang *et al.* [56] have prepared magnetic nanoparticles using chitosan attached on Fe_3O_4 nanoparticles in view to immobilize cellulase and observed that this specific immobilization technique had occasioned increased stability in the operational conditions of the reactions for a wider span of pH and temperature, along with ensuring a reusability of the immobilization nanoparticles. Kumar *et al.* [57] have equally synthesized magnetic Fe_3O_4 nanoparticles following an alternative route involving precipitation and silanization and subsequently using these nanoparticles to produce the corresponding chitosan-based beads. Kumar *et al.* (2013) reported that the lipase *Rhizopus oryzae* had been well immobilized on these functionalized beads that had exhibited a high stability for potential industrial applications. Song *et al.* [58] have formulated magnetic chitosan microspheres by a combined emulsification cross-linking and precipitation approach and observed that immobilized formate dehydrogenase exhibited an improved stability to heat effects and acidic-alkaline conditions stability, and finally reusability. Han *et al.* [59] used a one-pot technique to develop calcium phosphate-mineralized chitosan beads and reported that the antiswelling characteristics of the beads had been significantly enhanced, and when used as an immobilization support for yeast alcohol dehydrogenase, the chitosan-based beads had much improved stability toward heat effects, changes in pH, potential for recyclability, and storage capacity. Vieira *et al.* [60] have used agarose beads and chitosan-based structures to immobilize β-galactosidase derived from the species *Kluyveromyces fragilis* in view to promote the batch catalysis of the hydrolysis of whole milk lactose. Vieira *et al.* [60] noted that the support material used here had produced a peak and much more stable immobilization of β-galactosidase to the tune of 21 mg enzyme/g chitosan-based support, and the immobilized enzyme could be reused nearly 3 months later by virtue of an 80% retention of the primary enzymatic activity. Vieira *et al.* [60] reported that the immobilized β-galactosidase had been very effective for the hydrolysis of the lactose to efficiencies exceeding 94%. Ivanova *et al.* [61] have immobilized *Saccharomyces cerevisiae* cells on a magnetite-chitosan complex and magnetic nanoparticles coated with cellulose to study the production of ethanol by fermentation and remarked that the kinetics of ethanol synthesis was dependent on each type of carrier. Badgujar and Bhanage [62] have tested a green support material for immobilizing lipase (*Pseudomonas cepacia*), where the carrier was based on chitosan and polyvinyl alcohol. Badgujar and Bhanage [62] found that their new support material had produced significantly heightened catalytic performance of the lipase and could also be readily recycled in potential industrial applications whereby biological processes could be enhanced for their biokinetics. Liu *et al.* [63] have tested Na-alginate-chitosan and Ca-alginate-chitosan to study the enzymatic performance of immobilized lipase, and thereafter concluded on the variability in enzymatic activity with respect to synthetic conditions for preparing the enzyme carriers. Ghadi *et al.* [64] have recently prepared chitosan-based magnetic core-shell nanoparticles to immobilize lipase and equally observed a notable enhancement in the stability and overall effective enzymatic activity of the lipase when immobilized when so done. Srivastava *et al.* [65] demonstrated an increase in thermal stability of Fenugreek β-amylase enzyme when immobilized on a chitosan-based carrier attached onto polyvinyl chloride beads and additional bead carriers fabricated from a mix of chitosan and polyvinylpyrrolidone. Srivastava *et al.* [65] highlighted the green characteristics of the novel immobilization support materials in them being not toxic, readily amenable to complex immobilization schemes, and being reusable.

9.5 Outlook and Concluding Notes

Immobilization of the biohydrogen systems has proved the significant improvements in the production performances. Figure 9.3 shows the different aspects and types of immobilization systems used in the production of biohydrogen from biomass sources. The quantum of research efforts, findings, and correspondingly the number of research publications and reviews published in the last couple of decades on the use, application, and potentials of nanoscience have gained a steady increase in interest worldwide. Indeed, the core of nanoscience has been smoothly adapted and integrated with a number of other disciplines (e.g., medical science, mechanical engineering, food science, surgery, chemical engineering, environmental engineering, metallurgy, polymer science and engineering, to name but a few) to work out strategies and workable solutions for solving a number of technical issues. The complete set of historic data in the literature on the application of nanoscience and subsequently nanotechnology

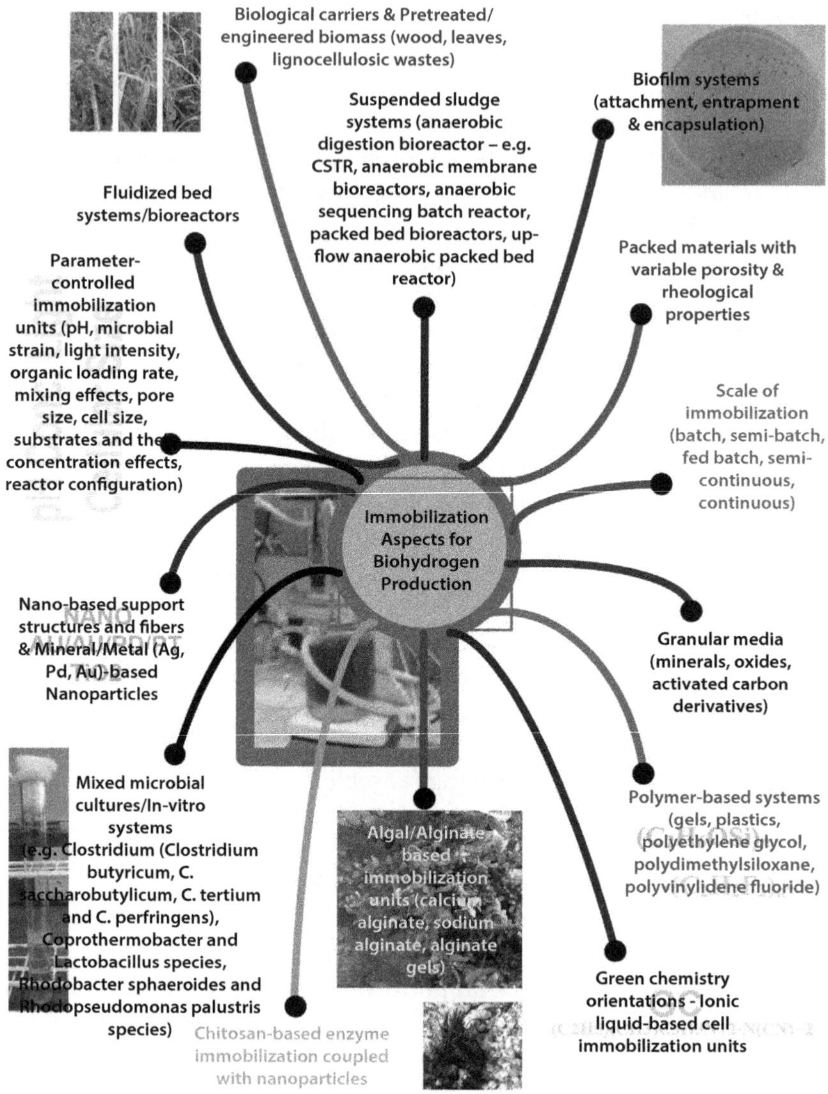

Figure 9.3 Different aspects and types of immobilization systems used in the production of biohydrogen from biomass sources.

has, hence, and will continue to advocate the merits, by large and by far, of this fresh multidisciplinary discipline. Nevertheless, besides the umpteen merits, nanotechnology rightfully claims in a number of specific fields, and there is also a need to work out the detailed case history of its environmental impacts through properly designed lifecycle assessment studies. As mentioned earlier, the invasive, and in many occasions disruptive, nature of nanotechnology has proven to be beneficial in a number of ways. In the very context of the topic addressed in this review that falls most suitably under the "biotechnology" and "bioenergy" banners, the tests run to investigate the possibilities of using nanoparticles and nanotubes, as evidenced by the review of the pool of works and findings described earlier in this paper, have all revealed the promise and merits of nanotechnology in improving the biokinetics of biohydrogen production from a number of synthetic and real biomass types.

Indeed, the use of nanoparticles has occasioned an enhanced biohydrogen production rate and yield, the latter being the major two kinetics-related improvements surveyed in several publications. Viewed from a strictly scientific standpoint, and in a first instance, irrespective of the scale of the reactions and size of the bioreactors used when testing the nanoparticles, nanoscience retains an earnest hope in making the biohydrogen "fuel economy" a forthcoming reality. Yet, the transition from the scale of "nanoscience" to a mature "nanobiotechnology" as adequately relevant and applicable to the production of biohydrogen from stabilized biomass types has to be well thought and thereafter designed taking a number of technical and economic considerations in perspective. This scaling up will naturally foster more research, the results of which will be fueling the development of new routes for promoting the application of nanobiotechnology for biohydrogen production. The shift from lab scale biohydrogen production to streamlined large-scale biohydrogen is essential, at least, to provide a robust and sustainable foundation for the "biohydrogen green economy".

In the specific context of harnessing the latent advantages of nano(bio) technology for elevating biohydrogen to the status of "green fuel" (as the goal of all research being done in this field is ostensibly to develop and secure a reliable biohydrogen fuel market model), the very first approach will be to translate the state of the "powdered nanoparticles" to "tubular, concentric, sheeted or a mixed arrangement of inert support materials embedded" with these nanoparticles. In effect, nanotubes or nanoparticles-embedded carbon tubes will be one way to generate larger, and maybe modular, bioreactors working on the basis of having immobilized enzymes or other adapted biohydrogen producing species on nano-engineered micro- or nanostructures. Hence, in this specific scope of upscaling biohydrogen production, the various configurations of nanotubes arrangements will have to be designed and pilot-scale tested for the following optimized key parameter performance: range of biohydrogen production rates and yields, cycle and recycle times of substrates throughput, wash out and replacement of microbial cultures, extent of saturation of nanotubes till biohydrogen production rates and yields fall below both technically and economically accepted thresholds, structural support units for nanotubes, temperature and pressure considerations for optimum biochemical regimes to prevail but within controllable extents, and finally the level of modularization needed in the bioreactor unit design.

Acknowledgment

The author Dr. Periyasamy Sivagurunathan greatly acknowledged the financial assistance from Japan Society for Promotion of Science: JSPS ID: P15370 for this study.

References

1. Singh, L., Wahid, Z.A. Methods for enhancing bio-hydrogen production from biological process: a review. *J. Indust. Eng. Chem.*, 21, 70–80, 2015.
2. Bundhoo, M.A.Z., Mohee, R., Hassan, M.A. Effects of pre-treatment technologies on dark fermentative biohydrogen production: A review. *J. Env. Manag.*, 157, 20–48, 2015.
3. Kadier, A., Kalil, M.S., Abdeshahian, P., Chandrasekhar, K., Mohamed, A., Azman, N.F., *et al.* Recent advances and emerging challenges in microbial electrolysis cells (MECs) for microbial production of hydrogen and value-added chemicals. *Renew. Sust. Energ. Rev.*, 61, 501–25, 2016.
4. Sivagurunathan, P., Kumar, G., Kim, S.H., Kobayashi, T., Xu, K.Q., Guo. W., *et al.* Enhancement strategies for hydrogen production from wastewater: A review. *Cur. Org. Chem.*, 20, 2744–52, 2016.
5. Arimi, M.M., Knodel, J., Kiprop, A., Namango, S.S., Zhang, Y., Geißen, S.U. Strategies for improvement of biohydrogen production from organic-rich wastewater: A review. *Biomass. Bioener.*, 75, 101–18, 2015.
6. Kumar, G., Mudhoo, A., Sivagurunathan, P, Nagarajan, D., Ghimire, A., Lay, C.H., *et al.* Recent insights into the cell immobilization technology applied for dark fermentative hydrogen production. *Bioresour. Technol.*, 219, 725–37, 2016.
7. Das, D., Khanna, N., Dasgupta, C.N. *Biohydrogen Production: Fundamentals and Technology Advances*. CRC Press, Boca Raton, Florida, United States 2014.
8. Azwar, M.Y., Hussain, M.A., Abdul-Wahab, A.K. Development of biohydrogen production by photobiological, fermentation and electrochemical processes: A review. *Renew. Sust. Energ. Rev.*, 31, 158–73, 2014.
9. Rittmann, S., Herwig, C. A comprehensive and quantitative review of dark fermentative biohydrogen production. *Microb. Cell Fact.*, 11, 115, 2012.
10. Lin, R., Cheng, J., Ding, L., Song, W., Liu, M., Zhou, J., *et al.* Enhanced dark hydrogen fermentation by addition of ferric oxide nanoparticles using *Enterobacter aerogenes*. *Bioresour. Technol.*, 207, 213–9, 2016.

11. Han, H., Cui, M., Wei, L., Yang, H., Shen, J. Enhancement effect of hematite nanoparticles on fermentative hydrogen production. *Bioresour. Technol.*, 102, 7903–9, 2011.
12. Hsieh P-H, Lai Y-C, Chen K-Y, Hung C-H. Explore the possible effect of TiO_2 and magnetic hematite nanoparticle addition on biohydrogen production by *Clostridium pasteurianum* based on gene expression measurements. *Int. J. Hydrogen Energy*, 41, 21685–91, 2016.
13. Buzea, C., Pacheco, II., Robbie, K. Nanomaterials and nanoparticles: Sources and toxicity. *Biointerphases.*, 2, 17–77, 2007.
14. Bunker, C.E., Smith, M.J. Nanoparticles for hydrogen generation. *J. Mat. Chem.*, 21, 12173–80, 2011.
15. Das, D., Veziroglu, T.N. Advances in biological hydrogen production processes. *Int. J. Hydrogen Energy*, 33, 6046–57, 2008.
16. Rahman, S., Masdar, M., Rosli, M.I., Majlan, E., Husaini, T., Kamarudin, S., *et al.* Overview biohydrogen technologies and application in fuel cell technology. *Renew. Sust. Energ. Rev.*, 66, 137–62, 2016.
17. Liu, H., Grot, S., Logan, B.E. Electrochemically assisted microbial production of hydrogen from acetate. *Env. Sci. Technol.*, 39, 4317–20, 2005.
18. Rozendal, R.A, Hamelers, H.V., Euverink, G.J., Metz, S.J., Buisman, C.J. Principle and perspectives of hydrogen production through biocatalyzed electrolysis. *Int. J. Hydrogen Energy*, 31, 1632–40, 2006.
19. Cheng, S., Logan, B.E. Sustainable and efficient biohydrogen production via electrohydrogenesis. *Proc. Nat. Acad. Sci.*, 104, 18871–3, 2007.
20. Logan, B.E., Call, D., Cheng, S., Hamelers, H.V., Sleutels, T.H., Jeremiasse, A.W., *et al.* Microbial electrolysis cells for high yield hydrogen gas production from organic matter. *Env. Sci. Technol.*, 42, 8630–40, 2008.
21. Pant, D., Singh, A., Van Bogaert, G., Olsen, S.I., Nigam, P.S., Diels, L., *et al.* Bioelectrochemical systems (BES) for sustainable energy production and product recovery from organic wastes and industrial wastewaters. *Rsc. Adv.*, 2, 1248–63, 2012.
22. Kadier, A., Simayi, Y., Kalil, M.S., Abdeshahian, P., Hamid, A.A. A review of the substrates used in microbial electrolysis cells (MECs) for producing sustainable and clean hydrogen gas. *Renew. Energy* 71, 466–72, 2014.
23. Hu. H., Fan, Y., Liu, H. Hydrogen production using single-chamber membrane-free microbial electrolysis cells. *Water. Res.*, 42, 4172–8, 2008.
24. Wang, J., Xu, S., Xiao, B., Xu, M., Yang, L., Liu, S., *et al.* Influence of catalyst and temperature on gasification performance of pig compost for hydrogen-rich gas production. *Int. J. Hydrogen Energy*, 38, 14200–7, 2013.
25. Catal, T., Lesnik, K.L., Liu, H. Suppression of methanogenesis for hydrogen production in single-chamber microbial electrolysis cells using various antibiotics. *Bioresour. Technol.*, 187, 77–83, 2015.
26. Abreu, A.A., Tavares, F., Alves, M.M., Pereira, M.A. Boosting dark fermentation with co-cultures of extreme thermophiles for biohythane production from garden waste. *Bioresour. Technol.*, 219, 132–8, 2016.

27. Kumar, G., Bakonyi, P., Zhen, G., Sivagurunathan, P., Koók, L., Kim, S.H., *et al.* Microbial electrochemical systems for sustainable biohydrogen production: surveying the experiences from a start-up viewpoint. *Renew. Sust. Energ. Rev.*, 70, 589–97, 2017.
28. Wang, Y., Li, B., Zhang, C., Cui, L., Kang, S., Li, X., *et al.* Ordered mesoporous CeO_2-TiO_2 composites: Highly efficient photocatalysts for the reduction of CO_2 with H_2O under simulated solar irradiation. *Appl. Catal. B: Env.*, 130–131, 277–84, 2013.
29. Kadier, A., Simayi, Y., Logrono, W., Kalil, M.S. The significance of key operational variables to the enhancement of hydrogen production in a single-chamber microbial electrolysis cell (MEC). *Iran. J. Hydrog. Fuel Cell.*, 2, 85–97, 2015.
30. Khan, M., Nizami, A., Rehan, M., Ouda, O., Sultana, S., Ismail, I., *et al.* Microbial electrolysis cells for hydrogen production and urban wastewater treatment: A case study of Saudi Arabia. *Appl. Energy*,185, 410–20, 2017.
31. Fang, H.H.P., Liu, H., Zhang, T. Phototrophic hydrogen production from acetate and butyrate in wastewater. *Int. J.Hydrogen Energy*, 30, 785–93, 2005.
32. Wimonsong P, Nitisoravut R, Llorca J. Application of Fe–Zn–Mg–Al–O hydrotalcites supported Au as active nano-catalyst for fermentative hydrogen production. *Chem. Eng. J.*, 253, 148–54, 2014.
33. Gadhe, A., Sonawane, S.S., Varma, M.N. Enhancement effect of hematite and nickel nanoparticles on biohydrogen production from dairy wastewater. *Int. J. Hydrogen Energy*, 40, 4502–11, 2015.
34. Zhang, L., Zhang, L., Li, D. Enhanced dark fermentative hydrogen production by zero-valent iron activated carbon micro-electrolysis. *Int. J. Hydrogen Energy.*, 40, 12201–8, 2015.
35. Zhang, Y., Shen, J. Enhancement effect of gold nanoparticles on biohydrogen production from artificial wastewater. *Int. J. Hydrogen Energy.*, 32, 17–23, 2007.
36. Mullai, P., Yogeswari, M.K., Sridevi, K. Optimisation and enhancement of biohydrogen production using nickel nanoparticles – A novel approach. *Bioresour. Technol.*, 141, 212–9, 2013.
37. Tian, X., Liao, Q., Liu, W., Wang, Y.Z., Zhu, X., Li, J., *et al.* Photo-hydrogen production rate of a PVA-boric acid gel granule containing immobilized photosynthetic bacteria cells. *Int. J.Hydrogen Energy.*, 34, 4708–17, 2009.
38. Xie, G.J., Liu, B.F., Xing, D.F., Nan, J., Ding, J., Ren, H.Y., *et al.* Photo-hydrogen production by *Rhodopseudomonas faecalis* RLD-53 immobilized on the surface of modified activated carbon fibers. *Rsc. Adv.*, 2, 2225–8, 2012.
39. Xie, G.J., Liu, B.F., Ding, J., Xing, D.F., Ren, H.Y., Guo, W.Q., *et al.* Enhanced photo-H_2 production by *Rhodopseudomonas faecalis* RLD-53 immobilization on activated carbon fibers. *Biomass. Bioenergy.*, 44, 122–9, 2012.
40. Ren, H.Y., Liu, B.F., Ding, J., Xie, G.J., Zhao, L., Xing, D.F., *et al.* Continuous photo-hydrogen production in anaerobic fluidized bed photo-reactor with activated carbon fiber as carrier. *Rsc. Adv.*, 2, 5531–5, 2012.

41. Giannelli, L., Torzillo, G. Hydrogen production with the microalga *Chlamydomonas reinhardtii* grown in a compact tubular photobioreactor immersed in a scattering light nanoparticle suspension. *Int. J. Hydrogen Energy.*, 37, 16951–61, 2012.
42. Nasr, M., Tawfik, A., Ookawara, S., Suzuki, M., Kumari, S., Bux, F. Continuous biohydrogen production from starch wastewater via sequential dark-photo fermentation with emphasize on maghemite nanoparticles. *J. Ind. Eng. Chem.*, 21, 500–6, 2015.
43. Liao, Q., Wang, Y.J., Wang, Y.Z., Zhu, X., Tian, X., Li, J. Formation and hydrogen production of photosynthetic bacterial biofilm under various illumination conditions. *Bioresour. Technol.*, 101, 5315–24, 2010.
44. Li, X., Wang, Y.H., Zhang, S.L, Chu, J., Zhang, M., Huang, M.Z., *et al.* Enhancement of phototrophic hydrogen production by *Rhodobacter sphaeroides* ZX-5 using a novel strategy — shaking and extra-light supplementation approach. *Int. J. Hydrogen Energy.*, 34, 9677–85, 2009.
45. Rashid, N., Lee, K., Han, J.I., Gross M. Hydrogen production by immobilized *Chlorella vulgaris*: optimizing pH, carbon source and light. *Bioproc. Biosyst. Eng.*, 36, 867–72, 2012.
46. Zagrodnik, R., Laniecki, M. The role of pH control on biohydrogen production by single stage hybrid dark- and photo-fermentation. *Bioresour. Technol.*, 194, 187–95, 2015.
47. Guevara-López, E., Buitrón, G. Evaluation of different support materials used with a photo-fermentative consortium for hydrogen production. *Int. J. Hydrogen Energy.*, 40, 17231–8, 2015.
48. Hakamizadeh, M., Afshar, S., Tadjarodi, A., Khajavian, R., Fadaie, M.R., Bozorgi, B. Improving hydrogen production via water splitting over Pt/TiO_2/activated carbon nanocomposite. *Int. J. Hydrogen Energy.*, 39, 7262–9, 2014.
49. Markowska-Szczupak, A., Wang, K., Rokicka, P., Endo, M., Wei, Z., Ohtani, B., *et al.* The effect of anatase and rutile crystallites isolated from titania P25 photocatalyst on growth of selected mould fungi. *J. Photochem. Photobiol. B: Biol.*, 151, 54–62, 2015.
50. Taboada, E., Angurell, I., Llorca, J. Dynamic photocatalytic hydrogen production from ethanol–water mixtures in an optical fiber honeycomb reactor loaded with Au/TiO_2. *J. Catal.*, 309, 460–7, 2014.
51. Qiao, Y., Li, C.M., Bao, S.J., Bao, Q.L. Carbon nanotube/polyaniline composite as anode material for microbial fuel cells. *J. Power Sourc.*, 170, 79–84, 2007.
52. Fan, Y., Xu, S., Schaller, R., Jiao, J., Chaplen, F., Liu, H. Nanoparticle decorated anodes for enhanced current generation in microbial electrochemical cells. *Biosens. Bioelectron.*, 26, 1908–12, 2011.
53. Xu, S., Liu, H., Fan, Y., Schaller, R., Jiao, J., Chaplen, F. Enhanced performance and mechanism study of microbial electrolysis cells using Fe nanoparticle-decorated anodes. *Appl. Microbiol. Biotechnol.*, 93, 871–80, 2012.

54. Huang, Y.X., Liu, X.W., Sun, X.F., Sheng, G.P., Zhang, Y.Y., Yan, G.M., *et al.* A new cathodic electrode deposit with palladium nanoparticles for cost-effective hydrogen production in a microbial electrolysis cell. *Int. J. Hydrogen Energy.*, 36, 2773–6, 2011.
55. Xiao, L., Wen, Z., Ci, S., Chen, J., He, Z. Carbon/iron-based nanorod catalysts for hydrogen production in microbial electrolysis cells. *Nano Energy.*,1, 751–6, 2012.
56. Zang, L., Qiu, J., Wu, X., Zhang, W., Sakai, E., Wei, Y. Preparation of magnetic chitosan nanoparticles as support for cellulase immobilization. *Indust. Eng. Chem. Res.*, 53, 3448–54, 2014.
57. Kumar, V., Jahan, F., Raghuwanshi, S., Mahajan, RV., Saxena, R.K. Immobilization of Rhizopus oryzae lipase on magnetic Fe_3O_4-chitosan beads and its potential in phenolic acids ester synthesis. *Biotechnol. Bioproc. Eng.*, 18, 787–95, 2013.
58. Song, Y., Kong, W., Song, H., Hua, S., Xia, C. Preparation of magnetic chitosan microspheres and their application to immobilization of formate dehydrogenase. *Indust. Catal.*,. 8, 5, 2012.
59. Han, P., Song, X., Wu, H., Jiang, Z., Shi, J., Wang, X., *et al.* Enhancing catalytic activity and stability of yeast alcohol dehydrogenase by encapsulation in chitosan-calcium phosphate hybrid beads. *Indust. Eng. Chem. Res.*, 54, 597–604, 2015.
60. Vieira, D.C., Lima, L.N., Mendes, A.A., Adriano, W.S., Giordano, R.C., Giordano, R.L.C., *et al.* Hydrolysis of lactose in whole milk catalyzed by β-galactosidase from Kluyveromyces fragilis immobilized on chitosan-based matrix. *Biochem. Eng. J.*, 81, 54–64, 2013.
61. Ivanova, V., Petrova, P., Hristov, J. Application in the ethanol fermentation of immobilized yeast cells in matrix of alginate/magnetic nanoparticles, on chitosan-magnetite microparticles and cellulose-coated magnetic nanoparticles *Int. Rev. Chem. Eng.*, 3, 289–299, 2011.
62. Badgujar, K.C., Bhanage, B.M. Enhanced biocatalytic activity of lipase immobilized on biodegradable copolymer of chitosan and polyvinyl alcohol support for synthesis of propionate ester: Kinetic approach. *Indust. Eng. Chem. Res.*, 53, 18806–15, 2014.
63. Liu, B., Zhang, H.l., Xue, W., Qi, Z., Tian, Z., Tai, Q. Preparation of alginate/chitosan microcapsule with lipase immobilization. *Chem. Indust. Eng. Prog.*, 9, 1541, 2010.
64. Ghadi, A., Tabandeh, F., Mahjoub, S., Mohsenifar, A., Roshan, F.T., Alavije, R.S. Fabrication and characterization of core-shell magnetic chitosan nanoparticles as a novel carrier for immobilization of *Burkholderia cepacia* lipase. *J. Oleo. Sci.*, 64, 423–30, 2015.
65. Srivastava, G., Roy, S., Kayastha, A.M. Immobilisation of fenugreek β-amylase on chitosan/PVP blend and chitosan coated PVC beads: A comparative study. *Food. Chem.*, 172, 844–51, 2015.

66. Gadhe, A., Sonawane, S.S, Varma, M.N. Influence of nickel and hematite nanoparticle powder on the production of biohydrogen from complex distillery wastewater in batch fermentation. *Int. J. Hydrogen Energy.*, 40, 10734–43, 2015.
67. Beckers, L., Hiligsmann, S., Lambert, S.D., Heinrichs, B., Thonart, P. Improving effect of metal and oxide nanoparticles encapsulated in porous silica on fermentative biohydrogen production by *Clostridium butyricum. Bioresour. Technol.,* 133, 109–17, 2013.
68. Taherdanak, M., Zilouei, H., Karimi, K. Investigating the effects of iron and nickel nanoparticles on dark hydrogen fermentation from starch using central composite design. *Int. J. Hydrogen Energy.*, 40, 12956–63, 2015.

10

A Framework for Using Nanotechnology in Military Gear

Hlophe Nkosingiphile.Siphesihle, Mbatha Precious Hlengiwe and Shalini Singh*

Department of Operations and Quality Management, Durban University of Technology, Durban, South Africa

Abstract

Military personnel are exposed to various types of hazards and threats daily in the battle field. The external threats and hazards include fire, biological and chemical weapons, and harsh environmental conditions. Internally, the protective gear that is used is susceptible to various types of hazards and threats, and is bulky and uncomfortable for the soldier. The introduction of nanotechnology in the military gear could improve the protective gear. Nano-based materials are more durable due to their chemical, physical, mechanical, and electrochemical properties. Studies show that the use of nanotechnology yields higher protection, longer endurance, and better self-supporting capacities for the soldier. Dry dirt, water, coffee, and fatty substances cannot adhere to the material. This chapter developed a framework presenting factors to be considered when nano-based materials are used in military gear. The focus was on the following areas: UV protection properties, self-cleaning properties, antibacterial properties, energy storage properties, and ballistic properties. General consensus at this point is that nanotechnology in the military is of benefit. However, more work still needs to be done in determining the level of toxicity and the health and safety issues regarding nano-materials.

Keywords: Nanotechnology, nano-based materials, protective gear, military personnel, military gear

**Corresponding author*: Shalinis@dut.ac.za

Suvardhan Kanchi, Shakeel Ahmed, Myalowenkosi I. Sabela and Chaudhery Mustansar Hussain (eds.) Nanomaterials: Biomedical, Environmental, and Engineering Applications, (239–256)

10.1 Introduction

Studies show that nanotechnology promises great improvement to some of the existing technologies in the military [1–3]. These include the following fields in the military: smart fabrics (uniform), robotics, weapons, biological and chemical sensors, vehicles, communication methods, and medical systems.

It is known that military personnel are exposed to various types of hazards and threats daily in the battle field [4–6]. According to Castano and Rodriguez [7], these threats and hazards include attack from weapons, fire, biological and chemical weapons, and harsh environmental conditions, all of which are protected by highly specialized gear. Czerwinska [6] suggests that the main problems associated with current body gear include bulky equipment for the soldier, injuries suffered in the battlefield, and the enemy's advanced weapons. Drawing on Ramdayal and Balasubramanian [5] and Czerwinska [6], the performance and survivability of a soldier relies on the comfort, mobility, and protection provided by the protective gear recognizing that the gear should have unique characteristics that enable the soldier to perform under different hostile conditions. This chapter will focus on smart fabrics properties and health-monitoring sensors used in the military.

Due to the limitations of protective gear currently used, recent studies [4, 5, 8] show that the Department of Defence (DoD) is introducing nanotechnology (NT) in the soldiers' protective gear to improve its performance under various conditions. Tiwari [4] and Lele [8] cite NairoTaniguchi who in 1974 defined nanotechnology as the engineering of functional systems at the molecular scale.

According to Lele [8], the properties of nano-materials (NM) make them ideal to be used in the military because of their small particle size and large surface area. Argawal *et al.,* [9] and Kurahatti *et al.,* [2] affirm that the introduction of nanotechnology in military gear could improve body gear. Especially when considering that it yields stronger, less weight material, and material that stops bullets. Tiwari [4] states that NM are more durable due to their chemical, physical, mechanical, and electromechanical properties. Furthermore, Czerwinska [6] and Argawal [9] believe that the use of NT yields higher protection, longer endurance, and better self-supporting capacities for the soldier.

This chapter investigates the effectiveness and impact of NM used in military gear in order to get better understanding of the potential problems associated with hazards and threats that could manifest from its use. Nanotechnology is a new and emerging field in the military and extensive research is required for the successful production of nano-materials. This places restrictions on the methodology and findings.

10.2 Literature Review

10.2.1 Antibacterial and Self-cleaning Properties

Ramdayal *et al.*, [5] state that the fabric materials currently used in the military protective gear are vulnerable to diseases, high temperatures, and macro-organisms. Concomitantly, the military is developing fabrics infused with silver nanoparticles (Ag), zinc oxide nanoparticles (ZnO), and titanium dioxide nanoparticles (TiO_2). Chaudhari *et al.*, [10] recognize that these nanoparticles are favored due to their antibacterial activities and are chemically stable under exposure to high temperatures. They suggest that the antimicrobial properties can be infused into the fabric of the gear by incorporating functional agents. They agree that ZnO and Ag nanoparticles are mostly used due to their strong inhibitory and antibacterial properties. For wounds, Ramdayal *et al.*, [5] state that these materials restore the injured tissue by maintaining a moist environment, act as a barrier to macro–organisms, and remove excess exudates. They cite Fu Chu Yang *et al.*, (2012) and Ringot *et al.*, (2009) who performed successful experiments based on incorporating Ag nanoparticles onto a fabric. These experiments proved that Ag nanoparticles have the ability of killing 100% of gram-positive *S. aureus* bacteria that were present on the fabric.

10.2.2 Ballistic Protection Properties

According to Obradovic *et al.*, [11] fabrics made of energy-absorbing fibers are used in military for ballistics protection. The ballistics performance of a material relies on its capability to absorb energy and spread it out quickly. Materials that are currently used include Kevlar, Nomex, Spectra, Dyncena, and Zylon. Studies have shown that these materials do not absorb most of the energy from the projectile and the amount of impact force experienced by the body can cause subcutaneous damage [1].

Drawing on this, Czerwinska [6] states that nano-materials such as carbon nano-tubes (CNTs) are incorporated into these materials to better their performance. CNTs can sense the impact of projectile and automatically stiffens to prevent penetration. Thilagavathi [1] cited *Lee et al.*, (2003) who reported on a new liquid body gear based on nanotechnology for ballistic protection. The normal Kevlar body gear is impregnated with a shear-thickening fluid (STF) composed of colloidal dispersion of hard spherical silica nanoparticles (Si) in a polymer solution of ethylene glycol. Obradovic *et al.*, [11] clarified this by conducting test experiments to prove that STF-Kevlar yielded high ballistic protection. It is evident that CNTs and STF-Kevlar provide good ballistic protection; however, the challenge is that Yanez *et al.*, [12] believe that CNTs are toxic on impact and may be exposed to the human skin if it is damaged.

10.2.3 Biological and Chemical Protection Properties

Tomar [13] alerts that exposure of soldiers to hazardous conditions such as biological chemical and agents can lead to high casualties. These hazards may be due to exposure to toxic proteins, bacteria, viruses, and powerful chemical warfare agents [14]. Tomar [13] believes that protection of a soldier from exposure to these hazards is imperative for their well-being. According to Thilagavathi [1] and Tomar [13], metal nanoparticle-based clay, magnesium oxide (MgO), titanium dioxide (TiO_2), silver (Ag), and nickel (Ni) have been developed and proved to be capable of providing excellent biological and chemical protection for the soldier. Furthermore, Kumar *et al.*, [14] outlined that CNTs can also be used in this regard.

Tiwari [4] proposed that a nano-engineered artificial electronic “nose” can be trained to detect toxic vapors, gases, and biological and chemical agents. According to Singh *et al.*, [15], an electronic “nose” is a gas sensor that identifies odors.

Kumar *et al.*, [14] elucidate that a novel aspect of nanotechnology is the use of nanowires made from silver (Ag), nickel (Ni), and gold (Au). These wires can act as barcodes for detecting pathogens such as smallpox, anthrax, ricin, and botulinum toxin. This will help in detecting pathogens at an early stage and medical treatment can be offered to the soldier.

10.2.4 Health Monitoring Sensing Properties

Against this backdrop, Tomar [13] argues that it is important for a Commander in Operations to monitor the physical and mental health conditions of soldiers for better mission execution. Argawal *et al.*, [9] believe that nano-engineered biocompatible implants can monitor a wounded soldier’s vital signs, provide basic first aid, and communicate with Commander in Operations. Srikanth *et al.*, [16] acknowledge that some of the sensor systems will be installed in the soldier’s helmet. The sensors will enable the helmet to perform tasks as radar detection, radio frequency and audio communication, biological and chemical sensing, electroencephalography (EEG) monitoring, sniper detection, and digital signal processing.

In addition, Gupta [3] states that carbon-based electrochemical sensors attached on men's underwear will be developed to monitor the amount of hydrogen peroxide, pH, and conductivity of body sweat and naturally occurring biological substance nicotinamide adenine dinucleotide hydride (NADH). The NADH helps the body to produce energy and also acts as an antioxidant. These health-monitoring sensors will be of assistance in providing first aid and in notifying the Commander in Operations of any injuries. In this way, the body sweat and NADH levels will be monitored constantly and abnormalities will be detected at an early stage.

10.2.5 UV Protection Properties

Ramdayal *et al.*, [5] support that soldiers are exposed to high temperatures in the battlefield and thus need protection. The body gear should therefore have UV blocking properties. Acknowledging this, Li *et al.*, [17] and Gouda and Aljaafari [18] purport that materials made from nano-particles provide excellent UV-blocking properties. Inorganic UV blockers such as nano TiO_2, nano ZnO, nano SiO_2, nano aluminium oxide (Al_2O_3), and nano iron oxide (FeO) are used in this regard. Chaudhari *et al.*, [10] point that nano TiO_2 is mostly suitable because it is non-toxic and stable under exposure to high temperatures. In contrast, Abouzead [19] suggest that nano-TiO_2 may cause hazardous effects and toxicity when it comes into contact with the skin. This was based on the experiments conducted on rabbit skin, which concluded that exposure to nano-TiO_2 after 24 hours showed erythematous patches and moderate edemas on the skin. The studies conducted before 2015 showed that there was not enough information concerning the nano-TiO_2 level of toxicity. Further developments in research in this field are now advancing to give specifics about its toxicity.

10.2.6 Ethics, Safety, and the Enhancement of Soldier's Performance

Ethical considerations of human enhancement in the military raise many concerns and at this point there is no definite solution established to address them. Lin *et al.*, [20] and Shields [21] cited Juengst (1988) who defined enhancement as a biological or chemical intervention introduced to the body to improve performance, capability, appearance, capability, or restore health. They state that if human enhancement compromises the soldier's dignity, it should be avoided. In support, they also cited Gross (2004) who emphasized the need to avoid the loss of dignity of the soldiers. Shunk [22] concurs that ethical and safety issues in enhancing soldier's performance have not been addressed fully. Arguments state that the military sector must not only focus on enhancing the soldier's performance but it must also consider the ethical challenges associated with it. He was not clear whether the soldier should give consent for any type of enhancement. At present, the side effects, long-term effects, and emotional and physical health of the soldier are not addressed. It is evident that ethics and safety in enhancing soldier's performance in the military require further consideration. In the light of the current terrorist uprising, these issues need to be addressed in preventing the creation of a super soldier that is out of control.

10.2.7 Risks in Engineered Nanomaterials

Shvedova *et al.*, [23] and Mercer *et al.*, [24] reported that exposure to SWCNTs in mice led to transitory pulmonary inflammation, oxidative stress, reduced pulmonary function, and decrease in bacterial clearance. Shvedova *et al.*, [23] and Mercer *et al.*, [24] indicated that single walled carbon nanotubes (SWCNTs) which when given to mice by inhalation in doses differing from 0, 5–2 mg/kg had a high risk of inflammation. Gajewicz *et al.*, [25] suggested that CNTs could enter the human body through the skin, eyes, and lung, the respiratory area through air inhalation, and could spread quickly in the central and peripheral nervous system then into the lymph and blood vessels, and could rapidly distribute in heart spleen, kidney, bone marrow, and liver, thereby affecting humans negatively.

Poland *et al.*, [26] posit that exposure to CNTs could cause cancer and other ailments. Of concern, they too observed that these CNTs can be contacted through inhalation, dermal penetration, and ingestion. Lademann *et al.*, [27] suggested that skin exposure to nanomaterials basically happened during handling of consumer products that were dermal applied.

Further studies recognizing the route and effects of CNTs [26–28] are consistent that exposure to nanomaterials might occur through inhalation, dermal penetration, and oral ingestion. Shvedova *et al.*, [23] argued that based on the results in mice, workers might be at risk of budding lung lesions if they were exposed to SWCNTs over a period of 20 days. MWCNTs were shown by Poland *et al.*, [26] to cause soreness and tissue damage in mice as shorter MWCNTs caused fewer inflammations. The International Commission on Radiological Protection (ICRP) (1994) reported that ingestion could happen from accidental hand to mouth transfer of materials and could occur during handling. They, however, suggested that ingestion might also go with inhalation exposure because of particles that are cleaned from respiratory area through the mucociliary escalator might possibly be swallowed. Moos, Chung, Woessner, Honeggar, Cutler, and

Veranth (2010) in agreeing with the ICRP (1994) also observed that many inorganic foods contain nanoscale ingredients in their process. Further, they contended that food can become polluted with nanomaterials by coming into contact with surfaces containing them (packaging materials, kitchen utensils). Chaundry *et al.,* [29] reported that inhalation has been the most studied exposure while the effects of dermal contact and ingestion have not gained the similar detailed research.

Other risks worth considering, by Pritchard [30], suggested that the catalytic effects and fire or explosion were other hazards. DWAF [31] had earlier argued that hazardous waste needs to be considered because it must have been contaminated by toxic and combustive chemical waste that has harmful or chronic impacts on human health and environment. Kang [32] concluded that there should be the need for alert documentation of the physical and chemical characteristic of CNTs, when conducting their toxicity.

This brings to the fore that those who have the maximum risk of exposure to nanomaterials are those in manufacturing and removal of CNTs.

10.2.8 Control of Risks

Drawing from the American National Standards and American Industrial Hygiene Association [33] cited in NIOSH (2013) prescribed control measures for nanomaterials, dusts and other hazardous materials that should be monitored within the circumstances of a complete Occupational Health and Safety Management System. Aligned to this, the following steps are prescribed as specific documented operations to serve as a reference point for others working in similar circumstances:

- Chemical or materials that are being used in the process
- Production technique used through each step of production
- Process equipment and engineering controls employed
- Exposure potential to the ENMs from the job or operation

The point being this would help organizations to decide whether more complicated analytical methods are needed and arrange a list of risk and control measures needed for these risks. Brock [34] cited in NIOSH (2013) mentioned that a containment of hierarchy of controls should be implemented in order to design inherent safety into the process. Furthermore, he explained that Prevention through Design (PtD) also called "inherent safety," "safety by design," "design for safety," and "safe design" is useful in order to reduce hazards, early in the design process, implying that the PtD strategies are implemented through:

- Preventive process inventories by producing the ENMs as they are inspired in the process
- Operating a process at a smaller energy state such as smaller temperature that could result in lower escapee emissions, thus ensuring safer operations
- Using fail-safe devices whereby probable failure in a process ensures that the system would slip back to a safer condition.

Resonating from this, he proposed that controlling potential exposures to nanomaterials involves elimination of greatly hazardous materials during substitution, engineering controls, administrative or work practices, and PPE.

Several authors [6, 8, 9, 35] have indicated that countries like United States, Russia, Germany, France, the United Kingdom, Sweden, Japan, China, South Africa, and India have invested in research and development of nano-materials for military use. Furthermore, nanotechnology institutes like the Institute for Soldier Nanotechnology (ISN) and the Military Institute for Armament have been developed. The aim of these institutes is to conduct research and development based on military nanotechnology. In light of nanotechnology being a new and emerging field in the military, this chapter was based on understanding and interpretating information gathered from the literature [36].

10.3 Application of Nanotechnology in the Military

Nano-engineered health monitoring sensors and protective equipment have recently been developed to equip soldiers in the battlefield. Table 10.1 briefly summarizes the class, function, and description of the hazard from which the solider is being protected.

The main aim of the body gear is to ensure comfort and protection for the soldiers against hazardous conditions. Studies have shown that nano-engineered body gear provides protection and medical support to soldiers [6, 10, 11, 13, 16, 18].

10.3.1 Protective Properties

10.3.1.1 Environmental Hazard Protection

Environmental hazards that pose a threat to soldiers are associated with change in environmental conditions such as heat or cold, fire, rain, snow,

Table 10.1 Functions of nano-engineered body gear (Thilagavathi *et al.*, 2008 and Gupta, 2011).

Class	Functions	Description of hazards being protected
Protective Properties	Environmental hazard protection	Protection against extreme heat or cold, fire, rain, snow, dust, wind, and UV exposure
	Biological, chemical, and hazard protection	Protection against ingestion, penetration, or skin contact of hazard chemicals, toxic gases, body fluids, bacteria, viruses and germs
	Injury protection	Ballistic and blunt impact protection
Medical Properties	Tissue repair	Treatment of wounds, scars, and burn injuries
	Bio-sensing	Monitoring of physical parameters, heart rate, blood oxygenation, body temperature, telemedicine applications

dust, wind, and UV exposure. Various studies show that body gear made from nano-TiO_2, SiO_2, FeO, Al_2O_3, ZnO, and Ag protect soldiers from these environmental hazards [5, 10, 18]. Furthermore, nano-TiO_2 is highly favored because it is considered as being non-toxic (in some circles) and stable under high temperatures. There are some health issues associated with nano-TiO_2 regarding its toxicity when it is exposed to human skin. Abouzead [19] found that exposure to nano-TiO_2 for 24 hours and longer causes erythematous patches and moderate edemas on the skin. Additionally, the percentage of nano-TiO_2 imparted on the body gear should not exceed the maximum toxicity levels. According to Abouzead [19], exposure to 0.5% nano-TiO_2 fabric for 72 hours did not have any impact on rabbit skin as compared to 1% and 2% nano-TiO_2 fabric. They concluded that 0.5% TiO_2 was safer than 1% and 2% TiO_2 fabric as no skin irritations were observed on rabbits. This will help in preventing skin irritations when the soldier is exposed to hazardous environment.

10.3.1.2 Biological and Chemical Hazard Protection

In the battlefield, soldiers are exposed to biological and chemical hazards such as bacteria, viruses, and warfare agents. Various studies conducted indicate that nano-MgO, TiO_2, CNTs, Si, ZnO, Ag, and Ni-infused body gear provide protection from biological and chemical hazards for the soldier [4, 13,15]. These nano-particles are highly favored due to their antibacterial properties and stability against biological and chemical hazards.

10.3.1.3 Injury Protection

Ballistics is one of the most dangerous threats faced by soldiers that result in injuries or wounds. Nano-materials such as CNTs and STF-kevlar have been developed to provide resistance to bullet and bullet fragment penetration. The STF-kevlar is composed of Si nanoparticles. These materials have the capability to sense the bullet impact, absorb its energy, and spread it out quickly. Of concern, Yanez *et al.*, [12] believed that on impact CNTs may be exposed to the body.

10.3.2 Medical Properties

10.3.2.1 Bio-sensing

Much concern is on the importance of monitoring the health and physical strength of soldiers; concomitantly, nano-sensors have been developed to ensure that the physical and health conditions of soldiers can be monitored. For instance, nano-engineered drug delivery systems, diagnosis devices, and medical implants have been developed. Some of the nano-sensor systems are earmarked to be installed on the helmet due to its height and stability. A benefit is that this assists the soldier in communication with the commander at headquarters.

10.3.2.2 Tissue Repair

Treatment of wounds is vital to prevent major blood loss and microorganisms that may cause infection to the soldier. Nano Ag is widely used for its ability to repair skin and can serve as a pressure garment to prevent loss of blood and accumulation of bacteria. It is proposed that incorporating medical properties into the body gear will help in decreasing the number of casualties in the battle field as the body gear will provide first aid.

10.3.3 Ethics, Safety, and the Enhancement of Soldier's Performance

Drawing from the literature gathered, it is evident that nano-engineered body gear enhances the soldier's performance by providing protection and medical monitoring. This, however, has raised some ethical and safety concerns regarding the dignity of soldiers and the toxicity of nano-materials. The findings revealed that it is yet to be established whether a soldier should provide consent before being exposed to enhanced military gear or whether they could refuse to any form of enhancement, particularly if it is against their ethical beliefs or threatens their well-being. This brings to the fore World War II where the soldiers were given methamphetamine drugs to enhance their performance in terms of endurance and strength. Consequently, serious health problems, including fatal heart attacks and addictions, were experienced, and it was suggested that this was due to lack of research and medical monitoring in the field of nanotechnology. The health effects of using nanotechnology to enhance soldiers' performance must be addressed to prevent the re-occurrence of tragic events of World War II.

10.3.4 Key Transmissions of ENM Exposure

The work of Kegan *et al.*, (2010) cited by Yokel and MacPhaill [37] maintain that transmission due to the inhalation has caused the most concern (Figure 10.1) particularly because it is the most common transmission of exposure to airborne particles in the workplace. Furthermore, they reported that the results also indicated that the skin has a little to no transdermal ENMs absorption. They cite the work by Tan, Commens, and Snitch (1996) who advocate that once the nanomaterials get to the outermost epidemic layers of the skin, there is a small barricade for absorption into the circulatory and lymphatic systems.

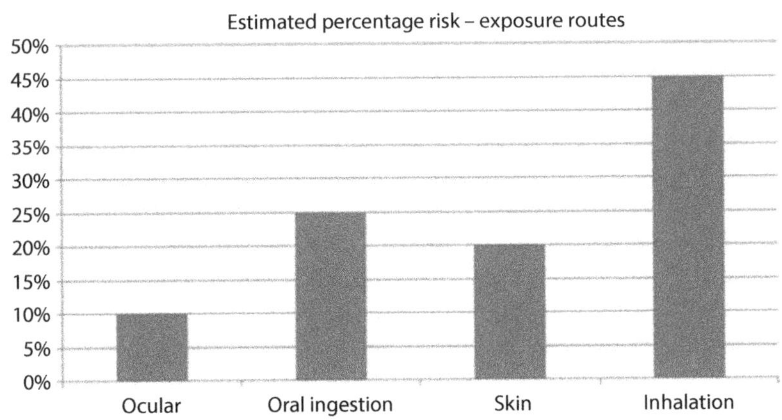

Figure 10.1 Estimated percentage of risk via exposure routes.

According to Keagan *et al.,* [38], oral (gastrointestinal) exposure can occur from intended ingestion, unintended hand-to-mouth movement, and inhaled nanomaterials that are cleared by the mucociliary escalator and of drainage from the eye hollow via the nasal cavity following ocular exposure. Furthermore, they suggested that some transmissions bypass the first clearance and metabolism that occur in the GI tract and liver, which include uptake (absorption) from the nasal cavity that goes directly into the brain, orotransmucosal and transdermal. (Some nanomaterials bypass the first pass clearance and metabolism–ingestion system because some white blood cells can fight with the nanomaterials but the problem is it will go directly into the brain, orotransmucosal and transdermal.) Therefore, they believed that transmissions might present a greater risk of ENM-inferred adverse effect because more ENMs are likely to get to the target organ(s) of toxicity. This could be of benefit also in the military by limiting the risk of exposure of soldiers to ENMs as some of the nano-materials used are considered to be toxic and they are also known as skin irritants. Several authors found that CNTs and TiO_2 are toxic on impact and may cause skin irritation if exposed to human skin [12, 19].

Studies of mice and rabbits exposed through inhalation and skin absorption to nanoparticles showed signs of pulmonary diseases and dermal irritations, respectively. Similarly it can be deduced that workers who inhaled ENMs during production processes risk the same fate. In addition using nano-engineered body armor in the military could pose the same threats as some of the nano-materials used can be transferred into the human body through inhalation and skin contact. As the respiratory tract is the route for inhalation, it is therefore the greatest concern for adverse health risks.

Results of studies show common risks to workers may include inflammation, granulomas, and pulmonary diseases such as asthma, lung disease, and cancer (Kagan *et al.,* 2010, cited by Yokel and MacPhaill [37]). The above findings necessitate a need for additional and adequate information and enlightenment on the use and handling of ENMs by workers.

In view of the above, it is suggested that the following activities: competence, training and awareness, control measures, hierarchy of controls, protection of workers, protection of consumers, emission into the atmosphere, and waste management, be considered in the risk reduction initiatives. These activities will further allow workers or organizations to ensure that protocols are in place to protect their workers from the risks identified. Furthermore, health and safety policy, objectives, emergency preparedness, and responsibilities would help employees to be observant and work safely. This will allow workers or soldiers to be trained in the safe use of ENMs.

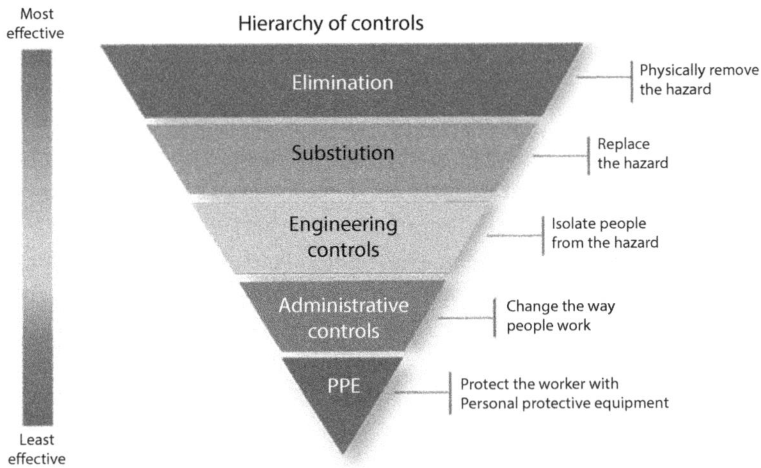

Figure 10.2 The hierarchy of controls for risk reduction and control when working with ENMs [33].

Figure 10.2 outlines a hierarchy of controls that can be used in risk reduction and control initiatives. Studies propose that users should follow the hierarchy of controls as it will guide them in the implementation of an essentially safer system, where the risk can be reduced when working or utilizing materials designed with ENMs. These hierarchies of controls could be of benefit to the Military Research Institute when they are developing new technologies for the military sector. This will aid in addressing the safety issues and reducing the risks of ENMs during manufacturing before they are dispatched to the soldiers for utilization.

10.4 Conclusions

This chapter showed that nano-based materials used in the military sector, particularly with body gear, can offer great benefits especially when it comes to enhancing the soldier's performance in terms of protective and medical properties. Although the body gear enhances the soldier's performance because it is lightweight, strong, and stable under hazardous environments, there is still uncertainty regarding its potential detrimental health issues. Furthermore, ethical and safety issues in enhancing the soldier's performance have not been explored in the literature. Therefore, further investigation is required to determine the level of toxicity and the health and safety issues regarding nano-materials. Ethical and safety issues need to be considered when developing new technologies in the military.

It was inferred that if organizational standards are put in place, SOPs could help in risk reduction on ENMs. SOPs can prevent workers from the illnesses or death because it will identify explicitly what needs to be done, and practice is standardized and concise where all employees have a clear understanding on tasks that are required to be carried out. Potential risks can be reduced among employees and the users of materials containing ENMs after the implementation of hierarchy of controls, suitable work practices, training of employees, health and safety policy, and appropriate protection of workers. Therefore, it could be inferred that risk reduction in ENMs could be achieved by following the SOPs and strict implementation of various recommended procedures and activities. The conclusions above are consistent with ANSI [33] and Brock [34] from the review of the literature.

10.4.1 Recommendations

As illustrated in Figure 10.3, the ethical and safety issues need to be addressed when developing technologies for soldier enhancement. This will help in preventing the loss of dignity of soldiers if ethical beliefs of soldiers are considered. Soldiers must be allowed to give consent, or refuse any form of enhancement if they feel it is against their religion or culture. Soldiers must be informed about health effects and side effects of using nano-engineered body gear. There must be a time frame for disposing used body gear. On retirement, a thorough medical examination must be

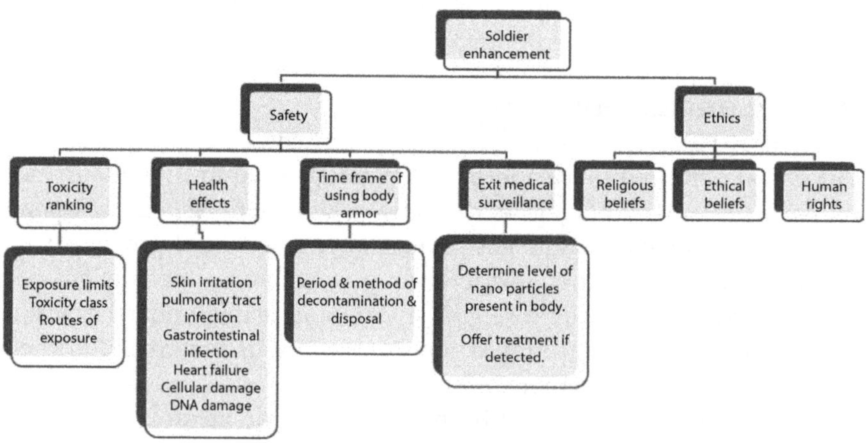

Figure 10.3 Safety and ethics issues to be addressed when new technology is developed to enhance the soldier's performance. Adapted from [20, 21, 22].

performed on a soldier to determine his health status. It is recommended that SOP and hierarchy of controls are the best solution in reducing risks in ENMs and selected safety standards promote the benefits of users who were exposed to them. This will also help to improve health conditions among users or organizations. Risks involved in processing and manufacturing ENMs should be managed as part of an occupational safety and health management plan. Environmental monitoring or industrial hygiene expertise is needed.

References

1. Thilagavathi, G., Raja, A., Kannaian, T. Nanotechnology and protective clothing for defence personnel. *Def. Sci. J.*, 58, 451, 2008.
2. Kurahatti, R., Surendranathan, A., Kori, S., Singh, N., Kumar, A., Srivastava, S. Defence applications of polymer nanocomposites. *Def. Sci. J.*, 60, 551, 2010.
3. Gupta, D. Functional clothing—Definition and classification. *Indian J. Fibre Text Res.*, 36, 321–326, 2011.
4. Tiwari, A. Military nanotechnology. *Int. J. Eng. Sci. Adv. Technol.*, 2, 825, 2012.
5. Ramdayal, Y., Balasubramanian, K. 2013. Advancement in textile technology for defence application. *Def. Sci. J.*, 63, 331, 2012.
6. Czerwinska, M. Military nanomaterials application. Military Institute of Armament Technology, *CHEMIK*, 68, 536–543, 2014.
7. Castano, V., Rodriguez, R. Nanotechnology for ballistic materials: From concepts to products. *Mater. Technol.*, 47, 267, 2013.
8. Lele, A. Role of nanotechnology in defence. *Inst. Def. Stud. Anal.*, 33, 229, 2009.
9. Argawal, S., Mahto, S., Argawal, R. Strengthening the growth of indian defence by harnessing nanotechnology—A prospective. *Def. Sci. J.*, 63, 46, 2013.
10. Chaudhari, S., Mandot, A., Patel, B. Effect of nano TiO_2 pretreatment on functional properties of cotton fabric. *Int. J. Eng. Res. Develop.*, 1, 24, 2012.
11. Obradovic, V., Stojanovic, D., Heinamann, R., Zivkovic, I., Radojevic, V., Uskokovic, P., Aleksic, R. Ballistic properties of hybrid thermoplastic composites with silica nanoparticles. *J. Eng. Fibres Fabrics*, 9, 97, 2014.
12. Yanez, Y., Munoz, B., Albores, A. Mechanisms of toxicity by carbon nanotubes. *Toxicol. Mech. Methods.*, 23, 178, 2013.
13. Tomar, S. Nanotechnology: Current global trends and future military applications for "Soldier as a System". *Inst. Def. Stud. Anal.*, 8, 55, 2014.
14. Kumar, O., Singh, Y., Rao, V., Vijayaraghavan, R. Carbon nanotubes: Detection of chemical and biological warfare agents. *Def. Sci. J.*, 58(5), 617, 2008.

15. Singh, K., Kumar, H., Kumar, A., Chaundary, G. Analysis and simulation of MEMS based multiple gases detection system using COMSOL. *Microelectron. Solid-State Electron.*, 2, 15, 2014.
16. Srikanth, D., Reddy, A., Praveen, V., Yenneti, S. Optimizing the nano technology in defence system for the future war fighter. *IOSR J. Electr. Electron. Eng.*, 9, 51, 2014.
17. Li, H., Deng, H., Zhao, J. Performance research of polyester fabric treated by nano titanium dioxide (Nano-TiO_2). *Int. J. Chem.*, 1(1), 57, 2009.
18. Gouda, M., Aljaafari, A. Augmentation of multifunctional properties of cellulosic cotton fabric using titanium dioxide nanoparticles. *Adv. Nanopart.*, 1, 29, 2012.
19. Abouzead, S., Fares, N., Mohamed, A., Mahmoud, Y. Impact of titanium dioxide used in processing military protection wears on the skin-ultrastructure and molecular study. *Life Sci.*, 12, 54, 2015.
20. Lin, P., Mehlman, M., Abney, K. Enhanced warfighters: Risk, ethics, and policy. California Polytechnic State University., 2013.
21. Shields, M. Personal augmentation—The ethics and operational considerations of personal augmentation in military operations. *Can. Milit. J.*, 15, 24–33, 2014.
22. Shunk, D. Ethics and the enhanced soldier of the near future. Army Capabilities Intergration Center, Future Warfare Division, Fort Eustis, VA, 2015.
23. Shvedova, A., Kisin, E., Mercer, R., Murray, A., Johnson, V., Potapovich, R., Tyurina, Y., Gorelik, O., Arepalli, S., Schwegler-berry, D., Antonini, J., Evans, D., Ku, B.-K., Ramsey, D., Maynard, A., Kagan, V., Castranova, V., Baron, P. Unusual inflammatory and fibrogenic pulmonary responses to single walled carbon nanotubes in mice. *Am. J. Physiol. Lung Cell. Mol. Physiol.*, 289, 698, 2005.
24. Mercer, R., Scabilloni, J., Waig, L., Kisin, E., Murray, A., Schwegler-berry, D., Shvedova, A., Castranova, V. Alteration of deposition pattern and pulmonary response as a result of improved dispersion of aspirated single walled-carbon nanotubes in a mouse model. *Am. J. Physiol. Lung Cell. Mol. Physiol.*, 294, 187, 2008.
25. Gajewicz, A., Rasulev, B., Dinadayalane, T.C., Urbaszek, P., Puzyn, T., Leszczynska, D., Leszczynski, J. Advancing risk assessment of engineered nanomaterials: application of computational approaches. *Adv. Drug Deliv. Rev.*, 64(15), 1663, 2012.
26. Poland, C., Duffin, R., Kinloch, I., Maynard, A., Wallace, W., Seaton, A., Stone, V., Brown, S., Macnee, W., Donaldson, D. Carbon nanotubes introduced into the abdominal cavity of mice show asbestos-like pathogenicity in a pilot study. *Nat. Nanotechnol.*, 3 423, 2008.
27. Lademann, J., Weigmann, H.J., Rickmeyer, C., Barthelmes, H., Schaefer, H., Mueller, G., Sterry, W. Penetration of titanium dioxide microparticles in a

sunscreen formulation into the horny layer and the follicular orifice. *Skin Pharmacol. Appl. Skin Physiol.*, 12(5), 247, 1999.
28. Helland, A., Wick, P., Koehler, A., Schmid, K., Som, C. Reviewing the environmental and human health knowledge base of carbon nanotubes. *Environ. Health Perspect.*, 115(8), 1125, 2007.
29. Chaundry, Q., Blackburn, J., Floyd, P., George, C., Nwaogu, T., Boxall, A., Aitken, R. A scoping study to identify gaps in environmental regulation for the products and applications of nanotechnologies. London: Department for Environment, Food and Rural Affairs, 10, 2006.
30. Pritchard, D.K. Literature review. Explosion hazards associated with nanopowders. United Kingdom: Health and Safely Laboratory, HSL, 12, 2004.
31. Department of Water and Forestry. Disposal sites for hazardous and general waste in South Africa: Baseline studies, DWAF, Pretoria, 1997.
32. Kang, S., Mauter, M., Elimelech, M. Physicochemical determinants of multiwalled carbon nanotubes bacterial cytotoxicity. *Environ. Sci. Technol.*, 42, 5843, 2008.
33. American National Standards Institute/American Industrial Hygiene Association, Occupational Health and Safety Management Systems. Fairfax, VA: AIHA, ANSI Z10, 2012.
34. Brock, B. Knowledge brief: containment hierarchy of controls. Tampa, FL: ISPE, 2009.
35. Krichevskii, G.E. Dual—Use technologies in production of XXI soldier combat uniform and civilian goods. *Russ. J. Gen. Chem.*, 83, 185, 2013.
36. Domegan, C., Flemming, D. Marketing Research in Ireland: *Theory and Practice. 3 ed.* Gill & Macmillan Ltd., Dublin, 2007.
37. Yokel, R.A., Macphaill, R.C. Engineered nanomaterials: exposures, hazards, and risk prevention. *J. Occup. Med. Toxicol.*, 6(7), 2, 2011.
38. Kegan, V.E, Shi, J., Feng, W., Shvedova, A.A., Fadeel, B. Fantastic voyage and opportunities of engineered nanomaterials: what are the potential risks of occupational exposure? *J. Occup. Environ. Med.*, 52, 943, 2010.

Part III

BIOLOGICAL APPLICATIONS

11

Plasmonic Nanopores: A New Approach Toward Single Molecule Detection

Gaurav Khandelwal[1], Sima Umrao[2], Narsingh R. Nirala[3], Sadhana S. Sagar[4] and Vinod Kumar[5*]

[1]*Indian Institute of Technology Delhi, Hauzkhas, New Delhi, India*
[2]*School of Electronics and Electric Engineering, Sungkyunkwan University (SKKU), Suwon, Korea*
[3]*School of Materials Science and Technology, IIT (BHU), Varanasi, India*
[4]*Rani Lakshmi Bai Central Agricultural University, Jhansi, India*
[5]*Department of Materials Engineering, Ben Gurion University of the Negev, Beer-Sheva, Israel*

Abstract

In recent years nanopores technology have been widely explored for single molecular detection of biomolecules. An integration of optical modalities with ionic current signals have found to be an attractive approach to receive more accurate information about target analyte. Assimilation of plasmonic detection with electrical read out signals of solid state nanopores has configured a new approach known as Plasmonic nanopores. Optical signals will help to reveal chemical states and properties of the specific analytes inside the nanopores with potential of multiplexed detection by multi-nanopore. Plasmonic nanopores hold immense possibilities for developing efficient sensing devices and thorough investigations are needed. The proposed book chapter will provide a detailed information about the fabrication of plasmonic nanopores, their recent application in single molecule analysis and future perspective.

Keywords: Nanopores, plasmonic, detection, sequencer, sensor

**Corresponding author*: mail2vinod2@gmail.com, vinod@post.bgu.ac.il

Suvardhan Kanchi, Shakeel Ahmed, Myalowenkosi I. Sabela and Chaudhery Mustansar Hussain (eds.) Nanomaterials: Biomedical, Environmental, and Engineering Applications, (259–284)

11.1 Introduction

In recent years, advancement of nanosciene and nanotechnology has enabled to develop smart detection systems at single molecular level. Among others, Nanopore-based devices have received significant interest due to their extremely high sensitivity, versatility, portability, etc. [1]. In general, a nanopore is a nanoscale pore (aperture/channel) in a membrane. A nanopore in a biological membrane is termed as a biological nanopore and if it is in a solid-state membrane, then it is named as solid-state nanopores. However, there is another class of nanopores, i.e. hybrid nanopores with combined characteristics of both biological and solid-state nanopores. Detection through nanopores is solely based on the working principle of Coulter Counter *technique* [2], which is employed to count small particles ranging from sub-micron to millimeters. Similar to Coulter counter, in nanopores techniques, the membrane with nanopores is held between the two reservoirs/chambers containing electrolyte. These two chambers are named as the *cis* and *trans* chamber (Figure 11.1). Analyte is introduced into the *cis* chamber and a transmembrane potential is applied that allows the translocation of analyte molecules through a nanopore. When an analyte molecule passes through the nanopore, it partially blocks the flow of electrolyte ions and induces a transient fluctuation in the ionic current, its amplitude, and duration, which can be used to probe the single molecule events including DNA interaction, DNA/RNA transport, virus sensing, and protein–receptor binding [3–5]. Microsecond time-scale characterization of nucleic acids is possible through such measurements without the need for complicated preparation, such as amplification, chemical modification, or probe and/or intercalator binding.

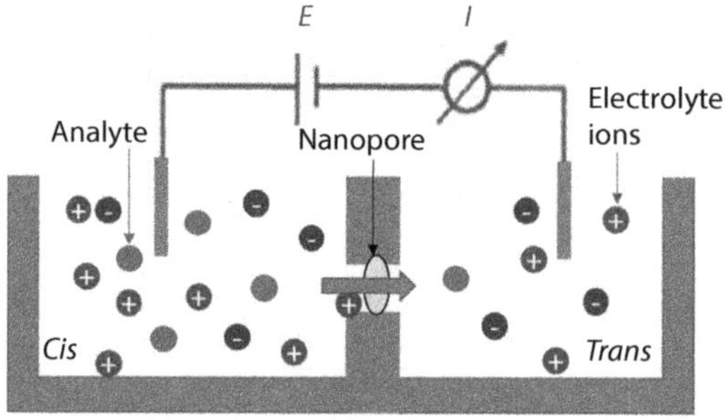

Figure 11.1 Schematic diagram showing working principle of nanopore.

11.1.1 Biological Nanopores

Inspired with natural protein channels that regulate molecular transport across the cell membrane and play vital roles in a variety of biological processes, the concept of biological nanopores is derived. Biological nanopores have shown immense capabilities for a single molecular level of biosensing. It is due to several unique features of biological nanopores, such as atomic-precision structural reproducibility and compatibility of pore sizes with many important bio-molecules. Biological nanopores can be further engineered in with various approaches like site-directed mutagenesis or incorporation of specific adaptors [6]. Alpha hemolysin (α-HL) embedded within a lipid bilayer was the first reported biological nanopore with a constriction of 1.4 nm at the narrowest point [7]. Apart from α-HL, numerous other membrane protein-based biological nanopores such as areolysin [8], MspA [9, 10], ClyA [11], FhuA [11], membrane-adapted phi29 motor protein [12], and SP1 [13] were explored and studied to detect different analytes, particularly in DNA sequencing. However, biological nanopores suffered with certain limitations, for example, the lipid bilayer is fragile and prone to rupture at harsh conditions of pH, salt, and temperature as well as lack of freedom to tune the protein pore size/geometry. In addition, the stochastic skipping and backstepping of enzyme motors (phi29) resulted in deletion and insertion of errors [14].

11.1.2 Solid State Nanopores

To overcome the associated problems of biological nanopores, solid-state nanopores have been introduced. Solid-state nanopore possess several unique advantages, including tunable pore size and shape with sub-nanometer resolution, mechanical robustness, superior thermal and chemical stability over a wide range of conditions (i.e., pH, temperature, concentration), parallel fabrication techniques that can easily produce many identical nanopore setups, and integration compatibility with sophisticated technology. The diameter of the solid-state nanopores can be precisely controlled ranging from sub-nanometers to hundreds of nanometers according to the experimental requirements. In general, solid-state nanopores in dielectric materials, such as SiN, exhibit superior chemical and thermal stability over lipid membranes. However, their stability is dependent on the conditions used to form these pores. [15]

Solid-state nanopores have emerged as a versatile concept for label-free detection and investigation of biomolecules at the single-molecule level. In brief, molecules that translocate through a small pore in a thin membrane can be electrically detected one by one, because they temporarily modulate the ionic conductance of the pore. The concept has proven useful for many applications, including molecular size discrimination, investigation of biomolecular interactions at the single-molecule level, and investigation of local structures along elongated molecules, such as protein bound to DNA [16]. Yet, solid state nanopores face challenges. For example, control over the translocation speed of the biomolecule [17–20] is crucial for base pair recognition on a DNA polymer, as already demonstrated using biological nanopores [21, 22].

11.1.3 Plasmoinc Nanopore

Furthermore, it would be advantageous to expand the nanopore approach with new measuring modalities (e.g., optical detection) beyond mere electrical probing. In last few years, considerable progress has been made to improve the efficiency of nanopore-based sensors, mainly in their ability to have much clear demarcation among very fine macromolecular properties [23]. For instance, designing and development of proficient nanopore sequencing devices with abilities of distinguishing among four different nucleotides of single-stranded DNA (ss-DNA) has been a major challenge in a number of studies. Real-life applications of solid-state nanopores have been limited by these major factors. (i) Noise and bandwidth: In nanopores, due to the limited signal bandwidth of each element involved in the current measurements, the temporal resolution is limited to 1–10 μs. In addition, the electrical signals are hindered by disturbed ion current noise spectra, which include low frequency (1/f) flicker noise and high frequency dielectric loss and capacitive noise, on top of the flat thermal noise (Johnson–Nyquist) and electronic shot noise [24–27]. All noise components play a key limiting role of the nanopore's ability to resolve fine molecular features, which are required in various sensing applications. (ii) Throughput: Simultaneous multiplexed readouts from hundreds if not thousands of nanopores, without compromising the detection bandwidth and sensitivity, are a central challenge in nanopore-based sensing [28]. (iii) Spatial information and spatial resolution: Very short nanopore channel is not sufficient for the spatial resolution of short DNA strands; thus, development of strategies to further improve the nanopore spatial resolution is another issue with nanopore-based technology. Several strategies have been projected to address these limitations. In many cases, the improved approaches involve supplementation of the electrical ion measurement with additional electrical measurements [29]. In another approach, the use of an atomically thin substrate, such as graphene, helped in improving the spatial resolution of the nanopore [30–33]. Furthermore, it would be advantageous to expand the nanopore approach with new measuring modalities (e.g., optical detection) beyond mere electrical probing. Recently, plasmonic solid-state nanopores were introduced [34–38], which presented new opportunities for biomolecular sensing. Here, a plasmonic nanoantenna enhances and focuses electromagnetic radiation to a nanoscale volume (hotspot) right at the nanopore through which biomolecules can be translocated (Figure 11.2) . Reports on plasmonic nanopores have so far mostly focused on nanoplasmonic heating [38–41]. However, great promise lies in also exploiting the capabilities of these plasmonic nanostructures for extreme light-concentration to local nanometer-sized hotspots.

This approach is very powerful, in terms that it provides a measurement that is fundamentally independent of the electrical sensing that relies on photons rather than electrons. Notably, the optical sensing can be performed at the far-field, as photons freely travel in the aqueous media surrounding the nanopores. This unique feature opens up vast opportunities for light excitations and broad spectral emission, which will cause minimal interference with the local electrical measurement performed at the nanopore itself. Further, integration of optical sensing in nanopores introduces the benefits of a wealth of high-performance reagents, such as high-brightness fluorophores covering a broad spectral range, high-sensitivity sensors, including Avalanche Photo Diodes (APDs), electron-multiplying and scientific CMOS CCD cameras, and ultracompact solid-state light sources spanning the near UV to the IR wavelength regimes and other components developed for single-molecule optical sensing.

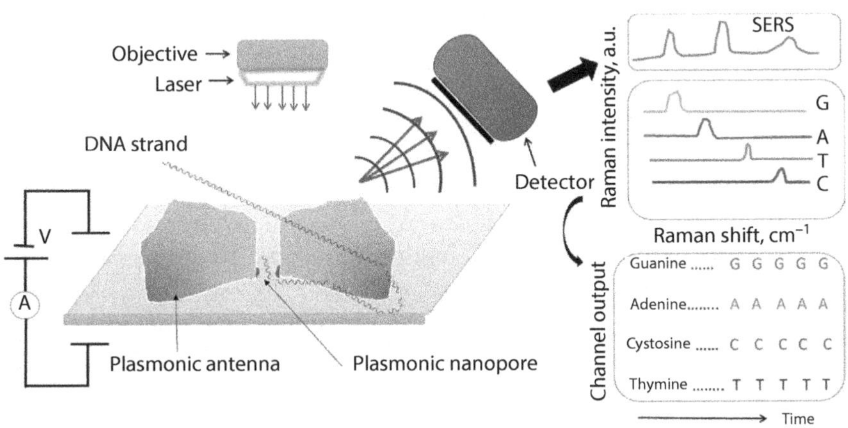

Figure 11.2 Schematic showing working principle of plasmonic nanopore.

In this book chapter, working principles of plasmonic nanopore are first explained followed by nanofabrication methods and optical properties of plasmonic nanopores. Recent applications of nanopores in special reference to DNA sequencing and others are then described. In last the future perspective of plasmonic nanopores are discussed.

11.2 Sensing Principles of Plasmonic Nanopore

Sensing principles of plasmonic nanopores are utilizing the same detection principles as in the conventional surface plasmon resonance (SPR) technique. It is a kind of a refractometric sensor [42].

Binding of molecules to the sensor surface brings about an increase to the local refractive index (RI), which leads to a redshift in the plasmon resonance that is detected by the spectroscopy technique. Using plasmonic nanopore, label-free and real-time analysis of biomolecular interactions can be studied. Brolo *et al.*, in 2004 were first to report on biosensing with nanohole arrays using relatively simple refractometric detection of protein adsorption [43]. In 2005, Dahlin *et al.*, studied protein–membrane interactions in real-time [44]. Käll group also studied refractometric sensing by a single nanohole using scattering spectroscopy in a dark field [45]. These pioneering studies were arguably not very interesting as there was no clever use of the nanopores. It is not until recently that plasmonic nanopores have started to be used for "more efficient" biosensor applications as explained in the following sections. In addition to refractometric detection, other optical "sensing" techniques (that somehow detect the presence of molecules) are also possible with plasmonic nanopores. Some examples are optical entrapment inside "double holes" [46, 47] (Figure 11.1E) and surface-enhanced Raman scattering [48] (SERS). Plasmonic nanopore traps have been suggested to offer the possibility to study biomolecular interactions on the single molecule level since the trapping event itself appears to generate a clearly detectable intensity change [47]. The trapping mechanism has been described as due to self-induced back-action [49]. In SERS, the vibrational modes from molecules very close (~1 nm) to the metal surface are detected through the enhanced electromagnetic fields that arise on metallic nanostructures in general. This excludes a proper recognition layer for specificity as it would move the targets too far away, but on the other hand one can get molecular fingerprints from the spectrum. In attempts to reach high and reproducible SERS signals, several types of plasmonic nanopores have been tested in recent years [50, 51] showing that the approach still attracts attention.

11.2.1 Fabrication of Plasmonic Nanopores

Most of the techniques used for making plasmonic nanopores contain some form of lithography, deposition, and etching steps, and they have been discussed briefly in following sections.

11.2.1.1 Materials of Choice

Plasmonic nanopores are generally prepared in a metal film on a dielectric support, which is always a silicon nitride membrane prepared by back-etching of a coated Si wafer [52] (TEM window). Junesch *et al.*, have exceptionally reported the preparation of plasmonic nanopores in a single suspended 20 nm gold film (Figure 11.3F) [53]. In all cases, for plasmonic activity, the nanopores must penetrate metal films. In majority, gold structures have been used due to their good optical properties (low optical losses and resonances at suitable wavelengths) and long-term chemical stability.

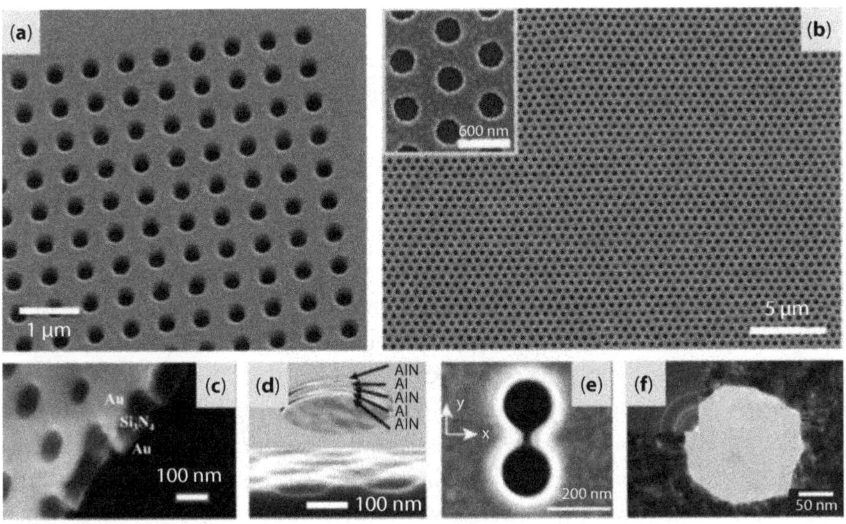

Figure 11.3 Electron microscopy images of plasmonic nanopores. (a) A square nanopore array in a 120 nm gold film on an 80 nm supporting silicon nitride membrane fabricated by electron beam lithography. (b) A long range ordered nanohole array in 50 nm silver prepared by colloidal self-assembly. (c) Nanopores in gold (20 nm) – silicon nitride (50 nm) – gold (20 nm) triple layers. (d) Nanoholes in multilayers of ultrathin aluminum and aluminum nitride films (with schematic). (e) A "double nanohole" in 100 nm gold fabricated by ion beam milling. (f) A nanopore in a single suspended 20 nm gold film imaged by transmission electron microscopy (inset showing diffraction pattern). (Reference: Dahlin, A.B., Analyst, 2015, 140, 4748–4759) [121].

Silver could be another option that provides even better optical properties and has been tried in some sensing work [46, 54]. However, tarnishing is the main drawback with silver metal, which can be overcome by surface passivation before use [53]. Aluminum has also been used [56], in part, as it offers the possibility to study important corrosion processes [56] and interband transitions.

11.2.1.2 Lithography

Numerous patterning techniques have been used to fabricate various types of plasmonic nanopores (Figure 11.3). Some of them are relatively complicated and expensive such as electron beam lithography [57] or ion beam milling [46, 58]. Electron beam lithography is used to generate a pattern in a resist coating on top of the thin films, which is then followed by deposition and dry etching steps to generate pores. This results in homogenous pore arrays (Figure 11.3A), with the possible disadvantage that the metal may also coat the interior of the pores in the supporting membrane. In ion beam milling, a nanopore can "drill" directly through the metal film and its supporting membrane, i.e., the etching comes with the lithography. This technique is naturally suitable for making single pores with special shapes (Figure 11.3E) [45]. However, the resulting pores tend to not have very vertical walls [45, 58]. Oh *et al.*, have used nanoimprint technology [39, 45] and template-stripping [55] in order to improve throughput. The use of colloidal self-assembly is an alternative to serial and costly nanolithography tools, where adsorbed polystyrene spheres represent the mask that defines the pattern of pores [60]. Interestingly, both long-range ordered and short-range ordered patterns are possible to generate. Nanosphere lithography is claimed as a more suitable technique for producing plasmonic nanohole arrays exhibiting long-range order in a hexagonal lattice originating from assembly of a 2D close-packed layer followed by glancing angle deposition [61] or plasma treatment to separate the particles from one another [54] (Figure 11.3B). Masson group has developed this fabrication approach [62–66], which gives relatively large diameters and void fractions in the metal. Sutherland [67–68], Sannomiya [53], and Dahlin [69–70] have produced a variety of nanoholes and nanopores with short-range order, typically with ~100 nm diameter and ~10 holes or pores per μm^2 "colloidal lithography." The definition of short-range order is that there is a characteristic spacing between the nearest-neighbor apertures manifested by a peak in the radial distribution function [69–71]. Typically, the characteristic center-to-center distance is twice the diameter of the colloids used.

11.2.1.3 Multilayers

Fabrication of nanohole arrays in multilayers of aluminum and aluminum nitride is reported by Ikenoya *et al.*, [56] (Figure 11.3D). Dahlin *et al.*, showed nanopores in a metal-insulator-metal (Au-Si_3N_4-Au) system [69] (Figure 11.3C). Multilayered structures offer new insights into the optical properties of coupled thin films and could also open up for new applications by having multiple isolated thin-film electrodes. Plasmonic nanopores are larger [72] than biological nanopores and it is due to limitations in fabrication methods. The most popular technique, i.e., colloidal patterning fails [70] to drill a low diameter nanopore as below 100 nm it resulted into much broader diameter distribution [69]. This can be overcome by post-fabrication electrode growth of the metal layer [54]. However, making nicely circular apertures on the order of 10 nm is still a general challenge for metals regardless of the fabrication method due to faceting at the edges [53, 69]. Plasmonic nanopores are not suitable for some types of sensor applications due to their wide diameters. For example, probing molecular translocation events by ion currents is likely not feasible when the pore diameter is much larger than the molecules [72, 73]. Even if smaller plasmonic pores can be fabricated in the future, they might not provide the possibility to do optical sensing since diameters on the order of 100 nm are preferable for efficient coupling to plasmon modes.

11.3 Optical Properties

Ebbesen *et al.*, [74] have studied the optical properties of single nanoholes and arrays in depth since the discovery of "extraordinary" transmission. More in-depth reviews are available describing the optical properties of plasmonic nanopores [76]. In brief, the optical properties of single nanoholes are in many ways similar to those of nanoparticles in many ways [77]. Similar to particles, individual holes support localized plasmon modes that depend strongly on the aperture shape [78]. In addition, the thickness of the metal is also important and for sufficiently thick films (100 nm) modes that propagate along apertures (perpendicular to the thin films plane) dominate the transmission [78]. Propagating surface plasmons are also possible to excite by single holes [79–80]. However, grating-type coupling (a.k.a. Bloch waves) to propagating surface modes is possible when multiple nanoholes are arranged periodically in a metal film [81]. The polarizability of each aperture is very important and a nanopore array resonance is an asymmetric spectral feature that has a transmission minimum accompanied by a maximum at a nearby longer wavelength [82]. Upon closer look into the literature, some inconsistencies regarding the optical properties of nanohole arrays were noticed. One such debate relates to whether the grating-type excitation mechanism primarily is associated with the transmission maximum or the nearby extinction (inverse transmission, absorption plus scattering) maximum. Although treating these spectral features as independent of one another is not possible, so studying their respective behavior in response to certain parameters such as aperture shape and periodicity is of great importance [71]. The original claim was that the transmission maximum was a resonance induced by the periodicity [74] which shows some deviations from experimental data which can be later explained by an interference effect [83, 84]. Data from multiple structures have also revealed that the extinction maximum agrees better with the predicted grating coupling resonance than the transmission maximum [82]. Particularly for thinner metal films (tens of nm), several papers report how the nanohole arrays reduce transmission by introducing coupling to surface plasmons [85, 86]. Predicting resonances is to some extent complicated by the fact that the presence of holes in a metal film alters the dispersion relation for surface plasmon modes [71, 87]. One can ask whether or not the optical properties of short-range ordered nanohole arrays are comparable to the long-range ordered ones. In some reports, a short-range ordered pattern generated by colloidal lithography are considered to be "random" and no grating-type mechanisms are discussed [68, 88]. An analogy between short-range and long-range order, both for thicker [82, 89] and thinner [71, 90] metal films have been reported by other studies. It is demonstrated that by using the characteristic spacing between short-range ordered holes as an effective periodicity and by calculating the dispersion relations for surface plasmons in thin film multilayers [56, 69, 70], good quantitative agreement with experimental data for the extinction peak is possible [56, 69–71]. This formalism is particularly for predicting the shift in the peak [56, 70, 91–93] caused by, for instance, molecular binding in a sensing experiment, which is explained as below.

11.4 Improving Performance

Sensing performance of plasmonic nanopores can be improved by incorporating following approaches. These approaches are more suitable for making the nanopore themselves more sensitive in order to detect smaller molecules and lower concentrations.

11.4.1 Use of a New Kind of Structures

Several groups have tried to fabricate slightly different types of nanopores using quite different methods, to reach better resolution for refractometric detection by them. Experimental investigations have linked the influence from pore shape [94], periodicity [95], film thickness [96], and roughness [97] as well as metal type [66] toward improving performances. In every case, the zero-incidence transmission spectrum is analyzed in hope to find plasmon resonances with higher wavelength shift and narrower spectral width. Sensitivity of plasmonic nanopores still remains an issue of debate. In some cases, only the resonance shift per RI change of the whole liquid environment is considered. In other cases, the peak width is introduced as a normalization factor, a so-called figure of merit [98]. Even peak magnitude has been taken into account [66]. In the final sensing application, one must also consider the extension of the plasmonic field in relation to the thickness of the molecular layer to be detected [99]. The refractive index sensitivity decreases approximately exponentially with the distance from the surface, following the decay of the transverse magnetic field [69] for plasmonic nanopore-based detection. Similar to that in conventional SPR, down to tens of nm for bonding surface plasmons in thin films [100, 71, 96] for plasmonic nanopores, the extension depends strongly on the nature of the plasmon mode and can vary from hundreds of nm.

11.4.2 Use of New Spectroscopy Techniques

The use of new spectroscopy technique can be a better alternative for efficient measurements with tuned shapes and dimensions of the nanopore structures. Yanik *et al.*, showed that narrow resonances can appear when a nanopore array is tilted slightly relative to the incident plane wave of light [98], leading to interference with sub-radiant modes that have no scattering losses, a so-called Fano resonance [101]. Same idea was also presented in earlier work [102]. Couture *et al.*, showed an important work to evaluate sensing with nanohole arrays in Kretschmann configuration (as in SPR) [64]. It was demonstrated that despite the longer field extension associated with the excitation of surface plasmons in this configuration, the bulk sensitivity factor is so much higher that the performance is better also for thin layers, as shown in Figure 11.4. However, one should keep in mind that the Kretschmann configuration is not straightforward to employ in nanopore structures with flow through, etc. The results in Figure 11.4 illustrate another example of how plasmonic nanopores are not superior compared to existing techniques (Kretschamnn SPR) in terms of direct sensor

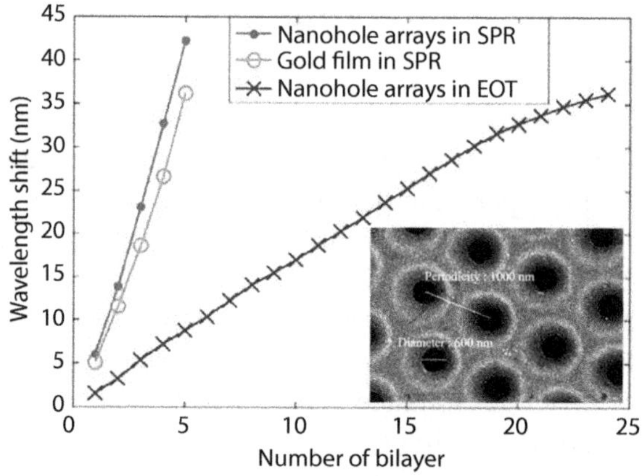

Figure 11.4 Using nanohole arrays as a conventional surface plasmon resonance sensor by excitation in the Kretschmann configuration (SPR). The response to polyelectrolyte multilayers is compared with a gold film without nanoholes and with excitation in transmission (EOT) (Ref. Couture *et al.*, [64]).

resolution. It has been reported to perform equally well in terms of bulk RI resolution [97], but this does not take into account differences in the evanescent field extension [99].

11.5 Surface Patterning

Patterning techniques can be a more useful approach for improving the sensing performance. Patterning techniques are such that only a part of the surface, the most sensitive, is activated for molecular binding. For functionalization of nanopores, thiol-based chemistry has long been used in a simple manner to specifically modify gold or silver [103]. Other materials, such as silica [104], titania [105], niobia [70], or silicon nitride [54] can then be left unaffected for further functionalization in subsequent steps. This makes it possible to direct molecular binding to certain regions, primarily the interior of nanoholes, in order to investigate the local field distribution or to improve performance [105–107]. The method can indeed improve the signal, but again mainly for reactions that do not reach equilibrium [105]. Once the surface starts to become filled up with its equilibrium coverage, the signal is instead higher if binding to the surface occurs everywhere in the structure [107]. Naturally, one can still argue that there is an "enhancement" in the sense that the signal per molecule is higher [106–107]. There seems to be a disagreement whether this is the correct measure of enhancement or if the signal per surface coverage is a more preferable measure [108].

11.6 Applications – Next-Generation DNA Sequencing and Beyond

The high need for low-cost and ultrafast sequencing technologies has driven the development of multiple, novel single-molecule methods [109]. Nanopore based DNA sequencing is widely considered to be a promising next-generation sequencing platform [110–111]. Protein pores (i.e., MspA) have already been shown to effectively sequence DNA strands [9, 16, 21]. It was achieved by reducing the translocation speed of the DNA strands by coupling them to ratcheting enzymes. Two primary challenges for the method still remain: First, improving the base calling accuracy and its ability to read any arbitrary sequence including long repeats. And second, realizing a drastic boost in the overall throughput of nanopore sequencing by simultaneous readout from hundreds if not thousands of nanopore. These challenges can be addressed by employing optical-based nanopore techniques with high-density nanopore arrays [27, 112]. Soni *et al.*, first introduced an optical-based nanopore sequencing approach that involves two steps [113]. In the first step, there is a sample preparation step in which the DNA is converted into an expanded form, followed by hybridization of fluorescently-labeled probes to each expanded base. In the second step, the fluorescent markers are optically detected, using an array of nanopores and TIRF illumination (Figure 11.5). The main benefit of the method is that it simplifies the readout procedure to involve only four different colored fluorophores. In contrast, the current electrical-based nanopore sequencing method involves a readout of 3 (or 4) nucleotide groups, which theoretically require discrimination among $4^3 = 64$ different current levels, although sophisticated algorithms can be used to reduce this number by exploiting the fact that DNA is ratcheted through the pore in discrete single-nucleotide steps and that each base is read 3 (or 4) times in a different sequence context [114–115]. However, the optical approach, in contrast, does not involve ratcheting enzymes and thus can theoretically achieve a higher strand loading efficiency and higher sequencing speed. These advantages, however, come at the price of an elaborate DNA preparation step, in which each of the four different nucleotides in the DNA strand is substituted with its own unique code oligonucleotide (typically ~15 nucleotide long). The substitution (or "DNA conversion") process involves cyclic ligations of the correct code oligonucleotide and digestion of the original bases. This off-line process can be simultaneously performed with a vast number of DNA molecules and does not require enzyme immobilization or an amplification step. After converting the DNA molecules, four different molecular beacons complementary to the four

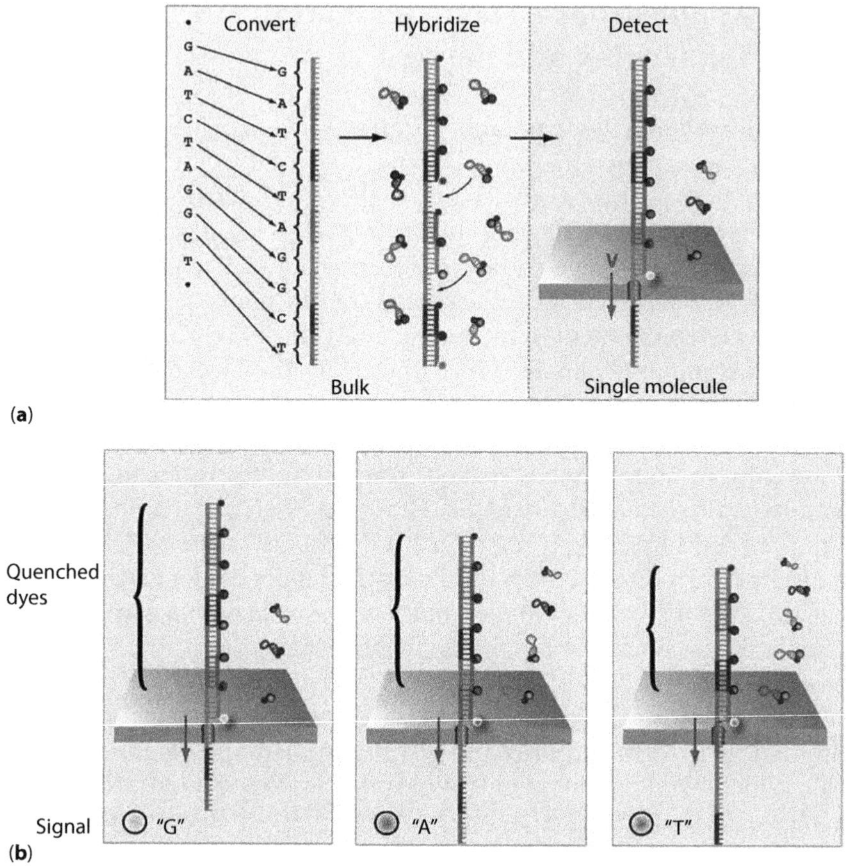

Figure 11.5 Schematic illustration of the optical sequencing method. Each base is converted into an extended sequence that is hybridized to a fluorophore–quencher beacon, where each base is represented by a different fluorophore color. The DNA/beacon complex is then threaded through a nanopore and the color barcode is detected optically. Each released beacon is automatically closed, quenching its own fluorescence while diffusing away from the vicinity of the pore (Ref. Glioba *et al.*, Analyst, 2015, 140, 4733–4747) [122].

possible oligonucleotide codes are specifically hybridized to the converted DNA. Each of the four beacons contains a different-color fluorophore on its 5′ end and a quencher on its 3′ end. The broad-spectrum quencher molecule quenches both fluorophores and the four different color fluorophores make it possible to distinguish between them.

The converted DNA strands and hybridized beacons are electrophoretically threaded through an array of nanopores, designed to bear a diameter that allows only one strand to translocate through it. The TIR mode of laser sources illuminates pores and optically monitors using EMCCD. Upon the entering of the DNA molecule through pore, the marked beacons are stripped off one at a time, creating a distinct burst of fluorescence. Each released beacon is automatically closed, quenching its own fluorescence while diffusing away from the vicinity of the pore (Figure 11.4, lower panel). Translocation speed of the DNA to approximately a few ms per unzipping event by using the stripping process and the unzipping time can be tuned by the voltage applied. McNally *et al.*, performed proof of concept experiments to validate this new sequencing method. To make larger pores applicable, the unzipping process will be more suitable (~2 nm), McNally *et al.*, covalently attached a "bulky" group (e.g., a protein or a nanoparticle) to the molecular beacons, which effectively increased the molecular cross section of the complex to 5–7 nm, enabling use of 3–5 nm pores. They have shown that each of the four possible nucleotides was represented by two successive beacons (or "bits"), allowing for use of two colors only. Further, to test the ability to observe the 2 bit signal, they prepared two samples: a 1 bit sample in which they attach an avidin (4 × 5 × 6 nm) to a biotinylated molecular beacon containing a fluorophore-quencher pair, in addition to a similar beacon without a fluorophore, both hybridized to a target ssDNA, and a 2-bit sample with a similar complex but with two beacons containing a fluorophore–quencher pair. The obtained optical signals clearly showed one- and two-photon bursts for the 1-bit and 2-bit samples, respectively. Next, they performed two-color unzipping experiments with two high quantum yield fluorophores A647 (ATTO647N) and A680 (ATTO680), simultaneously excited by the same red laser. The optical emission was split into two channels using a dichroic mirror and simultaneously imaged by a single EM-CCD camera. Due to the overlap between the emission spectra of the two fluorophores, they performed calibration experiments using 1-bit complexes labeled either with A647 or A680. Fluorescence intensities ratio of Channel 2 versus Channel 1 was 0.2 ± 0.06 for the A647 sample and 0.4 ± 0.05 for the A680 sample. The ratios for the accumulation of all the events were 0.2 and 0.4 for the A647- and A680-labeled sample, respectively. The control measurements have demonstrated that the color ratio can be used in order to determine the identity of individual fluorophores. The error in the determination of each of the two fluorophores was calculated from the overlap area between the distributions, yielding <9% for the A647 and <13% for A680. By using the calibration results, they tested their ability to discriminate between the 2-bit combinations representing the four different bases (Figure 11.6). An analysis of ~2000 events in which two distinct photon bursts were detected revealed a bimodal distribution of R with two

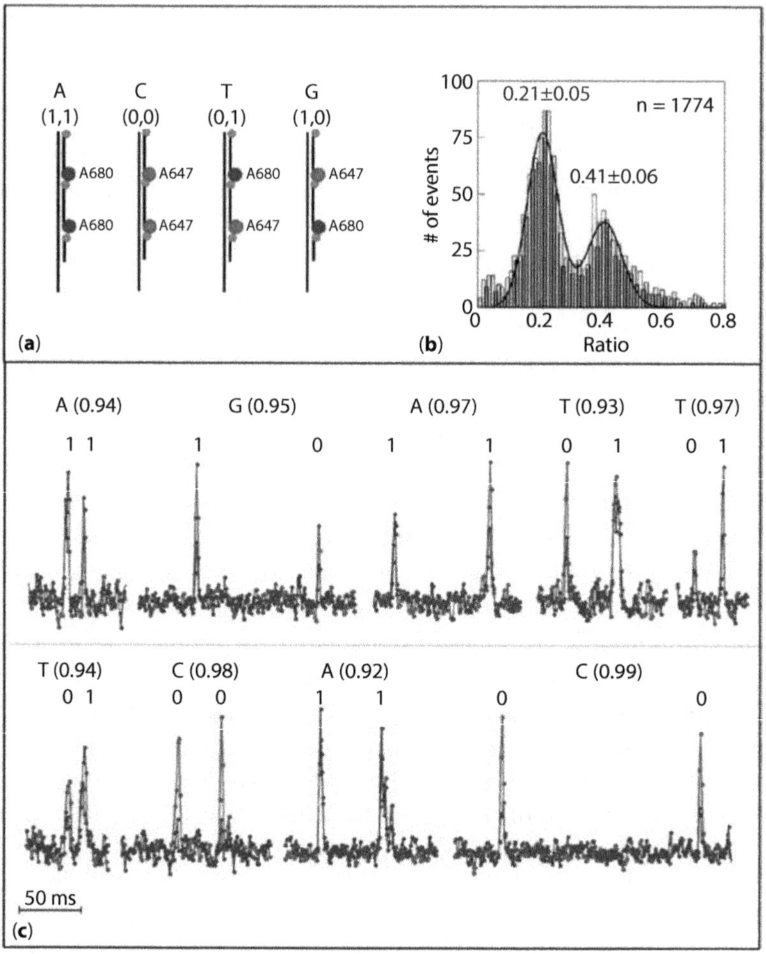

Figure 11.6 Optical detection of the four 2-bit combinations representing the four different nucleotides. (a) Illustration of the four samples labeled with two fluorophores correspond to the four bases. (b) The color ratio (*R*) distribution of 1774 events revealing two peaks corresponding to the two fluorophores. (c) Representative intensity-corrected fluorescence traces of unzipping events. Corresponding bit called, base called, and certainty score indicated above the event. The intensities in the two channels were corrected automatically by a computer code after each bit is called using a fixed threshold *R* value (Ref. Glioba *et al.*, Analyst, 2015, 140, 4733–4747) [122].

modes at 0.21 ± 0.05 and 0.41 ± 0.06, in agreement with the calibration results. Photon bursts with $R < 0.3$ were classified as 0 and those with $R > 0.3$ were classified as 1. Finally, they demonstrated multipore reading of the photon bursts using an array of 3 nanopores. Although plasmonic nanopore methodology provides a new approach for high throughput DNA sequencing, the SNR and error in barcode determination due to spectra overlap must be further improved. One of the possible ways in which the barcoding error can be reduced is by use of fluorophores with less overlap in their emission spectra. This could be achieved by simultaneously illuminating the nanopore with multiple laser lines. Assad *et al.*, opted the same idea and extended the range of usable fluorophores, by exploiting low PL nanopores fabricated in a thinned down silicon nitride membrane. Using such conditions, it was possible to detect DNA labeled with individual green-yellow (5-carboxytetramethylrhodamine, TMR) and red (Atto 647) fluorophores having λEM = 565 nm and 665 nm, respectively [116].

In this report, DNA barcode constructs consisting of five 16-nucleotide-long, fluorophore quencher beacons hybridized in a head-to-tail configuration along a template strand were used. Assad *et al.*, used two alternative constructs: a single-color barcode (TMR), and a dual-color barcode (TMR and Atto647, at a specific order) simultaneously excited by red and green lasers. Using confocal microscopy and 2 APDs in similar configuration as that used by Anderson *et al.*, [117], Assad and co-worker simultaneously recorded the electrical current and the optical current. The optic events showed five discrete photon bursts associated with the unzipping and fast diffusion of the five molecular beacons hybridized to the template DNA molecule (Figure 11.7). In both signals (using a single-color barcode and a dual-color barcode), the SNR was high, and no photon bursts were observed between events. The ability to use blue and green laser excitations, which was previously impossible due to low SNR, and the new understanding of the nature of PL in SiNx membranes, may significantly contribute to the improvement of nanopore-based, optical DNA sequencing methods as well as to other future applications.

11.7 Some Other Sensing Examples

In recent years, sensing applications of plasmonic nanopores have moved beyond studies of simple protein adsorption and protein–protein interaction using model protein as avidin-biotin. Wittenberg *et al.*, studied research on multiple sclerosis, measured the affinity of remyelating natural autoantibodies [39]. The antibodies were interacting with myelin-mimicking lipid bilayers formed on the nanopores. Interactions between lectins and polysaccharides [107] were reported by Lin *et al.*, Escobedo *et al.*, have showed simple intensity-based detection of the ovarian cancer marker r-PAX8 in an integrated microfluidic system, although not from a

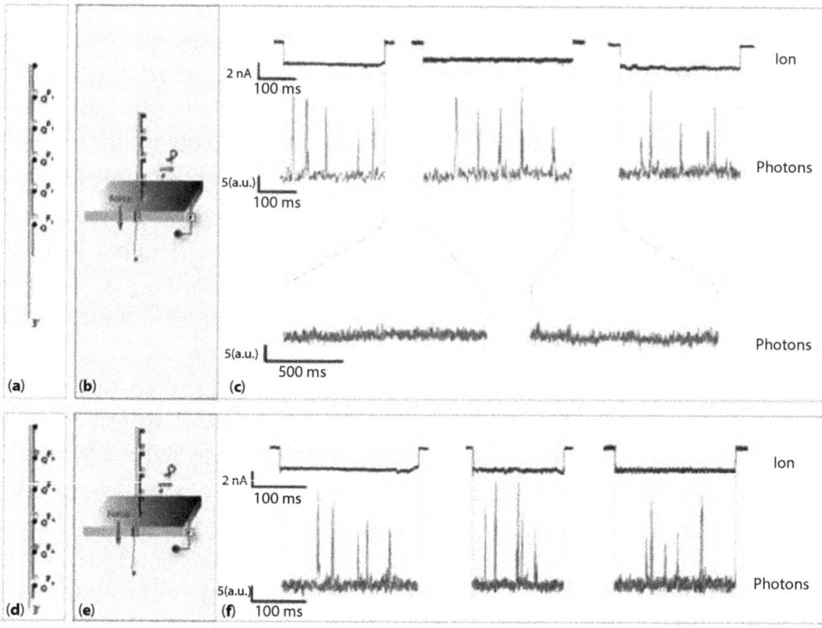

Figure 11.7 Single- and dual-color barcode detection using low PL nanopore. (a, d) Illustration of the ssDNA template consisting 16-mer binding sequences hybridized to molecular fluorophore-quencher labeled beacons. Each DNA strand is labeled with either five green ("F1") fluorophores (a) or specific sequence of green and red ("F1" and "F2", respectively) fluorophores (d) as well as a quencher oligo. The strands are threaded through a low PL, 3 nm nanopores. The marked beacons are stripped off one at a time creating a distinct fluorescent burst (b, e). The electrical and optical signals are measured simultaneously, showing five clear photon bursts per event in the green channel (c) or green and red channels (f) according to the sample. (Ref. Glioba *et al.*, Analyst, 2015, 140, 4733–4747) [122].

biological matrix [118]. Yanik *et al.*, have reported the detection of viruses from biological media, although spectra were recorded only after binding and washing steps [119]. Im *et al.*, have reported the detected proteins in exosomes using a multiplexed format (nanoplasmonic exosome assay), providing "molecular profiling" of cancer markers [120], which is the most highlighted recent sensing work with plasmonic nanopores (Figure 11.7). Because exosomes are currently a hot topic of research. In order to match the ~100 nm target exosomes, the authors have tuned the evanescent field of their plasmonic nanopores and the parallel binding was monitored by functionalizing different flow channels with different capture antibodies on a poly(ethylene glycol) background (Figure 11.8). Clear differences

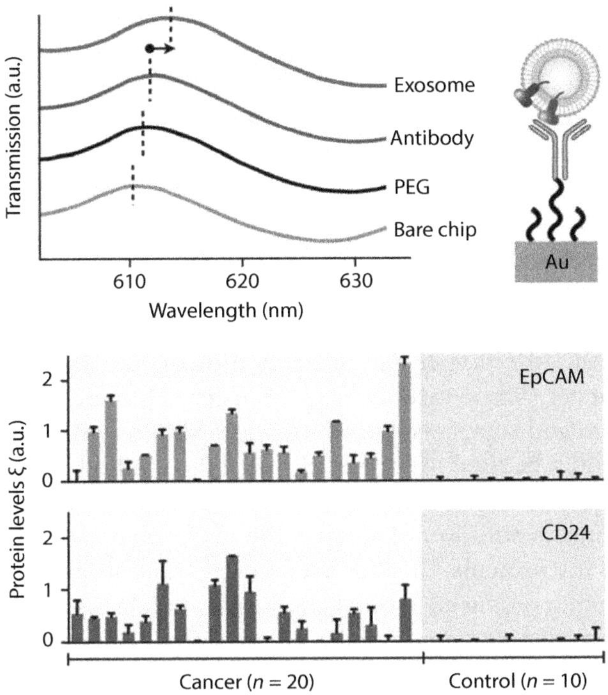

Figure 11.8 Detection of cancer markers in exosomes using plasmonic nanopores. The top shows the detection concept. Exosomes are captured by antibodies and the shift in the transmission maximum is measured. The resulting matrix for two cancer markers, 20 patients and 10 healthy controls, is shown below (Ref: Dahlin, A. B., Analyst, 2015, 140, 4748–4759) [121].

were noticed in the analysis of exosomes from cancer patients and healthy controls, using the epCAM and CD24 membrane proteins. This concept was, however, not combined with flow-through or any other nanopore-unique methodology, i.e., the sensor surface could probably just as well have been of another kind.

11.8 Future Perspectives

Single-molecule sensing by plasmonic nanopores has been evolving significantly in the last two decades generating new possibilities in biomedical research and in biotechnology. Applications of plasmonic nanopores for sensing purposes are still a very hot research field as it is a new approach that allows a high-bandwidth and high-throughput detection from multiple nanopores simultaneously. The advantages that nanopores can penetrate a supporting thin film make it possible to flow liquid through the surface and force molecules to the active detection sites. Complementarity of optical sensing in nanopores with electrical sensing is very useful in a number of ways. For instance, multi-color "bar-coding" of individual molecules can be used to tag specific DNAs and potentially allow precise quantifications of DNA/ RNA transcript at the single-molecule level. An integration of optical sensing in nanopores with nano-channels are very useful in efficient delivery long double-stranded DNA or other biopolymers. Further improvements of the optical SNR in solid-state nanopores, an additional sensing applications will be realized. Additionally, the incorporation of other optical approaches, such as Förster Resonance Energy Transfer, Fluorescence Correlation Spectroscopy, and super resolution strategies such as Stimulated Emission Depletion could be used to further enhance the method, providing it with superior spatial and temporal resolutions. Due to detection limits of plasmonic nanopores still do not surpass the performance of state-of-the-art commercial instruments; therefore, a focused application that is unique to plasmonic nanopores need to be taken into account. What would be the next avenue to plasmonic nanopores? How a plasmonic nanopore can be more helpful in sensing? Some interesting directions can be considered and they are not necessarily related to the detection of low concentrations of analytes in complex samples. It is imperative to consider the influence from negative surface curvature on molecular interactions, which remains an unexplored path, although this is relatively straightforward to investigate with plasmonic nanopores. Use of plasmonic nanopores as filtration devices, given the right surface functionalization, e.g., a polymer brush need to be considered. Selective permeability can be achieved by modification of the interior of the nanopores with a meshwork of macromolecules and receptors. This can be achieved by the use of other types of nanopores and more thinking about possible advantages can be made by using plasmonic nanopores, for which so many more sensing techniques can be instigated.

References

1. Gilboa, T., Meller, A. Optical sensing and analyte manipulation in solid-state nanopores. *Analyst.*, 140, 4733, 2015.
2. DeBlois, R.W., Bean, C.P. Counting and sizing of submicron particles by the resistive pulse technique. *Rev. Sci. Instrum.*, 41, 909, 1970.
3. Li, Y., *et al.* Asymmetric plasmonic induced ionic noise in metallic nanopores. *Nanoscale.*, 8, 12324, 2016.

4. van den Hout, M., *et al.* The passage of homopolymeric RNA through small solid-state nanopores. *Small.*, 7, 2217, 2011.
5. Liu, S., *et al.* Correlated electrical and optical analysis of single nanoparticles and biomolecules on a nanopore-gated optofluidic chip. *Nano Lett.*, 14, 4816, 2014.
6. Bayley, H.P., Prestwich, G.D. Interaction, assembly and processing. *Curr. Opin. Chem. Biol.*, 3, 61, 1999.
7. Kasianowicz, J.J., *et al.* Characterization of individual polynucleotide molecules using a membrane channel. Proc. Natl Acad. Sci., 93, 13770, 1996.
8. Pastoriza-Gallego, M., *et al.* Dynamics of unfolded protein transport through an aerolysin pore. *J. Am. Chem. Soc.*, 133, 2923, 2011.
9. Manrao, E.A., *et al.* Reading DNA at single-nucleotide resolution with a mutant MspA nanopore and phi29 DNA polymerase. *Nat. Biotech.*, 30, 349, 2012.
10. Butler, T.Z., *et al.* Single-molecule DNA detection with an engineered MspA protein nanopore. *Proc. Natl. Acad. Sci.*, 105, 20647, 2008.
11. Mohammad, M.M., *et al.* Engineering a rigid protein tunnel for biomolecular detection. *J. Am. Chem. Soc.*, 134, 9521, 2012.
12. Wendell, D., *et al.* Translocation of double-stranded DNA through membrane-adapted phi29 motor protein nanopores. *Nat. Nano.*, 4, 765, 2009.
13. Wang, H.Y., *et al.* Single-molecule DNA detection using a novel SP1 protein nanopore. *ChemComm.*, 49, 1741, 2013.
14. Shi, W., Friedman, A.K., Baker, L.A. Nanopore sensing. *Anal. Chem.*, 89, 157, 2017.
15. Michiel van den, H., *et al.* Controlling nanopore size, shape and stability. *Nanotechnology.*, 21, 115304, 2010.
16. Haque, F., *et al.* Solid-state and biological nanopore for real-time sensing of single chemical and sequencing of DNA. *Nano Today.*, 8, 56, 2013.
17. Fologea, D., *et al.* Slowing DNA translocation in a solid-state nanopore. *Nano Lett.*, 5, 1734, 2005.
18. Smeets, R.M.M., *et al.* Salt dependence of ion transport and dna translocation through solid-state nanopores. *Nano Lett.*, 6, 89, 2006.
19. Keyser, U.F. Controlling molecular transport through nanopores. *J. Royal Soc. Interface.*, 8, 1369, 2011.
20. Plesa, C., *et al.* Velocity of DNA during translocation through a solid-state nanopore. *Nano Lett.*, 15, 732, 2015.
21. Clarke, J., *et al.* Continuous base identification for single-molecule nanopore DNA sequencing. *Nat Nano.*, 4, 265, 2009.
22. Rosenstein, J.K., *et al.* Integrated nanopore sensing platform with sub-microsecond temporal resolution. *Nat Meth.*, 9, 487, 2012.
23. Uram, J.D., Ke, K., Mayer, M. Noise and bandwidth of current recordings from submicrometer pores and nanopores. *ACS Nano.*, 2, 857, 2008.
24. Smeets, R.M.M., *et al.* Noise in solid-state nanopores. *Proc. Natl Acad. Sci.*, 105, 417, 2008.

25. Smeets, R.M.M., Dekker, N.H., Dekker, C. Low-frequency noise in solid-state nanopores. *Nanotechnology.*, 20, 095501, 2009.
26. Vincent, T.C., *et al.* Noise analysis and reduction in solid-state nanopores. *Nanotechnology.*, 18, 305505, 2007.
27. Ruby dela, T., *et al.* Fabrication and characterization of solid-state nanopore arrays for high-throughput DNA sequencing. *Nanotechnology.*, 23, 385308, 2012.
28. Traversi, F., *et al.* Detecting the translocation of DNA through a nanopore using graphene nanoribbons. *Nat. Nano.*, 8, 939, 2013.
29. Schneider, G.F., *et al.* DNA translocation through graphene nanopores. *Nano Lett.*, 10, 3163, 2010.
30. Merchant, C.A., *et al.* DNA translocation through graphene nanopores. *Nano Lett.*, 10, 2915, 2010.
31. Garaj, S., *et al.* Graphene as a subnanometre trans-electrode membrane. *Nature.*, 467, 190, 2010.
32. Venkatesan, B.M., *et al.* Stacked graphene-Al_2O_3 nanopore sensors for sensitive detection of DNA and DNA–protein complexes. *ACS Nano.*, 6, 441, 2012.
33. Nicoli, F., *et al.* DNA translocations through solid-state plasmonic nanopores *Nano Lett.*, 14, 6917, 2014.
34. Belkin, M., *et al.* Plasmonic nanopores for trapping, controlling displacement, and sequencing of DNA. *ACS Nano.*, 9, 10598, 2015.
35. Cecchini, M.P., *et al.* Rapid ultrasensitive single particle surface-enhanced Raman spectroscopy using metallic nanopores. *Nano Lett.*, 13, 4602, 2013.
36. Chen, C., *et al.* Enhanced optical trapping and arrangement of nano-objects in a plasmonic nanocavity. *Nano Lett.*, 12, 125, 2012.
37. Nam, S., *et al.* Graphene nanopore with a self-integrated optical antenna. *Nano Lett.*, 14, 5584, 2014.
38. Li, Y., *et al.* Photoresistance switching of plasmonic nanopores. *Nano Lett.*, 2015, 15, 776, 2015.
39. Crick, C.R., *et al.* Precise attoliter temperature control of nanopore sensors using a nanoplasmonic bullseye. *Nano Lett.*, 15, 553, 2015.
40. Jonsson, M.P., Dekker, C. Plasmonic nanopore for electrical profiling of optical intensity landscapes. *Nano Lett.*, 13, 1029, 2013.
41. Homola, J. Surface plasmon resonance sensors for detection of chemical and biological species. *Chem. Rev.*, 108, 462, 2008.
42. Brolo, A.G., *et al.* Surface plasmon sensor based on the enhanced light transmission through arrays of nanoholes in gold films. *Langmuir.*, 20, 4813, 2004.
43. Dahlin, A., *et al.* Localized surface plasmon resonance sensing of lipid-membrane-mediated biorecognition events. *J. Am. Chem. Soc.*, 127, 5043, 2005.
44. Rindzevicius, T., *et al.* Plasmonic sensing characteristics of single nanometric holes. *Nano Lett.*, 5, 2335, 2005.
45. Pang, Y., Gordon, R. Optical trapping of 12 nm dielectric spheres using double-nanoholes in a gold film. *Nano Lett.*, 11, 3763, 2011.

46. Pang, Y., Gordon, R. Optical trapping of a single protein. *Nano Lett.*, 12, 402, 2012.
47. Brolo, A.G., *et al.* Nanohole-enhanced Raman scattering. *Nano Lett.*, 4, 2015, 2004.
48. Juan, M.L., *et al.* Self-induced back-action optical trapping of dielectric nanoparticles. *Nat. Phys.*, 5, 915, 2009.
49. Kumar, S., *et al.* Millimeter-sized suspended plasmonic nanohole arrays for surface-tension-driven flow-through SERS. *Chem. Mater.*, 26, 6523, 2014.
50. Andrade, G.F.S., *et al.* Surface-enhanced resonance Raman scattering (SERRS) using Au nanohole arrays on optical fiber tips. *Plasmonics.*, 8, 1113, 2013.
51. Chen, X., *et al.* Nanogap-enhanced infrared spectroscopy with template-stripped wafer-scale arrays of buried plasmonic cavities. *Nano Lett.*, 15, 107, 2015.
52. Jonsson, M.P., *et al.* Locally functionalized short-range ordered nanoplasmonic pores for bioanalytical sensing. *Anal. Chem.*, 82, 2087, 2010.
53. Junesch, J., Sannomiya, T. Ultrathin suspended nanopores with surface plasmon resonance fabricated by combined colloidal lithography and film transfer. *ACS Appl. Mater. Interfaces.*, 6, 6322, 2014.
54. Lee, S.H., *et al.* Self-assembled plasmonic nanohole arrays. *Langmuir.*, 25, 13685, 2009.
55. Lee, S.H., *et al.* Linewidth-optimized extraordinary optical transmission in water with template-stripped metallic nanohole arrays. *Adv. Funct. Mater.*, 22, 4439, 2012.
56. Ikenoya, Y., *et al.* Optical resonances in short-range ordered nanoholes in ultrathin aluminum/aluminum nitride multilayers. *J. Phys. Chem. C.*, 117, 6373, 2013.
57. Schwind, M., Kasemo, B., Zorić, I. Localized and propagating plasmons in metal films with nanoholes. *Nano Lett.*, 13, 1743, 2013.
58. Yanik, A.A., *et al.* Integrated nanoplasmonic-nanofluidic biosensors with targeted delivery of analytes. *Appl. Phys. Lett.*, 96, 021101, 2010.
59. Im, H., *et al.* Membrane protein biosensing with plasmonic nanopore arrays and pore-spanning lipid membranes. *Chem. Sci.*, 1, 688, 2010.
60. Wittenberg, N.J., *et al.* High-affinity binding of remyelinating natural autoantibodies to myelin-mimicking lipid bilayers revealed by nanohole surface plasmon resonance. *Anal. Chem.*, 84, 6031, 2012.
61. Masson, J.F., Murray-Methot, M.P., Live, L.S. Nanohole arrays in chemical analysis: manufacturing methods and applications. *Analyst.*, 135, 1483, 2010.
62. Murray-Methot, M.P., Menegazzo, N., Masson, J.F. Analytical and physical optimization of nanohole-array sensors prepared by modified nanosphere lithography. *Analyst.*, 133, 1714, 2008.
63. Correia-Ledo, D., *et al.* Assessing the location of surface plasmons over nanotriangle and nanohole arrays of different size and periodicity. *J. Phys. Chem. C.*, 116, 6884, 2012.

64. Couture, M., *et al.* Tuning the 3D plasmon field of nanohole arrays. *Nanoscale.*, 5, 12399, 2013.
65. Couture, M., *et al.* EOT or Kretschmann configuration? Comparative study of the plasmonic modes in gold nanohole arrays. *Analyst.*, 137, 4162, 2012.
66. Gibson, K.F., *et al.* Correlated AFM and SERS imaging of the transition from nanotriangle to nanohole arrays. *ChemComm.*, 47, 3404, 2011.
67. Murray-Méthot, M.P., Ratel, M., and Masson, J.F. Optical properties of Au, Ag, and bimetallic Au on Ag nanohole arrays. *J. Phys. Chem. C.*, 114, 8268, 2010.
68. Bochenkov, V.E., Frederiksen, M., Sutherland, D.S. Enhanced refractive index sensitivity of elevated short-range ordered nanohole arrays in optically thin plasmonic Au films. *Opt. Express.*, 21, 14763, 2013.
69. Prikulis, J., *et al.* Optical spectroscopy of nanometric holes in thin gold films. *Nano Lett.*, 4, 1003, 2004.
70. Dahlin, A.B., *et al.* Plasmonic nanopores in metal-insulator-metal films. *Adv. Opt. Mater.*, 2, 556, 2014.
71. Junesch, J., Sannomiya, T., Dahlin, A.B. Optical properties of nanohole arrays in metal–dielectric double films prepared by mask-on-metal colloidal lithography. *ACS Nano.*, 6, 10405, 2012.
72. Sannomiya, T., *et al.* Investigation of plasmon resonances in metal films with nanohole arrays for biosensing applications. *Small.*, 7, 1653, 2011.
73. Dekker, C. Solid-state nanopores. *Nat. Nano.*, 2, 209, 2007.
74. Kowalczyk, S.W., Blosser, T.R., Dekker, C. Biomimetic nanopores: learning from and about nature. *Trends Biotechnol.*, 29, 607, 2011.
75. Ebbesen, T.W., *et al.* Extraordinary optical transmission through sub-wavelength hole arrays. *Nature.*, 391, 667, 1998.
76. Garcia-Vidal, F.J., *et al.* Light passing through subwavelength apertures. *Rev. Mod. Phys.*, 82, 729, 2010.
77. Genet, C., Ebbesen, T.W. Light in tiny holes. *Nature.*, 445, 39, 2007.
78. Degiron, A., *et al.* Optical transmission properties of a single subwavelength aperture in a real metal. *Opt. Commun.*, 239, 61, 2004.
79. Rockstuhl, C., *et al.* Enhanced transmission of periodic, quasiperiodic, and random nanoaperture arrays. *Appl. Phys. Lett.*, 91, 151109, 2007.
80. Park, T.H., *et al.* Optical properties of a nanosized hole in a thin metallic film. *ACS Nano.*, 2, 25, 2008.
81. Rindzevicius, T., *et al.* Nanohole plasmons in optically thin gold films. *J. Phys. Chem. C.*, 111, 1207, 2007.
82. Gao, H., *et al.* Rayleigh anomaly-surface plasmon polariton resonances in palladium and gold subwavelength hole arrays. *Opt. Express.*, 17, 2334, 2009.
83. Pacifici, D., *et al.* Universal optical transmission features in periodic and quasiperiodic hole arrays. *Opt. Express.*, 16, 9222, 2008.
84. Genet, C., van Exter, M.P., Woerdman, J.P. Fano-type interpretation of red shifts and red tails in hole array transmission spectra. Opt. Commun., 225, 331, 2003.

85. Sarrazin, M., Vigneron, J.P., Vigoureux, J.M. Role of wood anomalies in optical properties of thin metallic films with a bidimensional array of subwavelength holes. *Phys. Rev. B.*, 67, 085415, 2003.
86. Braun, J., *et al.* How holes can obscure the view: Suppressed transmission through an ultrathin metal film by a subwavelength hole array. *Phys. Rev. Lett.*, 103, 203901, 2009.
87. Spevak, I.S., *et al.* Resonantly suppressed transmission and anomalously enhanced light absorption in periodically modulated ultrathin metal films. *Phys. Rev. B.*, 79, 161406, 2009.
88. Kekesi, R., *et al.* The effect of holes in the dispersion relation of propagative surface plasmon modes of nanoperforated semitransparent metallic films. *J. Appl. Phys.*, 116, 134306, 2014.
89. Reilly, T.H., *et al.* Controlling the optical properties of plasmonic disordered nanohole silver films. *ACS Nano.*, 4, 615, 2010.
90. Przybilla, F., Genet, C., Ebbesen, T.W. Long vs. short-range orders in random subwavelength hole arrays. *Opt. Express.*, 20, 4697, 2012.
91. Junesch, J., Sannomiya, T. Reflection phase and amplitude determination of short-range ordered plasmonic nanohole arrays. *J. Phys. Chem. Lett.*, 5, 247, 2014.
92. Dahlin, A.B., *et al.* Electrochemical crystallization of plasmonic nanostructures. *Nano Lett.*, 11, 1337, 2011.
93. Dahlin, A.B., Zahn, R., Voros, J. Nanoplasmonic sensing of metal-halide complex formation and the electric double layer capacitor. *Nanoscale.*, 4, 2339, 2012.
94. Virk, M., *et al.* A thermal plasmonic sensor platform: Resistive heating of nanohole arrays. *Nano Lett.*, 14, 3544, 2014.
95. Lesuffleur, A., *et al.* Periodic nanohole arrays with shape-enhanced plasmon resonance as real-time biosensors. *Appl. Phys. Lett.*, 90, 243110, 2007.
96. Monteiro, J.P., *et al.* Effect of periodicity on the performance of surface plasmon resonance sensors based on subwavelength nanohole arrays. *Sens. Actuator B-Chem.*, 178, 366, 2013.
97. Dahlin, A.B., Tegenfeldt, J.O., Höök, F. Improving the instrumental resolution of sensors based on localized surface plasmon resonance. *Anal. Chem.*, 78, 4416, 2006.
98. Cervantes Tellez, G.A., *et al.* Atomically flat symmetric elliptical nanohole arrays in a gold film for ultrasensitive refractive index sensing. *Lab Chip.*, 13, 2541, 2013.
99. Yanik, A.A., *et al.* Seeing protein monolayers with naked eye through plasmonic Fano resonances. *Proc. Natl. Acad. Sci.*, 108, 11784, 2011.
100. Mazzotta, F., *et al.* Influence of the evanescent field decay length on the sensitivity of plasmonic nanodisks and nanoholes. *ACS Photonics.*, 2, 256, 2015.
101. Jonsson, M.P., *et al.* Nanoplasmonic biosensing with focus on short-range ordered nanoholes in thin metal films (Review). *Biointerphases.*, 3, FD30, 2008.

102. Luk'yanchuk, B., *et al.*, The Fano resonance in plasmonic nanostructures and metamaterials. *Nat. Mater.*, 9, 707, 2010.
103. Tetz, K.A., Pang, L., Fainman, Y. High-resolution surface plasmon resonance sensor based on linewidth-optimized nanohole array transmittance. *Opt. Lett.*, 31, 1528, 2006.
104. Marie, R., *et al.* Generic surface modification strategy for sensing applications based on Au/SiO_2 nanostructures. *Biointerphases.*, 2, 49, 2007.
105. Dahlin, A.B., Jonsson, M.P., Höök, F. Specific self-assembly of single lipid vesicles in nanoplasmonic apertures in gold. *Adv. Mater.*, 20, 1436, 2008.
106. Feuz, L., *et al.* Improving the limit of detection of nanoscale sensors by directed binding to high-sensitivity areas. *ACS Nano.*, 4, 2167, 2010.
107. Ferreira, J., *et al.* Attomolar protein detection using in-hole surface plasmon resonance. *J. Am. Chem. Soc.*, 131, 436, 2009.
108. Lin, J.Y., *et al.* Nanopatterned substrates increase surface sensitivity for real-time biosensing. *J. Phys. Chem. C.*, 117, 5286, 2013.
109. Dahlin, A.B. Size matters: Problems and advantages associated with highly miniaturized sensors. *Sensors.*, 12, 3018, 2012.
110. Gupta, P.K. Single-molecule DNA sequencing technologies for future genomics research. *Trends Biotechnol.*, 26, 602, 2008.
111. Branton, D., *et al.* The potential and challenges of nanopore sequencing. *Nat. Biotech.*, 26, 1146, 2008.
112. Cherf, G.M., *et al.* Automated forward and reverse ratcheting of DNA in a nanopore at 5-A precision. *Nat. Biotech.*, 30, 344, 2012.
113. Sawafta, F., *et al.* Solid-state nanopores and nanopore arrays optimized for optical detection. *Nanoscale.*, 6, 6991, 2014.
114. Soni, G.V., Meller, A. Progress toward ultrafast DNA sequencing using solid-state nanopores. *Clin. Chem.*, 53, 1996, 2007.
115. Comer, J., Aksimentiev, A. Predicting the DNA sequence dependence of nanopore ion current using atomic-resolution Brownian dynamics. *J. Phys. Chem. C.*, 116, 3376, 2012.
116. Timp, W., Comer, J., Aksimentiev, A. DNA base-calling from a nanopore using a viterbi algorithm. *Biophys. J.*, 102, L37, 2012.
117. Anderson, B.N., *et al.* Probing solid-state nanopores with light for the detection of unlabeled analytes. *ACS Nano.*, 8, 11836, 2014.
118. Escobedo, C., *et al.* Quantification of ovarian cancer markers with integrated microfluidic concentration gradient and imaging nanohole surface plasmon resonance. *Analyst.*, 138, 1450, 2013.
119. Yanik, A.A., *et al.* An optofluidic nanoplasmonic biosensor for direct detection of live viruses from biological media. *Nano Lett.*, 10, 4962, 2010.
120. Im, H., *et al.*, Label-free detection and molecular profiling of exosomes with a nano-plasmonic sensor. *Nat. Biotech.*, 32, 490, 2014.
121. Dahlin, A.B. Sensing applications based on plasmonic nanopores: The hole story. *Analyst.*, 140, 4748, 2015.
122. Gilboa, T., Meller, A. Optical sensing and analyte manipulation in solidstate nanopores. *Analyst.*, 140, 4733, 2015.

12

Catalytically Active Enzyme Mimetic Nanomaterials and Their Role in Biosensing

Narsingh R. Nirala[1], Sima Umrao[2], Gaurav Khandelwal[3] and Vinod Kumar[4*]

[1]*School of Materials Science and Technology, IIT (BHU), Varanasi, India*
[2]*School of Electronics and Electric Engineering, Sungkyunkwan University (SKKU), Suwon, Korea*
[3]*Indian Institute of Technology Delhi, Hauzkhas, New Delhi, India*
[4]*Department of Materials Engineering, Ben Gurion University of the Negev, Beer-Sheva Israel*

Abstract

In recent years, the emergence nanotechnology with biology has ignited extensive research efforts for designing functional nanomaterials that exhibit exciting intrinsic properties for enzymes mimetic. The catalytically active nanomaterials (nanozymes) showed several advantages over natural enzymes, such as low cost, tenability in catalytic activities, high stability against stringent conditions. Nanozymes catalyzes oxidation of a peroxidase substrate TMB (as efficiently as shown by natural enzymes) in presence of H_2O_2 to oxidized colored product. And this makes a basis of developing a simple, sensitive and selective colorimetric method for determination of biomolecules. Thus, nanozymes hold great promises for developing simple, cost effective, rapid and reliable colorimetric biosensors. The present book chapter provides a detailed informations about the existing nanozyme based colorimetric biosensor and future perspectives.

Keywords: Catalytically active enzymes, mimetic nanomaterials, nanozymes, active nanomaterials in biosensing

**Corresponding author*: mail2vinod2@gmail.com, vinod@post.bgu.ac.il

Suvardhan Kanchi, Shakeel Ahmed, Myalowenkosi I. Sabela and Chaudhery Mustansar Hussain (eds.) Nanomaterials: Biomedical, Environmental, and Engineering Applications, (285–300)

12.1 Introduction

Artificial enzymes, the term given by Ronald Breslow for enzyme mimics [1], is a very vital and exciting branch of biomimetic, which is inspired by nature and aims to imitate the essential and general principles of natural enzymes using alternative materials [2]. Enzymes are specifically catalyzing a variety of reactions with high substrate specificity, activities, and yields under mild reaction conditions [1]. As a consequence, there is significant interest in utilizing enzymes for applications in the biosensor, pharmaceutical processes, food industry, and agrochemical production. However, problems related to their low operational stability (denaturation), the sensitivity of catalytic activity to environmental conditions, difficulties in recovery and recycling, and high costs in preparation and purification greatly limit their applications [3, 4]. To circumvent aforementioned limitations, artificial enzymes have been established as low cost and highly stable alternatives to natural enzymes [1, 5, 6]. So far, the design of artificial enzymes has very rapidly emerged as a lively field of research.

Recently, the merging of nanotechnology with biology has also ignited intensive research efforts for designing functional nanomaterials that exhibit various properties intrinsic to enzymes [6, 11]. A variety of nanoscale materials, such as cerium oxide nanoparticles [10, 12], magnetic nanoparticles [3, 11], gold nanoparticles (AuNPs) [13, 14], V_2O_5 [15, 16], PtPd–Fe_3O_4 [17, 18], graphene oxide [19], and carbon nanotubes [20], have been discovered to possess unique enzyme-mimic catalytic activities. These nanomaterial-based artificial enzymes (nanozymes) have already found wide applications in numerous fields, including biosensing, immunoassays, cancer diagnostics and therapy, neuroprotection, stem cell growth, and pollutant removal. Here, to highlight enzyme-like activity of the nanomaterial, we adopt the term "nanozyme" to describe a man-made nanomaterial that is capable of simulating catalytic function demonstrated by a natural enzyme.

12.2 Different Types of Catalytically Active Enzyme Mimetic Nanomaterials

For ease of access, the examples treated in this account are classified according to the structural characteristics of enzyme mimetic nanomaterials: carbon-, metal, and metal-oxide-based nanomaterials.

12.2.1 Carbon Derivative-based Enzyme Mimetic Nanomaterials

Carbon-based nanomaterials have been discovered to possess peroxidase-like activity [19, 21] such as graphene oxide [19], graphene–hemin nanocomposites [22], carbon nanotubes [23], graphene quantum dots (GQDs) [24], and carbon nanodots [25]. As an atomically thick sheet of sp2-hybridized carbon atoms, the graphene-based material has recently emerged as a rapidly rising star [26].

12.2.1.1 Carbon Nanotubes

In recent years, carbon nanotubes (CNTs) have also attracted considerable attention [27]. They are classified into two main categories: single-wall carbon nanotubes (SWNTs) and multiwall carbon nanotubes (MWNTs), depending on the number of graphene layers [27]. Like COOH–GO, it is demonstrated for the first time that SWNTs possess intrinsic peroxidase-like activity [24]. Inspired by the intrinsic peroxidase property of CNTs, we further reported a label-free colorimetric detection system for disease-associated single nucleotide polymorphism (SNPs) in human DNA (Figure 12.1) [28].

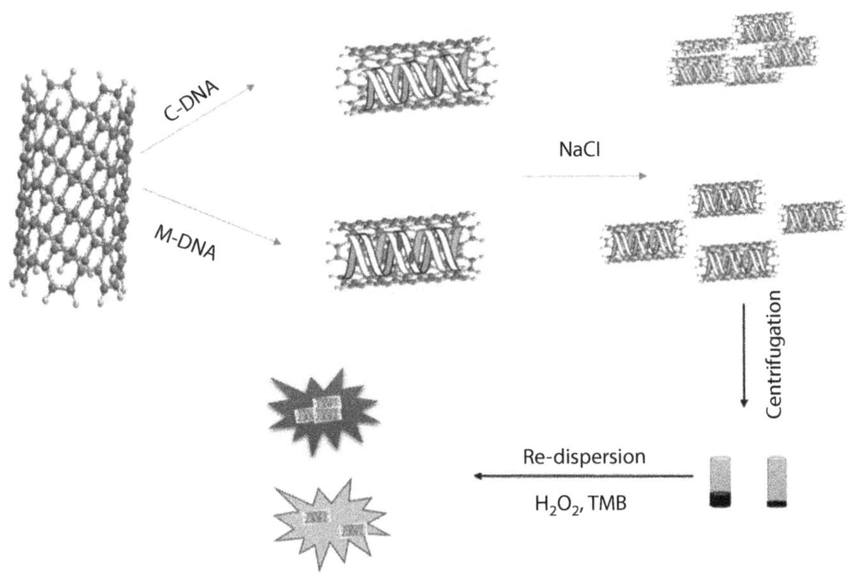

Figure 12.1 SNP detection of complementary (CDNA) and mismatched (M-DNA) duplex DNA based on enzyme mimetic.

At optimum salt concentration, single stranded DNA (ssDNA) could strongly adsorb on the SWNT surface and increase electrostatic repulsion due to the π–π stacking interaction, thus resisting salt-induced SWNT aggregation. In contrast, ds DNA could not stably adsorb on SWNT, resulting in large aggregates under the same salt concentration [20]. Afterward, the SWNTs settled on the bottom of the vial after centrifugation, and the precipitate redispersed in a phosphate buffer [20]. In the presence of TMB and H_2O_2, the colorimetric signal of the obtained SWNTs with double stranded DNA (dsDNA) was remarkably higher compared to that without target DNA.

In addition, the target response proved to be sensitive, and our colorimetric detection approach could be used to distinguish SNPs in human DNA [20, 28]. Besides the direct application of catalytic CNTs, we further developed a sensing and selective strategy for copper detection by click chemistry and combination of magnetic silica nanoparticles with CNTs.

12.2.1.2 Graphene Oxide

Intriguingly, the surprising discovery of carboxyl-modified graphene oxide (GO –COOH) can serve as an effective peroxidase mimic, which catalyzes the reaction of peroxidase substrate 3,3,5,5-tetramethylbenzidine (TMB) in the presence of H_2O_2 to produce a blue color reaction [19]. Similar to horseradish peroxidase HRP, the catalytic activity of the GO–COOH is dependent on pH, temperature, and H_2O_2 concentration [19]. The mechanism of catalytic graphene oxide has been investigated through studying the interactions between GO–COOH, H_2O_2, and TMB.

First, the different absorption spectra show that a bathochromic shift occurs for GO–COOH upon the addition of H_2O_2 [19]. The shifted absorbance suggests that electron transfer occurs from the top of the valence band of graphene to the lowest unoccupied molecular orbital (LUMO) of H_2O_2 [29]. Meanwhile, since TMB can be absorbed on the surface of graphene and donates lone-pair electrons in the amino groups to graphene, TMB will confer an increase in electron density and mobility in graphene [19]. Such a charge-transfer n-type doping of graphene increases the Fermi level and thus the electrochemical potential from the LUMO of H_2O_2 [30]. This accelerates the electron transfer from graphene to H_2O_2 [19]. As a result, nitrogen enrichment in this way provides a higher density of catalytically active centers with low stereo hindrance for binding redox species [19].

On the basis of the intrinsic peroxidase property of GO–COOH, Song *et al.*, designed a simple, cheap, and highly sensitive and selective colorimetric method for glucose detection by coupling graphene-based nanozyme with glucose oxidase (GOx) [19]. In this experiment, glucose could be detected as low as 1 μM, and the protocol exhibited excellent selectivity over other interferences. More significantly, our method has shown great potential for the analysis of glucose level in diluted blood and commercial fruit juices. Thereafter, Huang and co-workers used this catalytically active nanomaterial for colorimetric detection of cancer biomarker prostate-specific antigen. Apart from the intrinsic catalytic activity, graphene and its derivatives can also be utilized as good supports for heterogeneous catalytic processes due to their large specific surface area.

12.2.1.3 Graphene Quantum Dots

Graphene quantum dots (GQDs), a class of carbon nanomaterials containing one or few layered sheets with a lateral dimension less than 100 nm, have several unique properties over above-discussed micrometer-sized SWCNTs, graphene and GO sheets [31]. GQDs have been recognized as better electron transporters and acceptors, rendering them as optimal candidates for electrochemical sensing materials [32]. Due to their quantum confinement [33] and edge effects [34], they possess high surface area and extraordinary optical, electrical, and chemical properties [35–37] along with good solubility, robust chemical inertness, efficient stability against photobleaching, and excellent biocompatibility [38–40]. With such unique properties it is no wonder that GQDs have been explored for diverse applications in various sectors including biological imaging [41], electrochemical biosensors [42], organic photovoltaic devices [43], colorimetric detection [25], and catalysis [44]. GQDs with peroxidase-like activity were first reported [45] in the year of 2013, but this work involved a time-consuming multistep synthesis process using special equipment and expensive starting materials (such as carbon fibers and graphene oxide). The peroxidase-like activity of GQDs has been only used for H_2O_2 detection [45].

We report GQDs synthesized by a simple wet chemical method, as horseradish peroxidase (HRP) enzyme mimetic for enhanced free cholesterol detection [24]. The synthesis route using simple instruments is not only cost effective due to the usage of graphite powder as the starting material but is also fast and facile owing to one-step synthesis of large-scale graphene quantum dots (GQDs) with highly functionalized periphery carboxylic groups attached through acidic treatment of graphite powder. These as-synthesized GQDs show efficient catalytic activity toward the oxidation of peroxidase substrate 3, 3, 5, 5-tetramethylbenzidine (TMB) in the

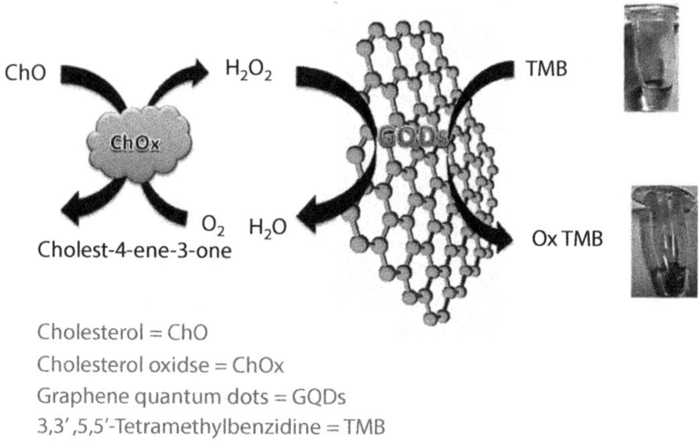

Figure 12.2 Schematic diagram showing oxidation color reaction of TMB by H_2O_2 catalyzed by GQDs.

presence of H_2O_2 to produce a blue-colored product used for the estimation of hydrogen peroxide and cholesterol (ChO) (Figure 12.2) [24].

12.2.1.4 Graphene–Hemin Nanocomposites

Recently, Song *et al.*, and coworkers reported a colorimetric assay for quantitative and fast detection of cancer cells based on the synergetic peroxidase-like activity of folic acid-conjugated graphene–hemin hybrid (GFH). Figure 12.3a,b [22] illustrates the basic procedure for the fabrication of GFH. Since folate receptors are overexpressed on the surface of different types of cancer cells, GFH could selectively bind to the surface of cancer cells by targeting folate receptors, such as human cervical cancer cells (HeLa) and human breast cancer cells (MCF-7) [46]. Owing to the large size and peroxidase mimicking the activity of GFH, selective GFH binding could be not only visualized under bright field microscopy but also quantitatively determined by a colorimetric method (Figure 12.2b) [22].

12.2.2 Nobel Metal Nanoparticle-Based Enzyme Mimetic Nanomaterials

12.2.2.1 Gold Nanoparticles

In addition to carbon-based nanomaterials, noble metal nanomaterials have also been explored to mimic the functions of natural enzymes [14]. Interests were mainly put into GOx- or/and peroxidase-mimicking

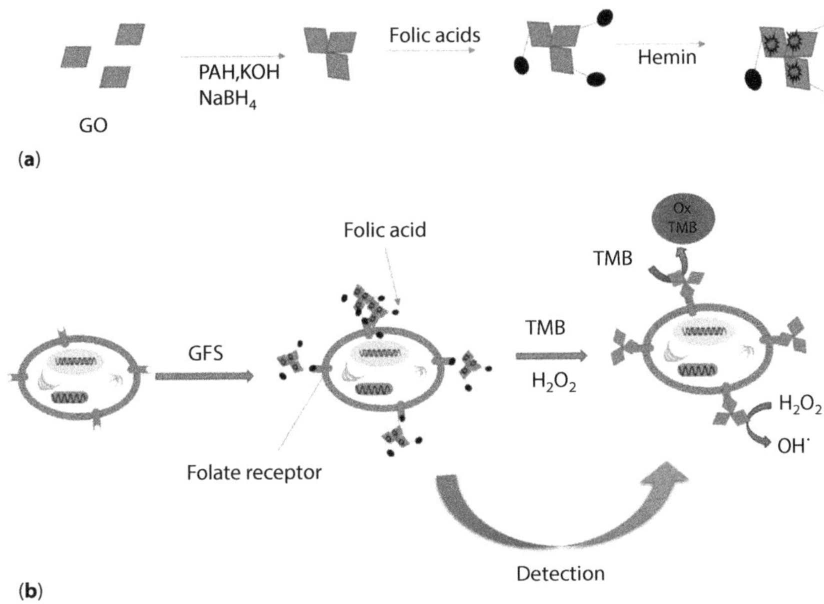

Figure 12.3 Schematic representation of (a) preparation of GFH and (b) cancer cell detection by using target-directed GFH.

activities of gold-based nanomaterials (i.e., mesoporous silica-encapsulated gold nanoparticles [47] and gold nanoclusters [48]. Gold colloids have fascinated scientists for over a century and now have been heavily utilized in various applications [49]. Historically, gold has been regarded as being chemically inert, but in recent years AuNPs with different surface modifications have been found to exhibit GOx-like peroxidase activity [14]. After that, Fan *et al.* have constructed a new sensor platform for sensitive detection of DNA and microRNA by utilizing this GOx-like activity [50]. However, the potential of AuNPs as enzyme mimics is limited by their relatively low catalytic activities and stability [50]. In addition, single-component AuNPs cannot simultaneously possess dual enzyme-like functionalities, as unsupported AuNPs with different surface properties only keep one enzyme-like functionality active while the other catalytic activity can be completely blocked (Figure 12.4).

Recently, noble metal nanoclusters have also become a burgeoning area of scientific interest [49]. Intriguingly, Wang *et al.*, discovered that bovine serum albumin-stabilized gold clusters (BSA-AuNCs) possess intrinsic peroxidase-like activity [50]. Inspired by these initial results, our group developed an easy-prepared fluorometric and colorimetric dual-channel probe for dopamine by using BSA-AuNCs [43].

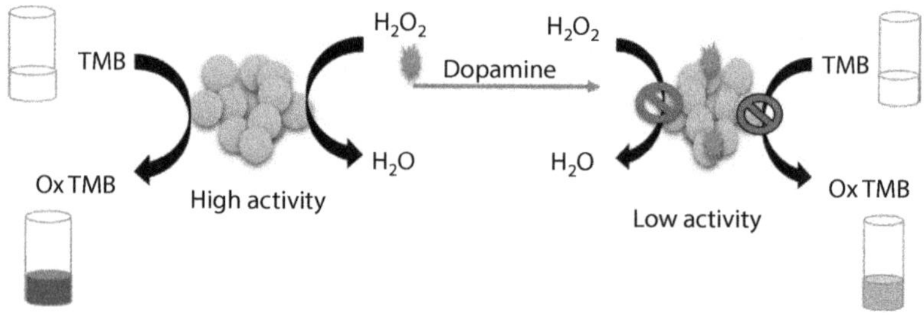

Figure 12.4 Schematic illustration of peroxidase-mimicking catalytic color reaction for sensitive sensing of dopamine.

12.2.3 Metal Oxide Nanoparticle-Based Enzyme Mimetic Nanomaterials

Like carbon- and metal-based nanomaterials, metal-oxide-based nanomaterials have also emerged as efficient enzyme mimics [3, 51]. Among them, cerium oxide nanoparticles [10] and magnetic nanoparticles [52] are two most widely used metal oxide catalysts. But this introduction will focus on our interests in making use of CeO_2 nanoparticle-based ones [53]. CeO_2 nanoparticles, which exist in a mixed valence state (Ce_3^+, Ce_4^+), possess many unique properties that have proven to be of high utility in biomedical and catalytic applications [54]. Recently, they have been reported to possess multienzyme, such as SOD [10], and catalase [9], mimetic properties. For instance, Perez's group reported that nanoceria has an intrinsic oxidase-like activity at acidic pH values, as it can quickly oxidize a series of colorimetric dyes without any oxidizing agent [8]. Following these early works, we found the pH-tunable oxidation ability of nanoceria to ferrocene carboxylic acid (Fc-COOH). After incubation of nano-CeO_2 with Fc-COOH solution at pH 7.4, there was no significant change in absorption or color.

12.3 Applications of Catalytically Active Nanomaterials in Biosensing

12.3.1 Biosensors

In recent time, horseradish peroxidase (HRP), which can catalyze the oxidation of a variety of substrates by H_2O_2, has been one of the most commonly used enzymes for the construction of biosensors. In spite of its high catalytic efficacy, HRP-based biosensors have critical problems, in that the catalytic activity of HRP is prone to degradation in long-term storage and harsh conditions, thereby leading to errors in the process of sensing. To solve this problem, peroxidase-like catalytically active nanomaterials that are highly robust against environmental conditions are utilized in place of HRP, providing a cost-effective method of fabrication of biosensors.

12.3.1.1 H_2O_2 Detection

H_2O_2 detection plays an essential role in the field of biology, medicine, environmental engineering, and food industry. Since H_2O_2, a product of an incompletely reduced metabolite of oxygen, is generated as a by-product of various biological pathways and is a contaminant in several industrial products and wastes, H_2O_2 detection is of practical importance in the field of biosensors. With substantial progress in biosensing technology, various methods for H_2O_2 detection have been reported. Among them is the colorimetric signal readout strategy, based on a redox reaction between HRP and colorimetric substrates such as 2, 2′ azino-bis (3-ethylbenzothiazoline-6-sulphonic acid) (ABTS) and 3,3′ 5,5′ tetramethylbenzidine (TMB). This strategy has been actively developed due to its high sensitivity, selectivity, and simplicity for detecting H_2O_2. However, since the colorimetric detection method using HRP has problems of low stability and high cost, nanozymes showing peroxidase-like activity have been intensively utilized to resolve these drawbacks.

Beginning with the remarkable discovery that MNPs exhibit intrinsic peroxidase-like activity [55], many researchers have focused on the development of novel H_2O_2 detection methods employing various nanozymes. Here, we discuss recent applications of various nanozymes in H_2O_2 detection. After Yan's report, H_2O_2 detection methods with MNPs (used as peroxidase-like nanozymes) were further developed by Wei and Wang [56]. This research outlined a colorimetric detection method for H_2O_2, in which MNPs were used to catalyze the oxidation of ABTS in the presence of H_2O_2. The catalytic oxidation of ABTS with H_2O_2 generates green colored products, by which H_2O_2 can be detected by the naked eye. They noted that ABTS could be oxidized by H_2O_2 in the absence of any catalysts but demonstrated that the presence of MNPs gave a 320% higher response of absorption spectra when compared with the absence of MNPs. Not only the peroxidase-like catalytic activity of Fe_3O_4 MNPs but also their high stability in harse conditions (pH and temperature) was confirmed with additional investigations.

Based on the colorimetric detection method above, many approaches have proceeded by varying the colorimetric substrates and nanozymes used. N,N-Dimethyl-phenyldiamine sulfate (DPD) was used as a colorimetric substrate in place of ABTS [45]. The DPD–MNPs analytical system showed several advantages (lower operating temperature and detection limit and higher sensitivity) over the system using ABTS, because DPD is more easily oxidized by H_2O_2 than ABTS and because oxidized DPD (DPD+) produces a colored product with a strong absorption maximum at 550 nm. Cao's studies reported that positively charged Au NPs can catalyze the oxidation of TMB by H_2O_2. Carboxyl-modified graphene oxide was shown to possess intrinsic peroxidase-like activity that can catalyze the reaction of TMB in the presence of H_2O_2 to produce a blue color reaction [23]. Concentrations as low as 5×10^{-8} mol L^{-1} H_2O_2 were detected with a linear range from 5×10^{-8} to 1×10^{-6} mol L^{-1}.

12.3.1.2 Glucose Detection Peroxidase-Like Nanozymes Coupled

Glucose oxidase (GOx) has been frequently employed in the construction of glucose biosensors. Wang *et al.*, developed a colorimetric glucose detection platform by combining the catalytic oxidation of glucose with GOx and the catalytic reaction of ABTS with MNPs [48]. Glucose concentrations as low as 30 μM were detected with a linear range from 50 μM to 1 mM in this study. There have been several reports of an electrochemical biosensing platform using GOx-coupled nanozymes. A highly efferent and robust electrochemical biosensing strategy employing a nanocomposite harboring GOx-coupled nanozymes was developed [49]. In this report, MNPs and GOx were entrapped in the pores of mesoporous carbon, in which GOx immobilized in the nanocomposite generates H_2O_2, which then is directly reduced to H_2O, with the electrocatalytic reduction mediated by MNPs (Figure 12.5). This system showed a linear range of (0.5 to 10) $\times 10^{-3}$ M and a detection limit of 0.2×10^{-3} M.

12.3.1.3 Immunoassays

Immunoassays have been used in hospitals, laboratory, medicine, and research to improve the health and well-being of humans and animals. Information gained by clinical immunoassay testing has shortened the length of hospital stays and decreased the severity of illness by identifying and assessing the progression of disease, thereby leading to improved therapeutic choices. In life science research, immunoassays are used in the study of biological systems for tracking different proteins, hormones, and antibodies. In industry, immunoassays are used to detect contaminants in food and water and in quality control to monitor specific molecules used during product processing. However, the most commonly used enzymes

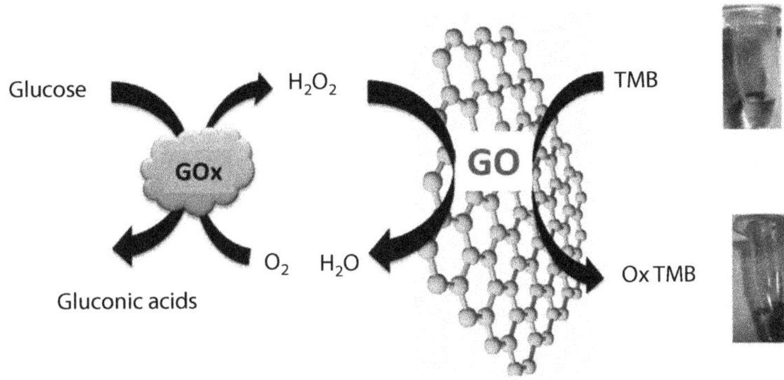

Figure 12.5 Colorimetric detection of glucose by using GOx and GO–COOH-catalyzed reactions.

in the immunoassay include horseradish peroxidase and alkaline phosphatase [57], which lose their enzymatic activities gradually over long-term storage [53].

To overcome these limits, various studies on replacing natural enzymes have been reported, and consequently, novel types of immunoassays using nanozymes in place of HRP have been developed Such as Sandwich or Antigen-Down Type Immunoassays. Gao and coworkers reported an immunoassay using chitosan-modified MNPs (CS-MNPs) as a replacement for HRP in the traditional immunoassay [50]. They provided protocols for antigen-down and sandwich immunoassays with CS-MNPs and detected mouse IgG and carcinoembryonic antigen (CEA), respectively. Chitosan modified on the surface of MNPs prevented aggregation of MNPs, so that MNPs were easily dispersed in aqueous solutions. Meanwhile, amino groups in the chitosan provided a convenient site for covalent linking of antibodies to MNPs, thereby replacing the linkage of HRP-conjugated antibodies to CS-MNP-conjugated antibodies in the immunoassay. Capture-detection immunoassay was also developed to detect CEA by employing the magnetic properties of CS-MNPs, which facilitate capturing, separating, and enriching antigens as well as re-dispersing the MNP aggregation in solution (Figure 12.6). This immunoassay generated significantly higher absorption intensity of color signal than the current ELISA and was able to quantify the argot antigen very rapidly within 3 minutes, while the conventional ELISA requires several tens of minutes for color signal development [45, 46]. It showed a limit of detection (LOD) for HER2 of 1.5 ng mL^{-1} in the linear range from 2.5 to 100 ng mL^{-1}. The nanocomposite was found to have 50 times higher catalytic efficiency than that of free MNPs, owing to the high catalytic action of Pt NPs.

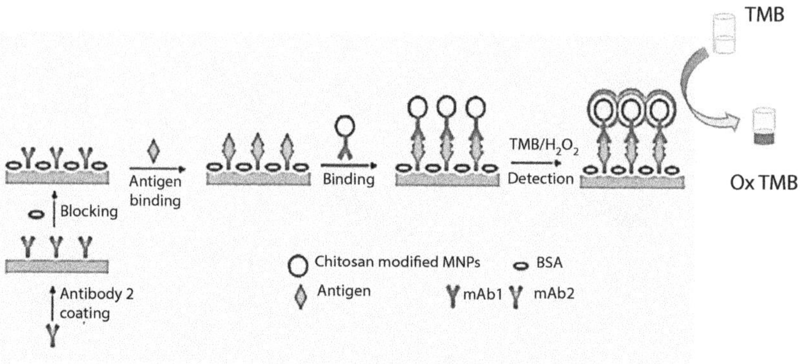

Figure 12.6 Fe_3O_4 MNPs as nanozymes for immunoassay.

Graphene oxide (GO) has been used in an immunoassay as a peroxidase-mimicking nanozymes [41]. Yan's group developed a sandwich-type immunoassay for the detection of a cancer biomarker prostate-specific antigen (PSA). In this work, a magnetic bead (MB) was used to immobilize the primary PSA antibody (Ab1) and then a GO-conjugated secondary antibody (Ab2) was applied in the presence of PSA. Subsequently, MB-Ab1 was separated from the immune complex by an external magnetic field, and GO catalyzed the oxidation of hydroquinone in the presence of H_2O_2 to generate a brown-colored product. Conjugating both MNPs and Pt NPs on the surface of GO enabled highly sensitive and rapid colorimetric detection of the target cancer cell [35]. In this work, it was notable that the electron transfer between MNPs and Pt NPs creates a synergistic effect, significantly enhancing the catalytic performance of MNPs-Pt NPs-GO nanohybrids. Using this immunoassay system, human breast adenocarcinoma cells (SKBR-3), which overexpressed HER2, were detected in 5 minutes with high specificity and sensitivity. The LOD for target SKBR-3 cells was found to be about 100 cells in the linear range from 100 to 1000 cells. Moreover, fluorescence imaging of SKBR-3 was successfully performed with MNPsPt NPs-GO nanohybrids.

References

1. Breslow, R. Biomimetic chemistry and artificial enzymes: Catalysis by design. *Acc. Chem. Res.*, 28, 146, 1995.
2. Garg, B., Bisht, T., Ling, Y.C. Graphene-based nanomaterials as efficient peroxidase mimetic catalysts for biosensing applications: An overview. *Molecules.*, 20, 14155, 2015.

3. Gao, L., Zhuang, J., Nie, L., Zhang, J., Zhang, Y., Gu, N., Wang, T., Feng, J., Yang, D., Perrett, S., Yan, X. Intrinsic peroxidase-like activity of ferromagnetic nanoparticles. *Nat. Nanotechnol.*, 2, 577, 2007.
4. Xie, J., Zhang, X., Wang, H., Zheng, H., Huang, Y., Xie, J. Analytical and environmental applications of nanoparticles as enzyme mimetics. *Trends Anal. Chem.*, 39, 114, 2012.
5. Kotov, N.A. Chemistry. Inorganic nanoparticles as protein mimics. *Science.*, 330, 188, 2010.
6. Breslow, R. Artificial enzymes. *Science.*, 218, 532, 1982.
7. Asati, A., Santra, S., Kaittanis, C., Nath, S., and Perez, J.M. Oxidase-like activity of polymer-coated cerium oxide nanoparticles. *Angew. Chem.*, 48, 2308, 2009.
8. Lin, Y., Ren, J., Qu, X. Catalytically active nanomaterials: a promising candidate for artificial enzymes. *Acc. Chem. Res.*, 47, 1097, 2014.
9. Pirmohamed, T., Dowding, J.M., Singh, S., Wasserman, B., Heckert, E., Karakoti, A.S., King, J.E.S., Seal, S., Self, W.T. Nanoceria exhibit redox state-dependent catalase mimetic activity. *ChemComm.*, 46, 2736, 2010.
10. Heckert, E.G., Karakoti, A.S., Seal, S., Self, W.T. The role of cerium redox state in the SOD mimetic activity of nanoceria. *Biomaterials.*, 29, 2705, 2008.
11. Park, K.S., Il Kim, M., Cho, D.Y., Park, H.G. Label-free colorimetric detection of nucleic acids based on target-induced shielding against the peroxidase-mimicking activity of magnetic nanoparticles. *Small.*, 7, 1521, 2011.
12. Asati, A., Santra, S., Kaittanis, C., Nath, S., and Perez, J.M. Oxidase-like activity of polymer-coated cerium oxide nanoparticles. *Angew. Chem.*, 48, 2308, 2009.
13. Pengo, P., Polizzi, S., Pasquato, L., Scrimin, P. Carboxylate–imidazole cooperativity in dipeptide-functionalized gold nanoparticles with esterase-like activity. *J. Am Chem. Soc.*, 127, 1616, 2005.
14. Comotti, M., Della Pina, C., Matarrese, R., Rossi, M. The catalytic activity of naked gold particles. *Angew. Chem. Int. Ed.*, 43, 5812, 2004.
15. André, R., Natálio, F., Humanes, M., Leppin, J., Heinze, K., Wever, R., Schröder, H.C., Müller, W.E.G., Tremel, W. V2O5 nanowires with an intrinsic peroxidase-like activity. *Adv. Funct. Mater.*, 21, 501, 2011.
16. Natalio, F., André, R., Hartog, A.F., Stoll, B., Jochum, K.P., Wever, R., Tremel, W. Vanadium pentoxide nanoparticles mimic vanadium haloperoxidases and thwart biofilm formation. *Nat. Nanotechnol.*, 7, 530, 2012.
17. Sun, X., Guo, S., Liu, Y., Sun, S. Dumbbell-like PtPd–Fe_3O_4 nanoparticles for enhanced electrochemical detection of H_2O_2. *Nano Lett.*, 12, 4859, 2012.
18. Sun, X., Guo, S., Chung, C.S., Zhu, W., Sun, S. A sensitive H_2O_2 assay based on dumbbell-like PtPd-Fe_3O_4 nanoparticles. *Adv. Mater. (Deerfield Beach, Fla.)*, 25, 132, 2013.
19. Song, Y., Qu, K., Zhao, C., Ren, J., Qu, X. Graphene oxide: intrinsic peroxidase catalytic activity and its application to glucose detection. *Adv. Mater.*, 22, 2206, 2010.

20. Song, Y., Wang, X., Zhao, C., Qu, K., Ren, J., Qu, X. Label-free colorimetric detection of single nucleotide polymorphism by using single-walled carbon nanotube intrinsic peroxidase-like activity. *Chemistry.,* 16, 3617, 2010.
21. Xue, T., Jiang, S., Qu, Y., Su, Q., Cheng, R., Dubin, S., Chiu, C.Y., Kaner, R., Huang, Y., Duan, X. Graphene-supported hemin as a highly active biomimetic oxidation catalyst. *Angew. Chem. Int. Ed.*, 51, 3822, 2012.
22. Song, Y., Chen, Y., Feng, L., Ren, J., Qu, X. Selective and quantitative cancer cell detection using target-directed functionalized graphene and its synergetic peroxidase-like activity. *ChemComm.,* 47, 4436, 2011.
23. Song, Y., Qu, K., Xu, C., Ren, J., Qu, X., King, P.W., Heben, M.J., Wogan, G., Tannenbaum, S., Strano, M.S., Yan, X. Visual and quantitative detection of copper ions using magnetic silica nanoparticles clicked on multiwalled carbon nanotubes. *ChemComm.*, 46, 6572, 2010.
24. Nirala, N.R., Abraham, S., Kumar, V., Bansal, A., Srivastava, A., Saxena, P.S. Colorimetric detection of cholesterol based on highly efficient peroxidase mimetic activity of graphene quantum dots. *Sens. Actuator B: Chem.*, 218, 42, 2015.
25. Shi, W., Wang, Q., Long, Y., Cheng, Z., Chen, S., Zheng, H., Huang, Y. Carbon nanodots as peroxidase mimetics and their applications to glucose detection. *ChemComm.,* 47, 6695, 2011.
26. Stankovich, S., Dikin, D.A., Dommett, G.H.B., Kohlhaas, K.M., Zimney, E.J., Stach, E.A., Piner, R.D., Nguyen, S.T., Ruoff, R.S. Graphene-based composite materials. *Nature.*, 442, 282, 2006.
27. Liu, Z., Tabakman, S.M., Chen, Z., Dai, H. Preparation of carbon nanotube bioconjugates for biomedical applications. *Nat. Protoc.,* 4, 1372, 2009.
28. Song, Y., Wang, X., Zhao, C., Qu, K., Ren, J., Qu, X. Label-free colorimetric detection of single nucleotide polymorphism by using single-walled carbon nanotube intrinsic peroxidase-like activity. *Chem. Eur. J.,*16, 3617, 2010.
29. Heller, D.A., Jin, H., Martinez, B.M., Patel, D., Miller, B.M., Yeung, T.K., Jena, P.V., Höbartner, C., Ha, T., Silverman, S.K., Strano, M.S. Multimodal optical sensing and analyte specificity using single-walled carbon nanotubes. *Nat. Nanotechnol.,* 4, 114, 2009.
30. Kim, J.H., Heller, D.A., Jin, H., Barone, P.W., Song, C., Zhang, J., Trudel, L.J., Wogan, G.N., Tannenbaum, S.R., Strano, M.S. The rational design of nitric oxide selectivity in single-walled carbon nanotube near-infrared fluorescence sensors for biological detection. *Nat. Chem.,* 1, 478, 2009.
31. Alivisatos, A.P. Semiconductor clusters, nanocrystals, and quantum dots. *Science.*, 271, 933, 1996.
32. Wu, Y., Zhou, J., Fishkin, N., Rittmann, B.E., Sparrow, J.R. Enzymatic degradation of A2E, a retinal pigment epithelial lipofuscin bisretinoid. *J. Am. Chem. Soc.,*133, 849, 2011.
33. Ponomarenko, L.A., Schedin, F., Katsnelson, M.I., Yang, R., Hill, E.W., Novoselov, K.S., Geim, A.K. Chaotic Dirac billiard in graphene quantum dots. *Science.,* 320, 356, 2008.

34. Zhu, S., Zhang, J., Qiao, C., Tang, S., Li, Y., Yuan, W., Li, B., Tian, L., Liu, F., Hu, R., Gao, H., Wei, H., Zhang, H., Sun, H., Yang, B. Strongly green-photoluminescent graphene quantum dots for bioimaging applications. *ChemComm.*, 47, 6858, 2011.
35. Zhu, Y., Murali, S., Cai, W., Li, X., Suk, J.W., Potts, J.R., Ruoff, R.S. Graphene and graphene oxide: synthesis, properties, and applications. *Adv. Mater.*, 22, 3906, 2010.
36. Terrones, M., Botello-Méndez, A.R., Campos-Delgado, J., López-Urías, F., Vega-Cantú, Y.I., Rodríguez-Macías, F.J., Elías, A.L., Muñoz-Sandoval, E., Cano-Márquez, A.G., Charlier, J.C. Graphene and graphite nanoribbons: Morphology, properties, synthesis, defects and applications. *Nano Today.*, 5, 351, 2010.
37. Geim, A.K., Novoselov, K.S. The rise of graphene. *Nat. Mater.*, 6, 183, 2007.
38. Chandra, S., Das, P., Bag, S., Laha, D., Pramanik, P. Synthesis, functionalization and bioimaging applications of highly fluorescent carbon nanoparticles. *Nanoscale.*, 3, 1533, 2011.
39. Cao, L., Wang, X., Meziani, M.J., Lu, F., Wang, H., Luo, P.G., Lin, Y., Harruff, B.A., Veca, L.M., Murray, D., Xie, S.Y., Sun, Y.P. Carbon dots for multiphoton bioimaging. *J. Am. Chem. Soc.*, 129, 11318, 2007.
40. Ray, S.C., Saha, A., Jana, N.R., Sarkar, R. Fluorescent carbon nanoparticles: Synthesis, characterization, and bioimaging application. *J. Phys. Chem. C.*, 113, 18546, 2009.
41. Sun, X., Liu, Z., Welsher, K., Robinson, J.T., Goodwin, A., Zaric, S., Dai, H. Nano-graphene oxide for cellular imaging and drug delivery. *Nano Res.*, 1, 203, 2008.
42. Gupta, V., Chaudhary, N., Srivastava, R., Sharma, G.D., Bhardwaj, R., Chand, S. Luminscent graphene quantum dots for organic photovoltaic devices. *J. Am. Chem. Soc.*, 133, 9960, 2011.
43. Gong, K., Du, F., Xia, Z., Durstock, M., Dai, L., Nitrogen-doped carbon nanotube arrays with high electrocatalytic activity for oxygen reduction. *Science.*, 323, 760, 2009.
44. Zhang, Y., Wu, C., Zhou, X., Wu, X., Yang, Y., Wu, H., Guo, S., Zhang, J. Graphene quantum dots/gold electrode and its application in living cell H2O2 detection. *Nanoscale.*, 5, 1816, 2013.
45. Su, L., Feng, J., Zhou, X., Ren, C., Li, H., Chen, X. Colorimetric detection of urine glucose based ZnFe2O4 magnetic nanoparticles. An*al. Chem.*, 84, 5753, 2012.
46. Song, Y., Chen, Y., Feng, L., Ren, J., Qu, X. Selective and quantitative cancer cell detection using target-directed functionalized graphene and its synergetic peroxidase-like activity. *ChemComm.*, 47, 4436, 2011.
47. Lin, Y., Li, Z., Chen, Z., Ren, J., Qu, X. Mesoporous silica-encapsulated gold nanoparticles as artificial enzymes for self-activated cascade catalysis. *Biomaterials.*, 34, 2600, 2013.
48. Tao, Y., Lin, Y., Ren, J., Qu, X. A dual fluorometric and colorimetric sensor for dopamine based on BSA-stabilized Au nanoclusters. *Biosens. Bioelectron.*, 42, 41, 2013.

49. Giljohann, D.A., Seferos, D.S., Daniel, W.L., Massich, M.D., Patel, P.C., Mirkin, C.A. Gold nanoparticles for biology and medicine. *Angew. Chem. Int. Ed.*, 49, 3280, 2010.
50. Zheng, X., Liu, Q., Jing, C., Li, Y., Li, D., Luo, W., Wen, Y., He, Y., Huang, Q., Long, Y.T., Fan, C. Catalytic gold nanoparticles for nanoplasmonic detection of DNA hybridization. *Angew. Chem. Int. Ed.*, 50, 11994, 2011.
51. Jung, J.H., Cheon, D.S., Liu, F., Lee, K.B., Seo, T.S. A graphene oxide based immuno-biosensor for pathogen detection. *Angew. Chem.*, 49, 5708, 2010.
52. Rossi, L., Quach, A., Rosenzweig, Z. Glucose oxidase–magnetite nanoparticle bioconjugate for glucose sensing. *Anal. Bioanal. Chem.* 380, 8, 2004.
53. Xu, C., Lin, Y., Wang, J., Wu, L., Wei, W., Ren, J., Qu, X. Nanoceria-triggered synergetic drug release based on CeO_2 -capped mesoporous silica host-guest interactions and switchable enzymatic activity and cellular effects of CeO_2. *Adv. Healthc. Mater.*, 2, 1591, 2013.
54. Kuchma, M.H., Komanski, C.B., Colon, J., Teblum, A., Masunov, A.E., Alvarado, B., Babu, S., Seal, S., Summy, J., Baker, C.H. Phosphate ester hydrolysis of biologically relevant molecules by cerium oxide nanoparticles. *Nanomed. Nanotech. Biol. Med.*, 6, 738, 2010.
55. Gao, L., Zhuang, J., Nie, L., Zhang, J., Zhang, Y., Gu, N., Wang, T., Feng, J., Yang, D., Perrett, S., Yan, X. Intrinsic peroxidase-like activity of ferromagnetic nanoparticles. *Nat. Nanotechnol.*, 2, 577, 2007.
56. Wei, H., Wang, E. Fe_3O_4 magnetic nanoparticles as peroxidase mimetics and their applications in H_2O_2 and glucose detection. *Anal. Chem.*, 80, 2250, 2008.
57. McReynolds, K.D., Hadd, M.J., Gervay-Hague, J. Synthesis of biotinylated glycoconjugates and their use in a novel ELISA for direct comparison of HIV-1 Gp120 recognition of GalCer and related carbohydrate analogues. *Bioconjug. Chem.*, 10, 6, 1021.

Index

Also of Interest

Check out these published volumes in the Advanced Materials Series

Advanced Materials for Wastewater Treatment
Edited by Shahid-ul-Islam
Published 2017. ISBN 1-119-40776-8

Advanced Magnetic and Optical Materials
Edited by Ashutosh Tiwari, Parameswar K. Iyer, Vijay Kumar and Hendrik Swart
Published 2016. ISBN 978-1-119-24191-1

Advanced Surfaces for Stem Cell Research
Edited by Ashutosh Tiwari, Bora Garipcan and Lokman Uzun
Published 2016. ISBN 978-1-119-24250-5

Advanced Electrode Materials
Edited by Ashutosh Tiwari, Filiz Kuralay and Lokman Uzun
Published 2016. ISBN 978-1-119-24252-9

Advanced Molecularly Imprinting Materials
Edited by Ashutosh Tiwari and Lokman Uzun
Published 2016. ISBN 978-1-119-33629-7

Intelligent Nanomaterials (2nd edition)
Edited by Tiwari, Yogendra Kumar Mishra, Hisatoshi Kobayashi and Anthony P. F. Turner
Published 2016. ISBN 978-1-119-24253-6

Advanced Composite Materials
Edited by Ashutosh Tiwari, Mohammad Rabia Alenezi and Seong Chan Jun
Published 2016. ISBN 978-1-119-24253-6

Advanced Surface Engineering Materials
Edited by Ashutosh Tiwari, Rui Wang, and Bingqing Wei
Published 2016. ISBN 978-1-119-24244-4

Advanced Ceramic Materials
Edited by Ashutosh Tiwari, Rosario A. Gerhardt and Magdalena Szutkowska
Published 2016. ISBN 978-1-119-24244-4

Advanced Engineering Materials and Modeling
Edited by Ashutosh Tiwari, N. Arul Murugan and Rajeev Ahuja
Published 2016. ISBN 978-1-119-24246-8

Advanced 2D Materials
Ashutosh Tiwari and Mikael Syväjärvi
Published 2016. ISBN 978-1-119-24249-9

Advanced Materials Interfaces
Edited by Ashutosh Tiwari, Hirak K. Patra and Xumei Wang
Published 2016. ISBN 978-1-119-24245-1

Advanced Bioelectronics Materials
Edited by Ashutosh Tiwari, Hirak K. Patra and Anthony P.F. Turner
Published 2015. ISBN 978-1-118-99830-4

Graphene
An Introduction to the Fundamentals and Industrial Applications
By Madhuri Sharon and Maheswar Sharon
Published 2015. ISBN 978-1-118-84256-0

Advanced Theranostic Materials
Edited by Ashutosh Tiwari, Hirak K. Patra and Jeong-Woo Choi
Published 2015. ISBN: 978-1-118-99829-8

Advanced Functional Materials
Edited by Ashutosh Tiwari and Lokman Uzun
Published 2015. ISBN 978-1-118-99827-4

Advanced Catalytic Materials
Edited by Ashutosh Tiwari and Salam Titinchi
Published 2015. ISBN 978-1-118-99828-1

Graphene Materials
Fundamentals and Emerging Applications
Edited by Ashutosh Tiwari and Mikael Syväjärvi
Published 2015. ISBN 978-1-118-99837-3

DNA Engineered Noble Metal Nanoparticles
Fundamentals and State-of-the-art-of Nanobiotechnology
By Ignác Capek
Published 2015. ISBN 978-1-118-07214-1
Advanced Electrical and Electronics Materials

Process and Applications
By K.M. Gupta and Nishu Gupta
Published 2015. ISBN: 978-1-118-99835-9

Advanced Materials for Agriculture, Food and Environmental Safety
Edited by Ashutosh Tiwari and Mikael Syväjärvi
Published 2014. ISBN: 978-1-118-77343-7

Advanced Biomaterials and Biodevices
Edited by Ashutosh Tiwari and Anis N. Nordin
Published 2014. ISBN 978-1-118-77363-5

Biosensors Nanotechnology
Edited by Ashutosh Tiwari and Anthony P. F. Turner
Published 2014. ISBN 978-1-118-77351-2

Advanced Sensor and Detection Materials
Edited by Ashutosh Tiwari and Mustafa M. Demir
Published 2014. ISBN 978-1-118-77348-2

Advanced Healthcare Materials
Edited by Ashutosh Tiwari
Published 2014. ISBN 978-1-118-77359-8

Advanced Energy Materials
Edited by Ashutosh Tiwari and Sergiy Valyukh
Published 2014. ISBN 978-1-118-68629-4

Advanced Carbon Materials and Technology
Edited by Ashutosh Tiwari and S.K. Shukla
Published 2014. ISBN 978-1-118-68623-2

Responsive Materials and Methods
State-of-the-Art Stimuli-Responsive Materials and Their Applications
Edited by Ashutosh Tiwari and Hisatoshi Kobayashi
Published 2013. ISBN 978-1-118-68622-5

Other Scrivener books edited by Ashutosh Tiwari

Nanomaterials in Drug Delivery, Imaging, and Tissue Engineering
Edited by Ashutosh Tiwari and Atul Tiwari
Published 2013. ISBN 978-1-118-29032-3

Biomedical Materials and Diagnostic Devices Devices
Edited by Ashutosh Tiwari, Murugan Ramalingam, Hisatoshi Kobayashi and Anthony P.F. Turner
Published 2012. ISBN 978-1-118-03014-1

Intelligent Nanomaterials (first edition)
Processes, Properties, and Applications
Edited by Ashutosh Tiwari Ajay K. Mishra, Hisatoshi Kobayashi and Anthony P.F. Turner
Published 2012. ISBN 978-0-470-93879-9

Integrated Biomaterials for Biomedical Technology
Edited by Murugan Ramalingam, Ashutosh Tiwari, Seeram Ramakrishna and Hisatoshi Kobayashi
Published 2012. ISBN 978-1-118-42385-1

CPSIA information can be obtained
at www.ICGtesting.com
Printed in the USA
BVHW03*0014310518
517777BV00004B/31/P

9 781119 370260